REPERTORY
BASED ON
ALLEN'S KEY NOTES
AND
NASH'S LEADERS

Including
Relationship of Remedies

Captain K.K. Sirker
M.B. (California University), I.M.S. (Late)

B. Jain Publishers (P) Ltd.
USA — EUROPE — INDIA

A
REPERTORY
BASED ON
ALLEN'S KEY NOTES
AND
NASH'S LEADERS

including

Relationship of Remedies

Captain K.K. Sirker
M.B. (California University), I.M.S. (Late)

A REPERTORY BASED ON ALLEN'S KEYNOTES AND NASH'S LEADERS

Revised Edition: 2005
5th Impression: 2015

Published by Kuldeep Jain for

B. JAIN PUBLISHERS (P) LTD.
1921/10, Chuna Mandi, Paharganj, New Delhi 110 055 (INDIA)
Tel.: +91-11-4567 1000   Fax: +91-11-4567 1010
Email: info@bjain.com   Website: **www.bjain.com**

Printed in India

ISBN: 978-81-319-0076-5

PREFACE

Dear readers,

This book has been undertaken under the belief that it would serve most useful purpose to students and practitioners of homoeopathy for ready reference. The book is a small one but the task has been a herculean one. Very often difficulties arise in working out a repertory as to where the different symptoms are to be found. Those who do not have the sufficient knowledge to classify symptoms, I would advice them to go through this book once or twice so as to be acquainted thoroughly with the different sections contained in the book.

I have not given a separate chapter on aggravations and ameliorations. The general aggravations and ameliorations will be found in the chapter of generalities, and the particulars will be found in different sections.

As regards the relationship I have put them in a tabular form for the convenience of the readers.

Besides what are found in the Allen's Keynotes and Nash's Leaders, there have been some important additions to give this little work a completeness so far as possible.

CAPT. K. K. SIRKER
M.B. (California University)
I.M.S. (Late)

"..... the subject is well presented and admirable ....."

Boericke and Tafel

CONTENTS

CONTENTS

ABDOMEN

ABSCESS, inguinal gland : **Hep**, *sil*.

ASCITES : (See Dropsy).

BAND, tight, intolerance of : **Lach**.

BEARING down sensation : (See Pain, dragging).

BIG-BELLIED : (See Enlarged).

BORBORYGMI : (See Rumbling).

BURNING : colch.

CLOSED, bowels : (See Intussusception).

CLOTHING, sensitive to : *carb-v*, **Lach**, *tab*.
   wants to loosen, around abdomen : *carb-v*, **Lach**.
   uncover : **Tab**.

COLDNESS : **Ambr**, *calc*, colch, elaps, *lach*, **Meny**, *tab*, **Verat**.
   fever during : *meny*.

CONGESTION, liver : **Sulph**.

COVERING, agg : *camph*, *sec*, *tab*.

CRAMP : (See Pain).

CROAKING : (See Rumbling).

CRYING, as if an animal : thuj.

DISCHARGE from umbilicus : *abrot*, *calc-p*.
   bloody fluid : *calc-p*.
   urine, of : *hyos*.

DISTENSION : bell, **Calc**, **Carb-v** (upper abdomen), **Chin** (whole of
   abdomen), Cocc, **Colch**, coll, **Lyc** (lower abdomen), nux-m, *sil*,
   Ter.
      burst, as if it would : **Colch**.
      children, in : **Bar-c**, **Calc**.
      eating, after : **Carb-v**, **Chin**, **Lyc**, *nux-m*, **Nux-v**.
      flatus, passing, amel : **Lyc**.
      painful : bell, lach.
      tympanitic : **Carb-v**, **Chin**, **Colch** (as if it would burst), lach,
         Lyc, ph-ac, **Ter**.

pit of stomach, inverted saucer like : **Calc**.

hypochondria, right : podo.

DROPSY, ascites : acet-ac, **Apis**, **Apoc**, **Ars**, dig, *hell*, **Ter**.

intermittents, after : hell.

quinine, after abuse of : apoc.

suppressed exanthamata, from : *apis*, *hell*, **Zinc**.

EMPTINESS : cocc, **Phos**, **Podo**.

ENLARGED : **Calc**, *iod*, **Sanic**, **Sep**, **Sulph**.

children, in : **Bar-c**, **Calc**, *sanic*, *sars*, **Sil**, *staph*, *sulph*.

mothers, in : **Sep**.

liver : **Chin**, **Lyc**, **Mag-m**, tarax.

mensenterics : **Calc**, *iod*.

spleen : *anthr*, **Cean**, **Chin**, **Iod**.

epidemic spleen disease of cattles : anthrac.

FERMENTATION (See Rumbling) : **Chin**, **Lyc**.

fruit, after : **Chin**, puls.

menses, during : **Lyc**.

FLABBY : *calc-p*.

FLATULENCE (See Rumbling) : *ant-c*, **Arg-n**, **Asaf** (all pressing upward), *calc-p*, **Carb-v**, **Chin**, **Colch**, coll, *dios*, ip, *kali-c*, **Lyc**, *mag-m*, **Nux-m** (after meal), *raph* (no flatus up or down), sabad, **Ter**.

belching does not amel : **Chin**.

bursting : **Carb-v**.

drink, after : carb-v.

eating, after : *carb-v*, *dios*, *kali-bi*, **Lyc**, **Nux-m**.

amel : *calc-p*.

eructations, amel : (See Eructations under Stomach).

fruit, after : **Chin**, puls.

lying, agg : carb-v.

tea drinkers, of : *chin*, *dios*.

upper abdomen : **Carb-v**.

lower abdomen : **Lyc**.

entire abdomen : **Chin**.

FULLNESS, sensation of : **Aloe, Chin, Kali-c, Lyc, Nux-v**.

  hypochondria, right : *podo*.

    left : *cean*.

GALL-STONE colic : (See Pain in Liver).

GRUMBLING : (See Rumbling, Gurgling).

GURGLING : **Aloe**, *lyc*, ph-ac.

  stool, before : **Aloe**.

HANGING down, as if intestines were : agar, **Ign, Ip, Staph**, *tab*.

  as if stomach were : *sul-ac*.

HARD : **Bar-c, Calc**, *raph*, **Sil**.

  liver : *chel*, **Chin, Iod, Mag-m**, *merc*, tarax.

HARDNESS, inguinal glands, no tendency to suppurate : *merc-i-f*, merc-i-r.

  Mesenteric glands : **Calc**, con.

HEAVINESS, as from a load : aloe, bry, **Graph, Lyc**, *mag-m*.

  hypochondria, right : *podo*.

   hepatic region : *bry, ptel*.

    dragging sensation on turning to left : bry, *ptel*.

    lying on right side, amel : *bry, ptel*.

     left side, agg : bry, *ptel*.

HERNIA, femoral : *lyc*.

  inguinal : **Lyc, Nux-v**.

   strangulated : **Bell, Nux-v, Op**, *plb*.

   children, in : **Aur**, lyc.

    right : lyc.

    left : nux-v.

   inclination : cocc.

   inflammation, with vomiting : *tab*.

   sensitive : *bell*, **Lach**.

  umbilical : cocc (after nux-v failed), **Nux-v**.

   strangulated : *plb*.

INDURATION : (See Hard).

INFLAMMATION (peritonitis, enteritis, etc.) : Apis, Ars, Bell, Bry, Colch,
　　Lach, Lyc, Pyrog, Rhus-t, *sil*, Ter.
　　　　appedicitis : Bell, Bry, *hep*, *lach*, Merc-c, *plb*, Sil, *terb*.
　　　　inguinal glands : *merc*, merc-i-r., rhus-t, *sil*.
　　　　liver : Chel, *merc*.

INTUSSUSCEPTION : Op, Plb.

LIVER and region of : Bell, Bry, Calc, Card-m, Chel, Chin, *coloc*, Kali-c,
　　Lyc, Mag-m, Merc, Nat-s, Nux-v, Phos, Podo, Sulph.

METEORISM : (See Distension).

MOVEMENTS in : Croc, *lyc*, lyss, sulph, **Thuj**.
　　　　alive, as if something : *thuj*.
　　　　arm of a foetus, like : Croc, *nux-m*, *sulph*, Thuj.

MOVEMENTS of the foetus, like : Croc, belon, *lyss*, murx, sulph, **Thuj**.
　　　　somersaults, violent : *lyc*, op, psor, *sil*.

OEDEMA : (See Dropsy).

OOZING from navel of infants, of bloody fluid : calc-p.
　　　　urine : hyos.

PAIN, aching, dull pain : *all-c*, *bell*, Bry, **Cham**, *chel*, *chin*, Coloc, Cupr,
　　dios, **Ip**, lil-t, lyc, merc, *merc-c*, *nux-m*, nux-v, Op, plb, Podo,
　　rheum, *stann*.
　　　　morning : Nux-v.
　　　　afternoon, 4 p.m. : coloc, Lyc.
　　　　night, 5 a.m. : kali-br, Merc, Nit-ac.
　　　　bending backward, amel : *bell*, *dios*.
　　　　bend double, must : *cham*, Coloc, *mag-p*.
　　　　　　agg : dios.
　　　　　　amel : *chin*, Coloc, *mag-p*, *stann*.
　　　　clothing, agg : *bell*, Lach.
　　　　coffee, after : *cham*, *nux-v*.
　　　　cold drinks, after : *calc-p*.
　　　　cold, from taking : all-c, Cham, Chin, *coloc*, Dulc.
　　　　colic : (See Pain, Cramping).
　　　　　　　　comes gradually and goes gradually : plat, stann.
　　　　　　　　quickly and goes quickly : Bell, Kali-bi.
　　　　　　　　constipation, from : op, plb.

cough, during : **Bell, Bry, Dros, Nux-v.**

damp weather, from : *dulc, nat-s.*

diarrhoea, during (colic) : **Cham**, *chin,* **Coloc, Dios**, *mag-c,* **merc, Podo.**

drinking, after : *bell,* **Coloc,** *podo.*

eating, while : *nux-v.*

on every attempt, to : *calc-p.*

after : *chin, coloc,* **Graph,** *nux-m, nux-v.*

amel : *chel,* iod, *psor.*

eructation amel : carb-v.

PAIN, fruit, after : *chin,* **Coloc.**

ice cream, after : **Ars,** calc-p, *puls.*

indignation, after : staph.

lying, while : *bell.*

on abdomen amel : **Bell,** *coloc, stann.*

menses, before : *am-c, bell,* **Calc-p,** *cocc, coloc, croc,* **Kali-c,** *mag-c, mag-p, nux-v,* **Puls.**

during : *bell, borx,* **Calc, Calc-p,** *cham, comic, coloc, cycl,* **Graph,** *kali-c, murx,* **Nux-v,** *plat,* **Puls.**

when flow becomes free, amel : *lach.*

heat, amel : **Ars,** *coloc, mag-p, nux-v.*

motion on : **Bell, Bry,** *gels,* **Ip,** *kalm,* mag-p, *nit-ac,* **Nux-v.**

paroxysmal : *bell,* berb, **Coloc, Cupr,** *dios, mag-p, plb.*

periodical : **Cham,** *chin, coloc,* **Cupr, Nux-v.**

pressure, agg : **Bell,** *nux-v.*

amel : **Coloc,** *mag-p, stann.*

radiating : *dios,* **Mag-p, Plb.**

to all parts of body : **Plb.**

retraction of umbilicus, with : **Plb.**

rheumatism of abdominal muscles : *cimic.*

stool, before : **Aloe, Am-c, Arg-met,** *chin, coloc,* **Mag-c,** *nux-v,* plb, **Podo.**

during : **Bry, Sulph.**

after : **Nit-ac, Sulph.**

amel : **Colch, Coloc, Nux-v.**

suppressed haemorrhoidal flow : **Nux-v.**

vexation, after : **Coloc**, *staph*.

violent : *ars*, *colch*, *coloc*, *cupr*, merc-c, *nux-v*, **Plb**.

wandering : *puls*.

shifting suddenly to distant part : **Dios**.

warm drink, amel : *chel*, lyc, *mag-p*.

warmth, amel : **Ars**, **Cham**, *coloc*, **Mag-p**, **Nux-m**, **Nux-v**, plb, *podo*, *puls*, **Rhus-t**.

extending to all parts of body, to : **Plb**.

hypochondria : **Lyc**, **Merc**.

right : **Bell**, **Chel**, *chin*, **Lyc**, **Podo**, **Ptel**.

extending to back : **Chel**, **Lyc**.

afternoon, 4 p.m. : **Lyc**.

PAIN, ilio-caecal region: **Bry**.

right : **Bell**.

touch agg : **Bell**.

bed cover intolerable : **Bell**.

liver : *berb*, *card-m*, **Chel**, **Chin**, **Lyc**, **Mag-m**, **Podo**.

colic, gall-stones : **Bell**, **Berb**, **Card-m**, **Chel**, **Lyc**.

jaundice, followed by : *berb*.

lying on back, amel : mag-m.

right side, on : *bell*, kali-c, *mag-m*, *merc*.

left side, on : *mag-m*.

rubbing, amel : **Podo**.

touched, when : mag-m.

walking, while : *mag-m*.

extending, back, to : **Chel**, **Lyc**, **Mag-m**.

spleen, chill, during : **Podo**.

PAIN (colic), cramping, griping : all-c, **Aloe**, *am-c*, **Am-m**, bar-c, **Bell**, *berb*, caul, **Cham**, **Chel**, **Chin**, **Coloc**, Coll, **Cupr**, **Dios**, Ip, **Lyc**, *mag-c*, **Mag-p**, *merc*, *merc-c*, mill, **Plb**, *rheum*, **Stann**.

morning, every day, 5 a.m. : kali-br.

afternoon, daily 4 p.m. : *coloc*, *lyc*.

night : *chin*.

abdominal section, after : bism, hep, *staph*.

anger, from : *cham*, *coloc*, **Staph**.

bending backward, amel : dios.

bending double, must : **Coloc**, mag-c, *mag-p*.

    amel : bov, *chin*, **Coloc**, mag-p.

    agg : *dios*.

biliary : (See Colic, Gall-stone).

cheese agg : *coloc*.

children, of : *all-c*, *bar-c*, *coloc*, jal, kali-br, *lyc*.

cold, from getting feet wet : all-c.

        taking : all-c, **Cham**, **Chin**, *coloc*, dulc.

colic, gall-stone : *berb*, **Card-m**, **Chel**, **Chin**.

    periodical : *card-m*, **Chin**.

constipation, preceded by : **Aloe**.

cucumbers, from : all-c.

drinking, after : **Coloc**.

eating, overeating, from : *all-c*.

    while : *calc-p*.

        every attempt, to : *calc-p*.

      after : bov, *chin*, *coloc*.

flatulent : cocc, **Mag-p**.

    of horses and cows, after failure of coloc : **Mag-p**.

fixed hour daily, at : *chin*.

heat, amel : **Mag-p**.

haemorrhoidal : all-c.

lead : *alum*.

lithotomy, after : staph.

lying while agg : dios.

    on abdomen, amel: *coloc*, *stann*.

menses, before : *am-c*.

moving about, amel : all-c.

ovariotomy, after : staph.

paroxysmal : **Cupr**.

periodical : **Cupr**.

pressure, amel : **Coloc**, *mag-p*, plb, *stann*.

rubbing, amel :

salad, from :

sitting, from :

standing, when : rheum.

standing erect, amel :

stool, before : **Aloe**, dulc, *mag-c*, rheum.

    during : **Aloe**.

      after, amel : *aloe*, mag-c, **Nux-v**.

uncovering arm or leg : rheum.

liver : *berb*.

umbilicus, region of : am-m, **Coloc, Dios, Ip**.

    leucorrhoea, before : am-m.

inguinal region : *aloe*.

right : aloe.

PAIN, cutting : **Aloe**, *cham*, **cocc**, **Coloc, Dios**, *iod*, **Ip, Mag-c, Merc-c, Nux-v, Puls**, *staph*, **Verat**.

bending double, amel : **Coloc**, mag-c, staph.

diarrhoea, before : *mag-c*.

menses, before : mag-c.

movement, on : cocc.

stools before : **Aloe**, dulc.

    during : **Aloe**.

      after : **Coloc**, *merc*, *merc-c*.

        amel : aloe, **Nux-v**.

extending from right to left : **Lyc**.

    left to right : *ip*, **Lach**.

umbilicus, region of : **Coloc, Dios, Ip, Nux. v**.

spleen, in region of : *cean*.

PAIN, dragging, bearing down : **Bell, Lil-t**, *lyss*, *murx*, sanic, **Sep**.

crossing limbs, amel : **Lil-t**, sanic, **Sep**.

PAIN, pressing : *bell*, **Calc, Lyc, Nux-v**.

hypochondria,

    right : **Lyc, Mag-m**.

    touching agg : *lach*, *mag-m*.

walking, while : *mag-m.*

hypogastrium : **Bell, Lil-t, Lyc, Sep.**

morning : **Lil-t,** murx, **Sep.**

downwards : lil-t.

genitals, towards : **Bell, Lil-t, Sep.**

sitting and standing erect, amel : **Bell.**

stool, during : **Lil-t,** *podo.*

urinating, during : *lil-t.*

PAIN, rubbing sharp stones, as of : *cocc.*

PAIN, sore, bruised, tenderness : **Apis, Arn, Ars, Bell, Bry,** *canth,* **Cham, Colch,** *ham,* **Lach, Lyc,** *nux-m,* **Ter.**

bed cover, touch of, agg : **Bell, Lach.**

bowels feel sore, as if bruised : ferr.

injury, after : ham.

jarring, on : **Bell, Bry.**

menses, before : *bell, bry.*

during : *bell, ham.*

motion, on : **Bell, Bry.**

pregnancy, during : *nux-m.*

walking, while : *bell.*

hypochondria, right : **Bell, Bry,** *chin,* **Lyc,** nat-s.

ilio-caecal region : bapt (right), **Bell, Bry.**

hypogastrium : **Ter.**

inguinal region : **Arn.**

walk bent, must : **Arn.**

PAIN, stitching : **Bry,** *cimic,* **Ip,** *kali-c.*

across abdomen : *cimic.*

extending downwards : **Ip.**

umbilicus : **Ip.**

extending to uterus : **Ip.**

PAIN, twisting : *dios* (as if grasped and twisted by a powerful hand), *staph,* **Verat.**

paroxysmal : *dios.*

PARALYSIS of intestines : **Op, Plb.**

PERISTALSIS reversed : *op.*

POT-BELLY : (See Enlarged).

PROTRUSION of transverse colon : bell.

RETRACTION : Plb.

        sensation, of : **Plb.**

        umbilicus : **Plb.**

RUBBING : (See Shaking).

RUMBLING (See Gurgling) : *aloe*, bapt. **Chin**, gamb, **Lyc**, nat-s (in rt. ileo-caecal region), ph-ac, puls.

        stool, before : *aloe*.

        ascending colon, in : *podo*.

        iliac region, right : bapt.

        hypochondria, left : lyc.

SHAKING, rubbing, liver region, with hands : podo.

SUNKEN : *calc-p*.

SUPPURATION, inguinal glands : **Hep, Lach, Merc**.

SWASHING, stool, before : **Crot-t**.

SWELLING, colon, transverse, protrude like a pad : *bell*.

        inguinal glands : *bar-c*, *carb-an*, *merc-i-r*, *mere.i-f*, **Merc, Sil**.

        mesenteric : **Iod**.

SWOLLEN, pit of stomach, like an inverted saucer : **Calc**.

TENSION : Bar-c.

ULCERS : Ter.

WEAKNESS : Phos, *podo*, *sep*.

❑❑❑

Alternation of States

Asthma and eruption : **Calad**, rhus-t.

Cheerfulness and melancholy : acon, *coff*, **Croc**, ign, plat, *nux-m*.
         and rage : **Croc**.

Canine hunger and loss of appetite : **Cina, Ferr**.

Chill and heat : ars, merc.

Congestion of head and congestion of heart : *glon*.

Cough and eruption : **Crot-t**.

Dancing and singing and melancholy : *croc*.
                and rage : *croc*.

Depression and exaltation : lach.

Delerium and colic : **Plb**.

Diarrhoea and constipation : **Abrot, Ant-c**, chel, coll, ptel, **Nux-v**, *sulph*, verat.
        and eczema : **Crot-t**.
        and headache : aloe, **Podo**.

Diarrhoea (in summer) and eczema (in winter) : **Petr**.

Diarrhoea (in summer) and headache (in winter) : *podo*.

Eczema and internal ailments : **Graph**.

Fistula in ano and chest symptoms : *berb, calc-p, sil*.

Gastric symptoms (in spring) and rheumatism (in fall) : *kali-bi*.

Glowing red face and pale face : **Cina**.

Headache and foot sweat : **Merc, Sil**.

Headache and gastralgia : arg-n, *bism*.
        and lumbago : aloe.

Laughing and weeping : *coff, ign*, **Nux-m**, *puls*.

Mental and physical : *cimic, plat*.
        and uterine : **Lil-t**.

Pulse, slow and quick alternate : dig.

Pain (sciatic) and numbness : **Gnaph**.

F-2

Palpitation and piles : **Coll.**

and suppressed menses : *coll.*

Rheumatism and dysentery : *abrot, kali-bi.*

and haemorrhoids : *abrot.*

and heart symptoms : *kalm.*

Stool, black and white alternate : aur-m-n.

Sciatica (in summer) and croupy cough (in winter) : staph.

Urticaria and croupy attack : *ars.*

Violent mania and disposition to silence : verat.

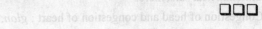

Back

AIR, cannot bear a draft of : *hep*, *sil*.

BREAK, as if it would : *ham*.

CARBUNCLES : (See Eruption).

CARIES of spine : (See Curvature).

COLDNESS (including Chill) : *am-m*, **Caps**, **Eup-per**, *gels*, **Puls**, **Sil**, **Sulph**.
   extending down the back : **Agar**.
      up the back : *gels*.
         up and down the back : **Gels**.
      cervical region : **Sil**.
      dorsal region, between scapulae : *am-m*, *lach*, pyrog.
      spine : *gels*.

COLD air, back sensitive to : **Sil**.

CONCUSSION of spine : **Hyper**.
   chronic effects of : *cic*, **Hyper**.

CONGESTION, spine : *verat-v*.

CONTRACTION (See Spasm, Drawing Pains, Tension, Spasmodic Drawing) : *cimic*, *med*.

CURVATURE of spine : **Calc**, **Calc-p**, *ther*.
   left, especially to : **Calc-p**.
   dorsal : plb.

DISTURBED functional activity of spinal cord, from exhausting disease : *caust*.
   mental shock, from, resulting in paralysis : **Caust**.

EMACIATION : *sars* (neck), tab.
   cervical region : *lyc*, **Nat-m**, *sanic*.
   dorsal region : plb.

EMISSION, agg : cob.
   amel : zinc.

ERUPTIONS : **Mez**, nat-m, **Psor**, **Sulph**.
   carbuncle : **Anthraci** (malignant type with terrible burning and sloughing), ars, *crot-h*.
      discharge, acrid and offensive : *anthraci*.

cervical region : *anthraci*, *hep*, **Lach**, **Sil**, sulph.

dorsal region : *hep*, *lach*.

herpes, cervical region : nat-m.

FLABBINES of skin : **Nat-m**, *sanic*.

skin hangs loose : **Nat-m**, *sanic*.

HANGS, loose, skin of neck : (See Flabbiness).

HEAT : helon (lumbar region), **Phos**.

extending up the back : **Phos**.

Heaviness, sensation of : *aesc*, helon.

INFLAMMATION, cord : **Gels**, plb.

membranes, spinal meningitis : **Apis**, **Bell**, **Gels**, *nat-s*, *plb*.

INJURIES of spine (See Concussion of Spine also) : *arn*, **Hyper**, *led*, **Nat-s**.

coccyx : **Hyper**.

IRRITATION of spine : (See Pain, Sore).

ITCHING, coccyx, tip of, intolerable : *borx*.

must scratch until raw and sore : bov.

LAMENESS, sensation of : *aesc, cimic*.

lumbar region : **Berb**, dulc, helon.

NUMBNESS : berb.

Lumbar region : **Berb**.

OPISTHOTONUS : **Cupr**, **Cic**, **Hyos**, nat-s, plb, *verat-v*.

PAIN : *act*, **Aesc**, *agar*, *arg-met*, **Arn**, *berb*, *chel*, **Calc**, *cimic,* cob, dulc, **Eup-per** (affecting bones), *gels*, *hyper*, **Kali-c**, **Lac-c**, **Lyc**, mag-c, *mag-m*, *med*, **Nat-s**, **Nux-m**, **Nux-v**, phyt, plb, **Psor**, **Puls**, **Rhus-t**, *ruta*, **Sep**, *staph*, *zinc*.

morning, before rising : staph.

night, bed, in : staph.

abortion, after : *kali-c*.

back gives out : **Aesc** (during leucorrhoea, pregnancy prolapse, walking, stooping), *kali-c* (walking while).

must lie down : kali-c.

damp weather : **Rhus-t**.

eating, after : *kali-c*.

emission, after : *staph*.

exertion, from : *agar*.

fever, during : *eup-per*.

labor, during : **Kali-c**, *nux-v*.

lifting, from : **Rhus-t**.

lying, while : *berb*, *rhus-t*.

    amel : kali-c.

    on back, amel : **Nat-m, Ruta**.

lying, on something hard, amel : **Nat-m**, *rhus-t*.

manual labour, from : *sulph*.

masturbation, from : **Nux-v**.

menses, before : **Kali-c**, *mag-c*.

      during : *kali-c*, *mag-m*.

metrorrhagia, after : *kali-c*.

motion, on : **Aesc**.

    amel : lac-c, **Rhus-t**.

move, beginning to : lac-c, **Rhus-t**.

pressure, amel : caust, **Kali-c**.

rheumatic : *Cimic*, Rhod, **Rhus-t**.

riding in a carriage : **Nux-m**.

    on horse back : ars.

rising from a seat : **Rhus-t**.

sexual excess, from : **Nux-v, Ph-ac**.

sitting, while : **Agar,** cob, *puls*, **Rhus-t, Zinc**.

stooping, when : aesc, **Sulph**.

swallowing, on : *kali-c*.

turning, when : *nux-v*.

    in bed, when : *nux-v*.

    must sit up to turn over : **Nux-v**.

urination, amel : **Lyc**.

walking, while : **Aesc, Kali-c**, *mag-m*.

    amel : cob, *puls*, **Rhus-t**, *zinc*.

extending to, other parts of body : sabin.

      back from other parts : *sep*.

      forwards and downwards : arg-met.

      thighs, to : mag-m.

cervical region : all-c, berb, cimic, eup-per, **Gels**, *nat-s*, *sil*. ,

    neuralgic : all-c.

rheumatic : **Cimic, Ran-b, Rhus-t**.
extending, eye, to : **Sil**.

right : **Sil**.
left : **Spig**.
head, to : **Sil**.
all over : **Gels**.
extending, occiput, to : **Sil**.
vertex, to : **Gels, Sil**.

dorsal region : berb, nux-v, **Sulph**.

scapulae : **Chel**, *kali-c*, merc.
right : **Chel**, *kali-c*, merc.
under : **Chel**.
left : chen-a, sang.

lumbar region : **Aesc**, *agar*, **Arg-met, Berb, Bry, Calc, Chin**, cob, **Eup-per**, *ferr*, *ham*, ip, med, *kali-c*, lyc, **Nux-v**, *psor*, **Rhus-t**, *ruta*, sabin, **Sep**, *staph*, ter, *zinc*.

abortion, after : *kali-c*.
back 'gives out' : (See Back, Pain).
break, as if it would : *ham*.
chill, before : *eup-per*.
cold, taking from : aesc.
emission amel : **Zinc**.
exertion, from : *agar*, berb.
jarring, from : berb.
labor, after : kali-c.
lie down, must : **Aesc**.
laying, while : **Berb, Rhus-t**.

on back : **Rhus-t**.
amel : *nat-m, ruta*.
on something hard, amel : **Nat-m, Rhus-t**.

masturbation, from : **Nux-v**.
motion, during : **Aesc**.

amel : **Rhus-t**, zinc.

red sand in urine, amel by passage of : **Lyc**.
rising from a seat : arg-n, **Rhus-t**.
sexual excess : cob, **Nux-v**, *zinc*.
sit must : **Aesc**.
sitting while : **Agar, Berb**, *cob*, *puls*, **Rhus-t**, *zinc*.
stool, after : ferr.

stooping : *aesc*.

turning when, must sit up in bed : **Nux-v**.

walking while : **Aesc**.

  amel : cob, puls, *rhus-t*, *zinc*.

extending, pubis to : **Sabin**.

  down the thighs : **Cimic**.

lumbo-sacral : **Aesc**.

sacral region : **Aesc**, **Agar**, **Berb**, *lac-c*, *med*, *psor*.

  exertion, during : agar.

  moving, first, on : lac-c, **Rhus-t**.

    amel : Lac-c, **Rhus-t**.

  sitting while : agar, *lac-c*, **Rhus-t**, zinc.

  cross super-sacral region : *lac-c*.

    extending to right natis and right sciatic nerve: *lac-c*.

    extending, downwards : *med*.

      running around : *med*.

coccyx : *hyper*, mag-c (coccydynia), lob, *med*.

  fall, after : **Hyper**.

spine : **Agar**, *berb*, hyper, med.

  fall, after : *hyper*.

  motion, on : *agar*.

  motion of arms or neck extorts cries : *hyper*.

  pressure, agg : *chinin-s*, *lac-c*, phos, zinc.

  turn, every, of body causes : agar.

  touch, agg : *chinin-s*, *lac-c*, phos, zinc.

  extending from base of brain to coccyx : lac-c.

PAIN, aching : *aesc*, agar, *berb*, **Bry**, **Eup-per**, ferr, lac-c, *kali-c*.

  chill, before : **Eup-per**.

  lumbar region : **Aesc**, agar, berb, ferr, *kali-c*, pic-ac.

    exertion, during : agar.

    sitting, while : *agar*, berb, zinc.

    stool, after : ferr.

  lumbo-sacral region : **Aesc**.

    constant : **Aesc**.

    sacrum : **Aesc**, **Agar**.

      sitting : **Agar**.

    spine : *lac-c*.

from base of brain to coccyx : *lac-c.*

nape of neck, when held in position too long : **Zinc**.

bearing down : *ham*.

break, as though the back would : **Bell**, ham.

haemorrhoids, with : ham.

broken, as if : **Eup-per**.

PAIN, burning : **Ars**, *kali-p,med*, **Phos**, *pic-ac*, **Sulph**, *zinc*.

cervical region : *med*.

extending down spine : *med*.

dorsal region : *zinc*.

scapulae between : **Phos**, *sulph*.

spots, in : *phos*, *sulph*.

spine : kali-p, **Phos**, *pic-ac*, *zinc*.

as of a piece of ice : lachn.

in spots: *phos*.

mental exertion : kali-p, *pic-ac*.

lumbar region : helon.

PAIN, crushed as though, base of brain : *nat-s.*

drawing : **Cimic**.

cervical region : **Cimic**, med.

dorsal region : **Cimic**.

scapulae, between : **Cimic**.

lumbar region : **Sabin**.

extending to pubic bone : **Sabin**.

round the body to pubis : vib.

gnawing, base of brain : *nat-s*.

pressing : **Bell**, berb.

lumbar region : berb.

sore, bruised, beaten : aesc, *agar*, **Arn**, **Eup-per**, nat-m, ph-ac, ther, *zinc*.

dorsal region, scapulae, between : chinin-s, ther.

jar of foot : ther.

noise agg : ther.

sitting sideways in chair, amel : chinin-s, ther.

lumbar region : **Agar, Arn, Bry, Eup-per**, med.

exertion, during : agar.

sitting, while : *agar*, berb, zinc.
touch agg : med.
sacral region : *lob*, **Rhus-t**.
exertion, during : agar.
moving, amel : **Rhus-t**
rest, agg : **Rhus-t**.
sitting, while : agar, zinc.
touch of clothing, sensitive to : **Lob**.

sore, spinal, spinal irritation : **Agar**, **Chinin-s**, cimic, hyper, *lac-c*, *med*, **Nat-m**, **Phos**, *tarent*, **Ther**, **Zinc**.
morning : agar.
piano-playing : agar, cimic, ran-b.
sexual excess, after : agar, **Kali-p**, **Nat-m**.
sewing machine, from using : cimic.
type-writing, from : cimic.
touch agg : *agar*, Chinin-s, hyper, *med*, *tarent*, **Ther**, **Zinc**.
vertebra, single, sensitive to touch : **Agar**.

PARALYSIS, spine : **Aesc**.

PARALYTIC weakness : cocc, sanic.

PERSPIRATION, cervical region : **Calc**, stann.

SENSITIVE to touch, spine : agar, **Hyper**, ther.
vertebra, single : agar.

SHIVERING : agar, chel, gels.
extending down the back : agar, chel, gels.
up the back : dig, gels.

SOFTENING of cord : **Kali-p**, *phos*, pic-ac, zinc.

SPASM (See Opisthotonus) : mag-m, *nat-s*.
menses, during : mag-m.

SPASMODIC drawing, cervical region (head bent back) : **Cimic**, **Cic**,
gels, *nat-s*.

STIFFNESS : **Berb**, **Caust**, **Cimic**, dulc, lachn (torticollis), med,
Nux-v, **Rhus-t**.
rising from seat : caust, **Rhus-t**.
sitting, while : **Rhus-t**.
stretching, agg : med.

cervical region : **Cimic**.
lumbar region : caust, **Rhus-t**.
    lying, while : **Rhus-t**.
        on something hard, amel : **Nat-m, Rhus-t**.
    motion, amel : **Rhus-t**.
    sitting, while : **Rhus-t**.

TENSION : med, nat-c.
cervical region : **Cimic**, med, *nat-c*.
menses, before : *nat-c*.

WEAKNESS (in spine) : **Calc-p, Ph-ac**, *pic-ac*, **Sel**.
emission, from : **Sel**.
sexual excess, after : **Nux-v, Ph-ac, Sel**.
typhoid, after : **Sel**.
neck weak, unable to support head : *abrot, aeth*, cocc, **Calc-p**, zinc.
unable to support body : **Calc-p**.
lumbar region : berb, cocc, helon.
nape of neck, when held in one position too long : **Zinc**.

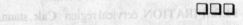

Bladder

BALL in, sensation of : *lach*.

CALCULI : Benz-ac, erig, **Lyc, Sars**.

CATARRH : Benz-ac, *ter*.

       gonorrhoea, suppressed from : *benz-ac*.

CONSTRICTION : *cact*, caps.

FULLNESS, sensation of : **Dig, Equis-h**, *ruta*.

       urination, after : *ruta*, sars.

       without desire to urinate : *op*.

GAS, passes from : *sars*.

HAEMORRHAGE (See Urine Bloody) : *cact*, *crot-h*, erig, *ham*, mill, *phos*.

INFLAMMATION : Acon, Bell, Canth, *chim*, **Sars, Ter**.

IRRITABLE : (See Urging to Urinate).

PAIN : *berb*, **Canth**, *caps*, **Equis-h**, *sars*, ter.

       coughing, when : caps.

       distension, as from : equis-h.

          urination does not amel : *equis-h*.

       violent : *canth*.

       neck : petros.

PAIN, burning : **Berb, Canth, Ter**.

       cutting : *berb*, *canth*, **Ter**.

       drawing : *berb*, canth, ter.

       sore : **Canth, Equis-h**, *sars*.

PARALYSIS : *arn*, **Caust, Gels**, *hyos*, **Nux-v, Op**.

       old people, in : *equis-h* (in women).

       over-distension, after : **Caust**.

       parturition, after, no desire : **Arn, Caust**, *hyos*, *op*.

PROLAPSE of bladder : staph.

RETENTION of urine (See Urination Retarded) : **Apis, Arn**, *cann-s*, **Canth, Caust**, *hyos*, **Op, Ter**.

       atony of fundus, from : *ter*.

       confinement, after : *arn*, **Caust**.

constipation, from : cann-s, *op*.

heat, during : op.

illness, in acute : op.

labor, after : **Arn**, *op*.

new born infants, in : **Acon**.

> after passion of the nurse : *op*.

paralysis, from : **Op**.

painful : **Canth, Caust, Nux-v**, *ter*.

spasmodic : ter.

tobacco, from : op.

urine passed by drops : (See Urination, Dribbling).

TENESMUS : Canth, *med*, **Merc-c, Nux-v**, puls, *sars*, **Ter**.

> urinating, when : *med*.

URGING TO URINATE : Apis, *arn*, **Berb**, borx, **Canth**, Equis-h, hyper, **Lil-t**, *lyc*, *lyss*, merc, **Merc-c**, ruta, **Sars, Staph, Thuj**.

> night : hyper.
>
> coition, after : staph.
>
> constant : **Apis, Canth**, caust, **Equis-h, Lil-t, Lac-c**, lyss, pareir (goes down on his knees).
>
> > passing a few drops at a time : *apis*, **Canth**.
> >
> > passing of large quantities, which does not amel : **Equis-h**.
> >
> > running water, at sight of : canth, *lyss*, sulph.
>
> frequent (See Urination Frequent) : **Apis**, *berb*, **Canth**, coloc, *equis-h*, **Lil-t, Merc, Merc-c**, *sars*, **Thuj**.
>
> ineffectual : **Arn**, caust, berb, **Canth**, *equis-h*, sars, **Thuj**.
>
> irresistible, intolerable : **Apis, Canth**.
>
> > can scarcely retain : **Apis**.
> >
> > have to urinate must or urine will escape : **Canth**.
>
> labor, difficult, after : op, staph.
>
> labor pain, with every : nux-v.
>
> lying when : **Puls**.
>
> married women, newly : **Staph**.
>
> painful : *apis*, **Canth**, pareir (pain runs down thighs).
>
> > child cries : **Borx, Lyc**, sanic, **Sars**.
>
> pressure in rectum, from : *lil-t*.
>
> sudden : apis, **Canth, Kreos, Petros**.
>
> > child jumps up and down with pain, if not gratified : petros.

cannot get of of bed quick enough : apis, **Kreos**, *petros*.
urination, before : *canth*.
   during : *canth*.
   after : *canth, staph*.
                  in prostatic trouble of old men : staph.

URINATION, dribbling (by drops) : *arg-n*, **Canth**, colch, *dulc*, Equis-h,
   Merc-c, *sars*, **Staph**, Ter.
   enlarged prostate, with : benz-ac.
   involuntary : *arg-n, arn, dulc, op, sel*.
      day and night : *nux-v*.
      confinement, after : *arn, op*.

URINATION, dribbling,
      sitting, while : *sars*.
      standing, when, passes freely : *sars*.
      vertically, urine drops : **Hep**.
      walking, while : sel.

URINATION, dysuria : *apis*, **Bell**, *con, hep*, **Lyc**, **Merc-c**, *nat-m*, **Nux-v**,
   Ter.
      married women, newly : **Staph**.
      painful, child cries before urine starts : **Borx**, *lyc*, nux-v, **Sars**.

URINATION, feeble stream (slow) : **Hep**, **Mur-ac**.
      drops vertically : *hep*.

URINATION, forked stream : **Thuj**.
      frequent : apis, caust (few drops at a time), *borx*, **Lyc**, **Merc**,
         Merc-c, *sars*, staph.
      impeded : *hep*.
      incomplete (See Unsatisfactory) : *alum*, **Clem**, **Hep**, sil.
      intermittent (interrupted) : **Clem**, **Con**.
      flows better when standing : *con*.
      involuntary : **Apis**, **Arg-n**, **Arn**, **Caust**, *cina*, **Dulc**, *equis-h*,
         hyos, kreos, murx, **Nat-m**, *op*, **Psor**, **Puls**, *ruta*, sanic,
         squil, *sel*, **Sep**, verat, zinc.
         daytime : *ferr*, **Fl-ac**.
                  and night : *arg-n*, **Caust**, equis-h.
         night (incontinence in bed) : **Apis**, **Arn**, **Benz-ac**, **Caust**,
         cina, **Equis-h**, hyos, **Kreos**, **Mag-p**, **Med**, **Nat-m**, *op*,
         psor, **Puls**, *sanic*, **Sep**.

difficult to awaken the child : *bell*, **Kreos**.

dreaming of urination, while : *kreos*.

eezema in the family, history of : psor.

first sleep, during : benz-ac, **Caust**, *kreos*, Sep.

full moon, during : psor.

heat and cold, from extremes of : med.

over-work or play agg : *med*.

URINATION, involuntary,

blowing the nose, when : **Caust**, puls, squil, verat.

catheterization, after : *mag-p*.

cold, becoming : *dulc*.

coughing, when : **Caust**, **Nat-m**, **Puls**, *rumx*, **Squil**, verat.

labor, after : *arn*, hyos, op.

laughing, when : **Caust**, *nat-m*, *puls*, **Squil**.

lying, while : kreos.

nervous irritation, from : mag-p.

old people, in : *sec*, *thuj*.

with enlarged prostate : *aloe*, *parier*, *sec*, *thuj*.

sneezing, when : **Caust**, *puls*, squil, verat.

walking, while : caust, **Nat-m**.

retarded, must wait for urine to start : **Arn**, **Caust**, **Hep**, *mur-ac*, *nat-m*.

alone, can only pass urine when : *nat-m*.

press must, before he begins : **Mag-m**, **Mur-ac**.

Press must, so that anus protrudes : **Mur-ac**.

sit for hours at urinal, has to : staph.

sitting, can only pass urine while : **Zinc**.

bent back-ward, can only pass urine while : zinc.

standing, can only pass urine, while : **Sars**.

slow : (See Feeble Stream).

split stream : (See Forked).

unconscious, urethra insensible : **Arg-n**, **Caust**.

unsatisfactory (See Incomplete) : *alum*, **Caust**, **Hep**, sil.

WEAKNESS : Caust, **Hep**, **Mag-m**, **Mur-ac**.

❏❏❏

Chest

ABSCESS,

　　axilla : **Hep, Merc, Nit-ac,** Sil.

　　lungs : **Calc, Hep,** *kali-c, merc.*

　　mammae : *bell, bry,* **Hep,** graph, *lach,* **Merc, Phyt, Sil.**

　　　　threatening : **Phyt.**

　　　　hastens suppuration : **Hep,** lach, *merc,* phyt, **Sil.**

AFFECTIONS, cartilage : *arg-met.*

　　　　heart : **Aur, Cact,** cimic, **Lach, Naja, Spig.**

　　　　reflex from uterus or ovaries : *cimic.*

　　　　rheumatism, from : led, **Naja, Spig.**

ANGINA pectoris : *aml-ns, kalm,* **Naja, Spig, Spong.**

ANXIETY, in : **Acon, Ars,** spong.

　　　　heart, region of : **Ars, Meny,** *naja, spong.*

　　　　　　apex, of : *lil-t.*

　　　　　　base, of : *lob.*

ATROPHY, mammae : **Con, Iod.**

BAND : (See Constriction).

CANCER, mammae : aster, **Con, Graph,** *kreos,* lach.

　　　　abscesses, repeated, after : **Graph.**

　　　　cicatrices, in old : **Graph.**

CATARRH : **Ant-t, Bry,** *dros,* **Dulc, Hep.**

　　　　whooping cough, after : *coc-c.*

CEASE, sensation as if heart would : aur.

　　　　fears unless constantly on the move the heart will cease : **Gels.**

　　　　fears if she moved, it would cease : **Cic, Dig.**

　　　　sudden : cimic.

CICATRICES, old, in mammae : **Graph.**

COLDNESS : med, *petr.*

mammae : *med* (cold as ice, rest of body warm).

menses, during : med.

nipple : *med.*

menses during : med.

COLDNESS, heart, region of : *carb-an, kali-m, nat-m, petr.*

COMPLAINTS after fistula operations : *berb, calc-p*, **Sil.**

CONGESTION (hyperaemia of chest) : **Acon**, *aur*, **Cact, Spong, Sulph,**
verat.

desire to urinate, if not satisfied : **Lil-t.**

exertion, after : aur.

lungs : dig.

CONSTRICTION : **Cact**, *caps, dros, iod, mosch, spong.*

band or cord tightly tied, as from : **Cact.**

heart : **Cact, Iod, Lil-t**, *naja.*

clasping and unclasping feels, by iron band: **Cact.**

grasping sensation : **Cact, Iod, Lil-t**, sulph.

no room to beat, as if bound : **Cact.**

walk erect, inability to : *lil-t.*

extending to back : *lil-t.*

CORD, sensation : (See Constriction).

CRACKS of nipples : **Caust,** *fl-ac*, **Graph, Phyt, Rat.**

DILATATION of heart : **Cact**, *naja.*

DISCOLOURATION,

redness : aster.

spots : **Led, Phos,** *sep.*

brown : **Sep.**

yellow : sep.

mammae, livid red : aster.

pale : bry.

DISTENSION,

mammae : aster (as before menses)

DRAWN in, feels, mammae : aster.

DROPSY : **Apis, Apoc, Ars**, dig, **Hell, Merc-sul**, *sulph* (facilitates absorption).

    acute : apoc.

    heart disease, from : **Merc-sul.**

    inflammatory : apoc.

    liver disease, from : **Merc-sul.**

    suppressed exanthamata, from : *apis*, *hell*, *zinc.*

    uncomplicated with organic disease : *apoc.*

    pericardium : *apis*, *apoc.*

DRYNESS, bronchi : *spong.*

EMPHYSEMA : Am-c.

EMPTINESS, sensation : phos, **Stann.**

ENLARGEMENT : (See Hypertrophy).

ERUPTIONS suppressed, causing respiratory ailments : hep.

ERUPTIONS : Ars, Carb-an, kali-br.

    pustules : kali-br.

EXPECTORATION, amel : *zinc.*

FAINT feeling about heart : (See Weakness).

FATTY degeneration of heart : **Aur, Kali-c,** lac-d, **Phos.**

FISSURES : (See Cracks).

FISTULA in mammae : *phyt*, **Sil.**

FLAT : *tub.*

FLUTTERING : cact, lith, **Lil-t, Naja, Nat-m.**

    faintness, after : **Nat-m.**

    lying, while : cact (on left side), lach, **Nat-m.**

GRASPING : (See Constriction).

HAEMORRHAGE (See Expectoration) : *acet-ac*, **Arn**, *bry*, **Cact, Calc,** coca, *croc*, crot-h, elaps, erig, ferr, **Ham,** *kreos*, merc, **Mill, Phos,** tril-p, ter.

    coagulated : *croc.*

    coughing, on : *ham.*

    effort, without : ham.

    exertion, after : *mill.*

    haemorrhoidal flow, after suppression of : mill.

F-3

fall from a height, after : **Arn**, *mill*.

menses, suppression, after : *bry*, mill.

monthly : *ham*.

passive : kreos.

pneumonia, result of : *kali-c*, merc.

venous : ham, *kreos*.

years, for : *ham*.

HARDNESS, mammae : (See Induration).

HEAT : Acon, Bell, *bry*, glon, sang (behind sternum), *spong*.

Heart, region of : **Glon**, *spong*.

flushes of : **Glon**.

extending to head : **Glon**.

HEAVINESS : (See Oppression).

HEAVY, mammae : **Bry**.

HYDROTHORAX : (See Dropsy).

HYPERTROPHY of heart : *brom, caust, naja*.

calisthenics in young girls, from : **Caust**.

gymnastics in growing boys, from : **Brom**.

mammae : *calc, con*, sang.

INDURATION, mammae (See Lumps and Nodules) : *bry* (pale but hot and painful), **Con** (stony hard), *iod, phyt*.

stony hard : *bry*, **Con**, phyt.

INFLAMMATION, bronchial tubes (bronchitis) : **Ant-t**, **Bry**, *calc*, cop, dulc, **Dros**, **Ferr-p**, **Hep**, *hyos*, **Ip**, *kali-bi, naja*, **Puls**, **Sil**, *sulph*.

old people, in : carb-v.

whooping cough, after : *coc-c*.

axilla, glands : *sil*.

heart : **Aur**, *kalm*, lach, *naja*.

endocardium : **Kalm**, *naja*.

gouty or rheumatic : **Kalm**.

pericardium : *kalm*.

lungs : **Ant-t**, **Bry**, *calc*, **Chel**, **Ferr-p**, **Hep**, *hyos*, **Lyc**, **Merc**, ran-b, **Sulph**, *ter*.

right : *ant-t, bell*, **Bry**, *chel, kali-c, lyc, merc*.

lower lobe : *kali-c, lyc,* phos.

upper lobe : ars, **Calc.**

left : myrt, *nat-s, sulph.*

lower lobe : *nat-s.*

upper lobe : *acon.*

infants : *ant-t,* **Ip.**

neglected or maltreated : **Lyc.**

pneumonia or pleuro : ars (after suppressed measles),
Ant-t, Carb-v (after ant-t), hyos.

cold, from sudden : **Acon,** arn, *ran-b.*

jaundice, with : ant-t.

sycotic pneumonia : **Nat-s.**

typhoid pneumonia : *hyos,* lach, *op,* **Phos.**

mammae : **Bell, Bry, Hep,** lac-c, **Phyt, Sil.**

nipples : *cham.*

tender to touch : cham, helon, *phyt.*

infant's breast tender to touch : cham.

pleura : **Acon,** *arn,* **Bry,** kali-c, phos, *ran-b,* **Sulph.**

cold, from : *acon,* arn, *bry,* ran-b.

overheated, when : ran-b.

right pectoral region : borx.

IRRITABLE, heart : *lil-t.*

ITCHING : con, iod, phos.

low down in lungs behind sternum : iod.

extends through bronchi to nasal cavity : coc-c, con,
iod, phos.

LABORED, heart's action : *glon.*

MILK, absent : *agn,* **Calc,** *lac-d, sec.*

bring back, to : *lac-d.*

child cannot bear milk : **Aeth,** *calc,* **Mag-c.**

child refuses mother's milk : *borx, calc,* **Calc-p,** cina, *merc,* sil.

difficult : *agn.*

disappearing : *asaf, lac-c.*

dry up, to, when necessary : *asaf, lac-c.*

flowing : cham (in nursing women), con (after weaning).

increased : **Bell, Bry, Calc, Puls.**

non-pregnant women : *asaf, cycl,* **Puls.**

at puberty : *puls.*

retardation of flow, of, from old cicatrices : **Graph.**

runs out : (See Flowing).

stringy : **Borx.**

suppressed : *agn, asaf,* **Bry,** lac-c, lac-d, **Puls,** *sec.*

thick and tastes bad : *borx.*

MURMURS : Cact, Dig, Kalm, Naja, Spig.

at apex : **Spig, Spong.**

NARROW : tub.

NODULES, mammae : **Phyt.**

OPPRESSION : Am-c, Bry, Cact, Calc, cocc, *glon,* **Ip,** lob, mill, *naja,* **Phos, Sep,** spong, **Sulph.**

iron band prevented normal motion, as if : **Cact.**

walking, rapidly, amel : *lob.*

weight, as from a great : **Cact, Phos.**

heart : *am-c, aml-ns,* **Cact,** *glon,* kalm, *naja.*

ORGASM of blood : **Aml-ns, Glon, Lach,** *lil-t,* **Phos, Sep, Sulph.**

PAIN : All-c, Am-c, Aml-ns, brom, **Bry, Cact, Calc,** *cham, chel,* crot-t, *lyc, mag-p, merc, naja,* **Phos, Phyt, Puls, Spig, Spong,** *sulph, tarent,* ther.

chill, from : **Phos.**

cough, during : **Bry,** *calc,* **Lyc,** nat-s.

inflammatory : *ran-b.*

inspiration, during : **Bry.**

lying, abdomen, on, amel : *bry.*

side, on : naja.

painful : **Bell.**

amel : **Bry.**

left : **Phos.**

right : **Merc.**

motion, agg : **Bell, Bry, Calc,** *ran-b.*

PAIN, myalgic : *ran-b*.

 neuralgic : all-c, **Ran-b.**

 paroxysmal : ran-b.

 paroxysmal : ran-b.

 pleuritic : **Bry**, *ran-b*.

 pressure agg : phos.

   amel : **Bry.**

 respiration : **Bry.**

 rheumatic : **Bry, Ran-b, Rhus-t.**

 riding in a carriage : naja.

 running upwards : **Brom.**

 spinal irritation, from : *agar*, ran-b.

 touched, when : *ran-b*.

 spine touched, when : tarent.

 turning : *bry*, **Ran-b.**

 weather, changing : **Ran-b.**

  stormy : *ran-b*.

  wet : *ran-b*, *rhus-t*.

 lower, right : *chel*, *kali-c*, *merc*.

 heart : *aml-ns*, **Cact**, **Kalm**, **Lach**, *lil-t*, lith-c, *lob*, *naja*, **Rhus-t**, *spong*, *tarent*.

  extending to back : sulph.

  gout, after : *kalm*.

  menses, during : *lith-c*.

  moving, agg : *mag-m*.

  rheumatism, after : *kalm*, **Naja**, *lith-c*.

  sitting, while : *mag-m*.

  touching spine : tarent.

  urinating, when : *lith-c*.

  apex, at : *lil-t*.

  base, at : *lob*.

 lungs, middle lobe : med.

  upper, left, right through to left shoulder blade : apis, arum-t, **Myrt**, *pix*, **Sulph**, ther.

   right : ars.

lower, left : nat-s.

Mammae : aster, **Bell**, **Bry**, **Con**, cimic, *lac-c*, **Merc**, **Phyt**, sang.

descending, on : *lac-c*.

menses, before : **Calc**, **Con**, *lac-c*.

during : *con,* lac-c, *merc-c*.

nurses, when child : *crot-t*, *phyt*, *puls*, **Sil**.

extending from nipple, to all over body : **Phyt**.

to back : crot-t.

to uterus : *puls*, **Sil**.

support the breast, must : **Bry**, **Phyt**.

nipples : con, *helon*, *lac-c*.

PAIN, infra-mammary, left : *aster*, cimic, ust.

sides : **Lyc**, phos, **Ran-b**, **Sulph**.

left : **Lach**, lil-t, naja, **Phos**, **Ran-b**, *sulph*.

left, upper, extending to shoulder : anis, myrt, pix, **Sulph**, ther.

right : **Bell**, **Chel**, *lyc*.

right pectoral region : *borx*.

intercostal space : *phos*, **Ran-b**.

motion, on : **Bry**, **Chel**, *ran-b*.

neuralgia : *mez*, *ran-b*.

herpes, before or after : *mez*, *ran-b*.

paroxysmal : *ran-b*.

sternum, behind : kali-i, sang.

PAIN, burning : **Apis**, canth, *carb-v*, merc, *phos*, ran-b, sang, spong, *sulph*.

extending to face : **Sulph**.

lungs : *phos*.

sides : **Phos**, **Ran-b**.

cutting, lancinating (sudden sharp pain) : **Kali-c**, *ran-b*.

mammae : aster.

heart : **Aur**, **Cact**, **Lach**, *spig*, syph.

night : med, *spig, syph*.

extending from, base, to apex : *syph*.

to clavical or shoulder : *spig*.

apex to base : *med*.

darting : (See Stitching).

drawing : aster, crot-t.

    mammae : aster.

        felt when child nurses : crot-t.

        extending to scapula : crot-t.

        nipple : crot-t.

           as with a string when child nurses : **Crot-t**.

gripping : *cact*.

    vise-like grip : *cact*.

  lancinating : (See Pain, Cutting).

  pressing : kalm, sang.

    extending downwards : cact, *kalm*.

        upward : *led*.

rawness (includes trachaea and bronchi) : **Caust**, spong.

sharp : (See Cutting).

shooting : (See Stitching).

PAIN, sore, bruised : **Bry**, **Caust**, crot-t, *eup-per*, **Chel**, **Hep**, nat-s, nit-ac, **Ran-b**, spong.

    coughing, from : **Bry**, *caust*, **Dros**, *nat-s*.

    hold chest during cough : **Bry**, **Dros**, *eup-per*, nat-c, *nat-s*

    inspiring : **Bry**.

    motion, on : *ran-b*.

    sitting upright, amel : **Bry**, nat-c, *nat-s*.

    touch : **Ran-b**.

    turning : **Ran-b**.

    mammae : *bry*, **Cham**, *con*, helon, **Lac-c**, med, merc, *phyt*.

        evening : *bry*, lac-c.

        infant's breast tender to touch : cham.

        jar, agg : **Bell**, *lac-c*.

        menses, before : **Con**, kali-c, *lac-c*.

           during : *con*, helon, kali-c, *lac-c*, merc.

        pregnancy, during : **Arn**.

        stairs, going up and down : **Bell**, *bry*, **Lac-c**.

           must hold firmly : bry, **Lac-c**.

    nipples : **Arn**, **Crot-t**, helon, med, *phyt*, cham.

        menses, during : *helon*.

touch, agg : *cham*, helon, med, *phyt*.

sides : *ran-b*.

touch, agg : **Ran-b**.

springing : cact.

sticking : kalm, phel (through right chest extending to back).

extending downward : cact, *kalm*.

upward : *led*.

sitching : **Bry**, *cact*, *carb-an*, *chel*, **Kali-c**, kali-i, *merc*, **Merc-c**, nat-m, ptel, **puls**, **Ran-b**, squil, **Spig**, ther.

change of weather : **Ran-b**.

coughing : **Bry**, *kali-c*, **Merc**, *puls*.

effusion, with or without : squil.

inspiring : **Bry**.

lying, while : chel.

back, can lie only on the : *acon*, *bry*, *phos*.

lying, side, on the affected : *kali-c*.

on the painful, amel ; **Bry**.

night, side, on : stann.

left, on : **Phos**, **Spig**.

motion, during : **Bry**, **Spig**.

pulse, synchronous with : *spig*.

remain after recovery of pleurisy : carb-an, **Ran-b**.

respiration : **Bry**.

weather, cold wet : spig.

extending, to back : *chel*, *kali-c*, kali-i, *merc*.

downward : cact, *kalm*.

upward : led

mammae : *bry*, *con*, *phyt*.

sides : **Bry**, **Chel**, **Kali-c**, **Ran-b**, squil.

right : **Bry**, **Chel**, **Kali-c**, merc, *ran-b*.

respiration, during : **Bry**.

left : **Phos**, *ran-b*, **Sulph**, *ther*.

upper : anis, myrt, pix, **Sulph**, *ther*, *tub*.

extending to neck : anis, myrt, pix, **Sulph**, *ther*.

nipple, just below : *nat-s*, *rumx*.

coughing : **Bry**, *kali-c*.

inspiration : **Bry, Kali-c.**

heart : **Bry, Kalm, Naja**, puls.

gout, after : *kalm*.

rheumatism, after : **Kalm.**

tearing : bry.

PALPITATION, heart : **Aml-ns**, *am-c*, apoc, **Aur**, *bov*, **Cact**, *calc-ar*, **Calc**, cimic, *coll*, conv (sympathetic), **Dig, Glon, Iod, Kalm**, ox-ac, *lil-t*, *mag-m*, *mill*, *mosch*, *mur-ac*, nat-m, **Naja, Spig, Spong, Tab**, tril-p.

day and night : *cact*.

midnight after, wakes up : **Spong.**

anxiety : **Acon**, *spong*.

ascending steps : am-c, *ars*, **Calc.**

audible : spig.

bending forward, when : **Spig.**

eating, after : lil-t.

emotion, slightest : **Calc-ar**, *lith-c*.

exertion, from : am-c, **Arg-n**, coca, **Dig, Iod, Naja, Spig.**

heart strain, from : **Arn**, borx, *caust*.

incarcerated flatus, from : coca, arg-n, nux-v.

intermits : nat-m.

lying, while : *cact*.

amel : *psor*.

side : *lil-t*.

right : *lil-t*.

amel : kalm, *lach*, nat-m, **Phos, Psor**, *tab*.

left : **Cact**, *lac-c*, *lach*, *lil-t*, nat-m, **Phos**, *tab*.

menses, before : *cact*, **Spong.**

during : spong.

mental exertion, from : *calc-ar*.

motion, least, from : *cimic,* **Dig, Spig.**

amel : mag-m.

reflex, from uterus or ovaries : cimic, *conv*.

sitting, while : *mag-m.*

tumultuous, violent, vehement : *aml-ns*, **Arg-n**, *aur*, *coca*, *nat-m*, nux-v, *spig*, *spong*, tab.

heart strain, from : **Arn**, borx, *caust*, coca.

incarcerated flatus, from : **Arg-n**, *coca*, nux-v.

overexertion, from : **Arg-n**, *coca*, nux-v.

shaking the whole body : *nat-m*, **Spig.**

visible : **Spig.**

walking, when : *cact*, naja.

amel : *mag-m.*

PARALYSIS,

heart : **Carb-v**, **Naja.**

post-diphthertic : *naja.*

lung : **Ant-t.**

suffocation from mucus in bronchi : **Ant-t.**

PERSPIRATION : Bov, Calc, sil.

upper part of body, and : **Calc,** *sil.*

axilla : *bov*, calc, **Sep, Sil.**

offensive : **Sep, Sil.**

onion-like : *bov.*

PHTHISIS : *bals-p*, **Calc, Calc-p,** *dros*, *kali-p*, **Kali-s, Lyc, Phos, Psor, Puls, Ther.**

apex, left : **Phos, Sulph,** *ther*, *tub.*

right : **Calc-ar.**

florida : **Ther.**

incipient : **Calc, Med,** tril-p, **Tub.**

injury to chest, after : mill, *ruta.*

last stage : **Calc.**

purulent and ulcerative : **Calc,** *dros*, tril-p.

young persons, nocturnal cough, in : *dros.*

PRESSURE in chest : (See Oppression).

PULSATION, heart : *aml-ns*, nat-m.

PURRING feeling in region of heart : *spig.*

RATTLING in : (See Respiration).

RETRACTION of nipples : *hydr*, **Sars**, *sil*.

RUSH of blood (See Heart, Flushes, Orgasm) : *calc-ar*, **Aml-ns**, **Glon.**

           left side : *calc-ar*, **Aml-ns**, **Glon.**

           heart, to : **Glon, Lil-t.**

                extending to head : **Glon.**

SENSITIVE : (See Pain, Sore).

SMALL, nipples : sars.

SPASM of : *cic*, **Mosch** (hysterical), *samb*.

           diaphragm : *cic*.

STONE cutter's complaints : sil.

SUFFOCATIVE spells about heart : **Laur.**

           agg. by sitting up : laur, **Psor.**

           amel by lying down : laur, **Psor.**

SUPPURATION of lungs : (See Abscess).

SUSPENDED, heart feels, as if by a thread : **Kali-c**, lach.

SUPPRESSED milk (See Milk) : **Bry.**

SWELLING,

           axillary glands : *carb-an*, *con*, **Hep**, **Merc**, **Sil.**

           mammae : *carb-an*, *con*, *helon*, *lac-c*, *phyt*, **Sil.**

                hard as old cheese : *bry*, *lac-c*, phel, phyt.

                heal or suppurate, no tendency to : phyt.

           menses, before : con, *lac-c*.

                    during : *con*, helon, lac-c.

           purple : phyt.

TENSION : sang (behind sternum).

TENDERNESS : (See Pain, Sore).

THROBBING : (See Pulsation).

TUMEFIED : (See Swelling).

ULCER, lungs : **Kali-c.**

ULCERATION of mammae : **Phyt**, **Sil.**

UNEXCITABLE, nipple : sars, sil.

WATER, drops of cold, were falling from heart, sensation as of : cann-s.

WEAKNESS : **Arg-met**, **Ant-t**, *calc,* carb-v, *dig, ph-ac, phos*, **Stann**, *sil, sulph.*

> left : *arg-met.*
> cough, from : *ph-ac*, **Stann.**
> growth, from too rapid : **Ph-ac.**
> laughing, when : *stann.*
> loss of vital fluid, from : *ph-ac.*
> lying left side : *arg-met.*
> mental emotion, from depressing : *ph-ac.*
> nervous : ph-ac.
> phthisis, in : *ph-ac.*
> reading aloud : *stann.*
> singing, when : **Stann**.
> speech, impending : dig, *stann.*
> talking, when : *ph-ac*, **Stann**, sulph.
> heart : **Dig** (without vulvular complications), lil-t, nat-m, **Naja**, pyrog.

WEIGHT : (See Oppression).

WITHERED, nipples : sars, sil.

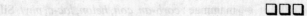

Chill

COLDNESS, in general : am-c, **Ars**, *bell*, *bry*, *calc*, *calc-p*, **Carb-v**, **Chel**, **Chin**, **Chinin-s**, **Eup-per**, **Gels**, **Ign**, **Led**, **Lyc**, **Meny**, **Mez**, **Nat-m**, **Nit-ac**, **Nux-m**, **Nux-v**, *podo*, **Psor**, **Puls**, pyrog, **Sep**, **Staph**, **Thuj**, **Verat**.

DAYTIME : Chin.

MORNING : Eup-per, *gels*, **Nat-m**, **Nux-v**.

FORENOON : Nat-m, **Nux-v**, **Sulph**.

AFTERNOON : Apis, **Ars**, **Bell**, **Chin**, **Chinin-s**, **Ferr**, **Gels**, **Lyc**, **Puls**, *sulph*.

       3 p.m. : *apis*, ign, thuj.

EVENING : Am-c, **Apis**, **Bell**, **Bry**, **Chin**, **Hep**, **Lyc**, **Merc**, **Puls**, **Rhus-t**, **Sulph**.

NIGHT : Merc, rhus-t, **Sulph**.

       3 a.m. : thuj.

AIR, in the open : **Ars**, **Calc**, **Chin**, **Hep**, **Nux-v**.

       the least draft of : **Calc**, **Chin**.

ANGER, after : **Bry**, *cham*, **Nux-v**.

ANTICIPATING : chin, **Chinin-s**.

       about two to three hours, each attack : *chinin-s*.

       every seven days : chin, **Chinin-s**.

       every fourteen days : chin, **Chinin-s**.

BEGINING in and extending from abdomen : **Apis**, **Ign**.

       arms : **Bell**.

       back : **Caps**, **Dulc**, *eup-per*, gels, **Lach**.

          between scapulae : **Caps**.

          dorsal region : **Lach**, **Eup-per** (up and down).

          lumbar region : **Nat-m**, **Eup-per** (up and down).

       chest : **Apis**.

       thigh : **Thuj**.

CHILLINESS (See generalities, Cold) : am-c, *arg-n*, **Bar-c**, **Bry**, **Camph**, caps, **Caust**, **Ferr**, **Hep**, *led*, *merc*, meny, **Nux-v**, **Puls**, pyrog, **Sep**.

       forenoon : **Nat-m**.

       evening : **Puls**.

cannot cover too warmly, but warmth does not amel : caust.

anger, after : aur, *bry*.

long lasting : *camph*.

menses, before : *mag-c*.

during : am-c.

movement, slightest : **Nux-v**.

pain, with : *ars, caust, puls*.

the more the pain, the more the chill : *puls*.

severe : *camph*.

stool, after : merc.

uncovered, when, yet feels smothered, if wrapped up : **Arg-n**.

warm room, when in a : *puls*.

bones, of : *pyrog*.

CREEPING : Merc.

CONGESTIVE (See Pernicious) : *camph*.

DRINKING, agg : **Eup-per, Ars, Nux-v, Calc, Caps, Verat**.

HEAT, external amel : **Ign**.

LONG LASTING (See Shaking) : **Camph**, verat.

PAIN, with : **Puls**.

PERIODICITY regular and distinct : **Aran, Cedr, Chinin-s**.

clock-like : *aran, cedr*.

PERNICIOUS : *camph*, **Nux-v, Psor, Verat**.

PERSPIRATION, with : *pyrog*.

SHAKING : **Ars, Camph**, *caps, chin,* **Ferr, Gels, Hep, Ign, Nat-m, Phos, Psor, Puls, Pyrog, Rhus-t, Sep**.

drinking, on : **Caps**.

pain, from : **Puls** (more pain, more shaking).

SHIVERING : (See Trembling).

SIDE, left side of body : caust, carb-v, lyc.

'SHIVERS', cold, from emotion : asar.

TREMBLING and shivering : cimic.

labor, first stage, during : **Cimic**.

UNCOVERING : *arg-n,* **Ars, Hep, Nux-v, Psor, Rhus-t, Sil**.

yet feels smothered when wrapped up : *arg-n*.

WARMTH, desire for, which does not relieve : **Aran, Nux-v**.

external, amel : **Ars, Bell, Caps,** *hep,* **Ign, Nux-v**.

Cough

DAYTIME : **Euphr**, ferr, **Nat-s**, *staph*.
        only : **Euphr**, *ferr*, nat-m, sang, *staph*.

MORNING : ambr, hep, **Nux-v**, *psor*, **Sulph**.
        waking, on : **Nux-v**, *psor*.
        expectoration, with : ambr, **Hyos**.

AFTERNOON, 4 p.m. daily : **Lyc**, mill.

EVENING : *ambr*, **Hep**, **Lyc**, *phos*, *psor*, **Puls**, spong.
        lying, agg : *phos*, *psor*, tub.
        expectoration, without : ambr, **Hyos**.
        twilight till midnight : phos.

NIGHT : **Acon**, **Bell**, **Cham**, *con*, *dros*, *eup-per*, *hep*, **Hyos**, med, **Merc**, **Puls**, sang, **Sil**, **Sulph**.
        midnight, before : hep.
            after : am-c, **Dros**.
                towards morning : **Hep**, **Dros**.
                      3 to 4 a.m. : *am-c*, **Kali-c**, thuj.
        phthisis, in : **Dros**.

AIR, changing : **Phos**, **Rumx**, spong.
        cold : **Acon**, **Hep**, **Phos**, **Rumx**, spong.
            slightest inhalation of : **Rumx**.
        draft of : **Acon**.
        dry : caust.
            cold : **Acon**, **Hep** (especially west wind), spong.
        open : *hep*.

ASTHMATIC (wheezing) : **Ant-t**, **Ars**, **Cupr**, **Dros**, **Ip**, *spong*, seneg.

AUTUMN : *cina*.
        and spring, damp weather agg : ant-t (before Ter), cina, **Ter**.

BARKING : **Acon**, **Hep**, **Dros**, iod, **Spong**, verb.

BATHING, agg : caust, nux-m, **Rhus-t**.

BED, in : (See Lying).
        warm, on becoming, in, agg or excites : dros, merc, *nux-m*.

BRONCHITIS, pneumonia, after : **Sang**.

BREATHING, deep : **Bry**.

BRUSHING teeth : staph.

CELLERS, living in : *nat-s*, *nux-m*.

CHILL, before : **Rhus-t**.
>   during : **Rhus-t**.

CHOKING (See Suffocation) : **Hep**, **Ip**, stann.

CLEANING the teeth : (See Brushing).

CHRONIC, in psoric children : **Bar-c**, *eup-per*, **Psor**.

COLD, air : (See Air).
>   becoming, on : **Ars**, **Hep**, **Phos**, **Rhus-t**, *sang*.
>>   arm or hand : **Hep**, **Rhus-t**.
>>   single part : **Hep**, **Rhus-t**.
>   damp places, living in : **Nat-s**, **Nux-m**.
>   drinks : *hep*, *spong*.
>>   amel : **Caust**, **Cupr**.
>   dry air : (See Air).
>   going from warm, to : *phos*.
>   standing, cold water, in : nux-m.
>   weather : cham.

CONCUSSIVE : (See Racking).

CONSTANT : **Alum**, **Caust**, kali-br, med, **Rumx**, **Stict**.

CONSTRICTION : **Cupr**, *Ip*.

COUGHING, agg : **Ign**.

CROAKING : acon,

CROUPY : *acet-ac*, **Acon**, *brom*, **Hep**, **Samb**, **Spong**, staph.
>   inhalation, with : acet-ac, **Spong**.
>   last stages, in : acet-ac.
>   winter, alternating with sciatica in summer : staph.

CRYING, agg : **Arn**, dros.

DAMP room, agg : (See Cellers).

DEEP : apoc, **Dros**, *hep*, lyc, med, *samb*, **Stann**, *verb*.

DEEP enough, sensation as though he could not cough, to start mucus :
>   **Caust**.

DEEP sounding : dros, *verb*.

DENTITION : *cham*.

DINNER, after : staph.

           only : staph.

DISTRESSING : **Caust**, **Nux-v**.

DRINKING, after : *bry*, **Dros**, hyos, *phos*.

           amel : *caust*, **Spong**.

DRY : **Acon**, am-c, apoc, **Brom**, **Bry**, *cham*, *cina*, caust, **Hyos**, ign, **Iod**, *ip*, kali-br, **Kali-c**, **Mang**, med, *merc*, myrt, naja, *rhus-t*, **Rumx**, *samb*, sang, **Spong**, squil, *stann*, ter.

           evening : **Hep**, **Puls**, rhus-t, stann.

           night : **Am-c**, *cham*, **Dros**, **Hep**, **Hyos**, **Lach**, **Phos**, **Puls**, *rumx*, *sang*, *stict*.

                3 to 4 a.m. : **Am-c**, *kali*, *c*.

                flatus, passage of, amel : sang.

                sitting up, amel : **Hyos**, **Puls**, sang, *stict*.

                though sounds loose : **Ant-t**, **Brom**.

                tickling in the throat, from : am-c, *rumx*.

                waking from sleep : sang, **Sulph**.

EATING, from or after : *bry*, dros, hyos, phos.

           amel : ferr, **Spong**.

ECZEMA, suppressed, after : psor.

ELONGATED uvula, from : (See Tickling).

ERUCTATIONS excite : *ambr*.

EXCITEMENT, from : **Spong**.

EXHAUSTING : *merc*, *rumx*, *stict*.

EXPIRATION : acon, **Caust**.

EXPLOSIVE : *caps*.

           escape of fetid, pungent air, with : caps.

FATIGUING : (See Exhausting).

FEATHER, as from (See Tickling) : dros.

FEVER during : **Acon**, **Ars**, **Ip**, **Nat-m**, **Nux-v**, rhus-t.

           intermittent, in : *rhus-t*.

         before : samb.

FISTULA operation, after : *berb*.

GAGGING : (See Gagging under Stomach).

GONORRHOEA suppressed, after : *med, thuj*.

GRASPING throat, during : *all-c*.

GURGLING : *cupr*.

HACKING : Alum, Ars, Lach, Phos, ter, **Tub**.
  daytime : *calc, samb*.
  morning : arn, *ars*, kali-c, thuj.
    rising, after : *arn, chin, ferr*.
  afternoon : **Sang**.
  evening : **Ign, Sang, Sep**.
    lying down, after : **Ign, Sang, Sep**.
  dryness in larynx, from : **Con, Sang**.
  lying down, while : **Hyos, Sang**.
  tickling in larynx, from : **All-c, Ars, Coc-c, Dros, Lach, Nat-m, Phos**.

HANDS, must hold chest with both : **Arn, Bry, Dros,** kreos, nat-s, sep.

HARD : acon, **Bry,** kali-br, **Kali-c**.

HEAD touches pillow as soon as : **Bell,** bry, crot-t, **Dros, Hyos,** *murx*.

HEADACHE, with, as if head would fly to pieces : **Bry**.

HEART, affections, with : **Lach,** *laur*, **Naja,** spong.

HEATED, on becoming : nux-m.

HOARSE : Acon, ambr, **Dros,** *verb*.
  night : **Dros**.
    midnight : dros.
      after : **Dros**.

HOLLOW : Caust, lyc, med (like coughing in a barrel), samb, stann, verb.

INCESSANT : (See Constant).

INDIGNATION, after : (See Vexation).

INSPIRATION : *brom*.
  deep : (See Breathing).

IRRITATING things, from, such as, salt, wine, pepper, vineger : **Alum**.

IRRITATION in air passages, from : **Acon, Cham, Iod, Nux-v**.
  in heart, from : naja.

ITCH, suppressed, after : psor.

ITCHING, in chest : con, iod.

> in larynx : con, iod.

LAUGHING : *arg-met*, dros, *phos*, *stann*.

LOOSE : apoc, dulc, eup-per, *kali-s*, nux-m, *nat-s*, sang, squil (more fatiguing than dry one in evening).

> morning : rhus-t, squil.
>
> eating, after : nux-m.
>
>> but dry after drinking : nux-m.
>
> expectoration, without : **Ant-t**, brom.
>
> hectic fever, with : eup-per.

LOUD : acon.

LYING agg : aral, **Caust**, **Con**, *dros*, **Hyos**, kali-br, *lach*, med, *phos*, **Rumx**, *spong*.

> daytime, amel : *dros*.
>
> evening : **Dros**, rumx.
>
> night : **Dros**, **Kali-c**, **Rumx**, *stict*.
>
>> as soon as head touches pillow : *bell*, crot-t, **Dros**, **Hyos**, rumx.
>
> amel : **Euphr**, *ferr*, kali-bi, **Mang-cact**.
>
>> on abdomen or stomach, amel : *med*.
>
> head low, with : spong.
>
> side : *acon*, phos, *stann*.
>
>> right : **Merc**.
>
>> left : dros, *phos*, *rumx*, stann.

MEASLES, during : *coff*, dros, *stict*.

> after : coff, **Dros**, *eup-per*, stict.

MEAT, after : *staph*.

MENSES, begins with and ends with : lac-c.

> before : lac-c.
>
> during : lac-c.
>
> suppressed, from : mill.

METALLIC : *kali-bi*.

MINUTE guns, short : cor-r.

> during day, and whooping at night : cor-r.

MOTION agg : *bry*, cina, spong.

MUCUS, chest in : **Ant-t**.

        raising large quantities does not amel : lyc.

NERVOUS : Caps, kali-br.

NOTES, from high : alum, arg-n, **Arum-t**.

PAIN in distant parts on coughing : *caps*.

PAROXYSMAL : *ambr*, *caps*, cimic, **Cina**, *con*, crot-t, **Cupr, Dros, Hyos, Ip**, *kali-c*, merc, **Stann**.

        morning early : **Coc-c, Dros**.

        night : *merc*.

        attack follow one another rapidly : **Dros**.

        breath, scarcely able to take : **Dros**.

        consisting of, few coughs : bell, calc.

                long coughs : **Cupr**.

                short coughs : *dros*.

                three coughs : *cupr*, stann.

                two coughs : merc.

        child cries before : **Arn**.

        dry spot, in larynx, caused by : *con*.

                in throat, caused by : cimic.

        epistaxis during every paroxysm : **Ind**.

        followed by copious mucus : **Coc-c**, *dros*.

                which amel : **Coc-c**, *dros*.

        head would fly to pieces, as if : *caps*.

        moving or speaking, from : *bry*, *cina*.

        sudden : *caps*.

PERIODIC : cina.

PREGNANCY, during : apoc, *caust*, *con*, kali-br, *nux-m*.

PRESSURE on larynx, from : **Lach**, rumx.

        throat pit, on : rumx.

RACKING : Bry, Merc, Stann, *stict*.

RASPING : Spong.

RATTLING : Ant-t, *brom*, *hep*, *kali-bi*, kali-s, squil, *seneg*.

READING aloud, agg : *ambr*, *dros*, **Phos**, spong.

RETCHING : (See under Stomach).

RINGING : acon, **Dros**, spong.

ROOM, change of, from : **Phos**, **Rumx**, spong.

ROUGH : acon, *hep*.

SAW-LIKE : (See Sibilant).

SEVERE : (See Violent).

SHATTERING : (See Racking).

SHORT : *apoc*, berb.

       fistula operation, after : *berb*, *calc-p*, **Sil**.

SIBILANT : *spong*.

       like a saw driven through a pine board : **Spong**.

SINGING, agg : *arg-met*, *arg-n*, **Arum-t**, *dros*, hyos, *phos*, spong.

SITTING, up, amel (See Lying) : **Dros**, *hyos*, nat-s, phel.

SLEEP, during : **Cham**, **Lach**.

       after : **Lach**, spong,

       going to, on : **Lach**, spong.

       preventing : **Lyc**, **Puls**, **Sep**.

       wakens from : **Caust**, **Phos**, **Sulph**.

       does not waken : *cham*, calc, *psor*, lach.

SMOKING, agg : spong, staph.

SPASMODIC (See Paroxysmal) : **Ambr**, bad, **Bell**, **Bry**, *caps*, *chel*, **Cina**, *con*, cor-r, crot-t, **Cupr**, **Dros**, **Hyos**, ign, **Ip**, *kali-c*.

       night : **Coc-c**.

       dry spot, in larynx, caused by : *con*.

       in throat, caused by : cimic.

       head touches pillow, as soon as : crot-t.

SPEAKING : phos.

SPRING, in : *cina*.

       and autumn, agg from damp weather : (See Cough, Autumn).

SPRINGS up, child, and clings to those around : *ant-t*.

STANDING agg : ign.

       still, during a walk : astac, ign.

       water, in : nux-m.

STRANGLING : (See Choking).

SUFFOCATIVE : acon, crot-t, **Cupr, Hep, Ip, Samb**.
        night : **Cham, Hep**.
          midnight : **Samb**.
        child becomes stiff and blue : **Cupr, Ip**.
        walk about, must, or sleep in a chair : *crot-t*.

SUPPRESSED intermittents : *eup-per*.

SWALLOWING : spong.

SWEETS agg : med, spong,

SYMPATHETIC : Lach, Naja, Spong.
        heart, from : **Lach, Naja**.

TALKING : *ambr, cupr,* **Dros**, hyos, *phos*, rumx, spong.

TEARING : *all-c*.

TICKLING : Acon, am-c, *bell, dros*, ham, **Hyos**, *rumx*.
        larynx : *am-c*, **Bell, Dros**, *hyos, rumx*.
           as soon as child touches pillow at nigtht : *bell*, **Dros,**
               Hyos, *rumx*.
        throat-pit, supra-sternal fossa or behind sternum : cham,
        rumx.

TITILLATING (See Tickling) : *dros*.

TORMENTING, or teasing : *rhus-t*, rumx, tril-p,

TOUCHING, the throat pit : *rumx*.

TRUMPET-toned : *dros, verb*.

UNCOVERING agg, (See Cold) : bar-c, **Hep**, *kali-bi*, **Rhus-t, Rumx**.
        feet : **Sil**.
        hand : bar-c, **Hep, Rhus-t**.
        head : **Rumx, Sil**.

VEXATION, after : **Cham, Ign, Staph**.

VIOLENT : Bell, Carb-v, Caust, Cupr, euphr, **Ip**, kali-bi, med, rumx.

WARM, fluid amel : **Ars, Lyc, Nux-v, Rhus-t, Sil**, *spong*.
        food amel : *spong*.
        room : *bry, dros*.
           entering, from open air : *bry*, nat-c.
           going from, to cold air : **Phos**.
           going from, to cold air and vice versa : *rumx*.

WEATHER, warm wet : iod.

WEEPING : (See Crying).

WHEEZING : (See Asthmatic).

WHISTLING : acon, *spong.*

WHOOPING cough, after : *caust, sang.*

WHOOPING : *ambr*, ant-c, *caust*, **Carb-v**, **Cina**, *cupr*, **Dros**, *ip*, *lob*, *samb*, *sang*, stann.

> night : cor-r (whooping at night but minute guns during day), **Coc-c.** (latter part of night).
>
> cataleptic spasm, with : cupr.
>
> child becomes blue and stiff : *cupr*, **Ip.**
>
> cold washing agg : *ant-c.*
>
> > amel : caust.
>
> crowing inspiration, without : *ambr.*
>
> epidemic, during : **Dros.**
>
> followed by copious mucus : **Coc-c.**
>
> long lasting : cupr.
>
> speak, unable to : cupr.
>
> suffocating : *cupr.*
>
> sun, overheated from, agg : *ant-c.*
>
> three attacks successively : *cupr*, stann.
>
> warm room, agg : ant-c.

WIND, in the : *acon*, **Hep.**

> cold dry : **Acon**, **Hep.**
>
> west : **Hep.**

WINTER every : cham, *psor.*

□□□

Ear

ABSCESS, boils, etc.

  behind : **Aur,** *caps,* **Sil.**

  inside : **Hep, Sil.**

    right : carb-ac.

      physical exertion, after : carb-ac.

  external : merc, pic-ac.

CARIES : Aur, Sil.

  mastoid process : **Aur, Caps, Sil.**

CATARRH : (See Discharge).

  eustachian tube : **Calc,** *kali-bi,* **Kali-s,** merc-d, **Puls, Sil.**

CHILBLAINS : (See Itching, Burning).

CONDYLOMATA : thuj.

DISCHARGE : *aur, crot-h,* **Calc, Calc-p, Calc-s, Carb-v, Graph, Hep,** Kali-bi, **Kali-s,** *merc, merc-d, nat-s,* **Psor, Puls, Sil, Sulph,** thuj.

  blood : **Crot-h.**

  bloody : *crot-h,* merc.

  children, in : **Merc-d.**

  excoriating : **Sulph.**

  fetid : **Aur.**

  gluey, sticky : **Graph.**

  ichorous : **Psor.**

  measles, after : psor.

  offensive : **Aur, Merc, Psor,** *thuj.*

    fish-brine, like : *graph,* **Tell.**

    putrid meat, like : **Psor,** *thuj.*

  purulent : **Merc-d,** thuj.

  scarlet fever, after : **Psor,** *tell.*

  sticky : (See Gluey).

  thick : **Calc, Hydr, Kali-bi, Kali-s, Puls.**

  thin : *psor.*

  transparent : *graph.*

  watery : *graph.*

yellow : **Kali-bi, Kali-s,** *nat-s,* **Puls.**

green : *kali-s,* nat-s, **Puls.**

DISCOLOURATION, redness : **Agar,** *sulph.*

chilblains : **Agar.**

DRYNESS : Graph.

ERUPTIONS : *graph,* **Psor.**

moist : **Graph,** *psor.*

scurfy : graph, **Psor.**

behind the ears : **Graph,** petr, **Psor,** sanic.

moist : **Graph, Psor,** sanic.

offensive : **Psor.**

viscid : **Graph,** sanic.

white : sanic.

scurfy : graph, **Psor.**

sore : *graph,* **Psor,** sanic.

around the ears : staph.

FUNGUS excrescences : *merc.*

HEAT : agar.

INFLAMMATION : Merc, Puls.

inside : **Bell, Graph, Hep, Sulph,** *thuj.*

middle ear : *kali-m,* **Merc-d, Sulph,** *thuj.*

eustachian tube : *merc-d.*

ITCHING : *agar,* **Petr, Sulph.**

burning : **Agar.**

frozen, as if : **Agar, Petr.**

behind the ear : **Graph, Nat-m.**

external ear : **Agar, Puls, Rhus-t, Sulph.**

MOISTURE behind the ear : **Graph,** tub.

NOISES : Bell, Cann-i, Caust, Chin, Chinin-s, ferr, **Graph,** *nit-ac,* tril-p.

menses, before : *kreos.*

during : *kreos.*

cracking : *graph,* **Nit-ac.**

masticating, when : *graph,* **Nit-ac.**

humming : arg-n, caust, **Chin,** *kreos.*

ringing : **Chin,** *ferr.*

menses, from : **Ferr.**

roaring : caust, **Chin,** ign, *kreos.*

menses, before : kreos.

during : kreos.

music, amel : *ign.*

tinkling : caust.

OBSTRUCTION, eustachian tube : **Merc-d.**

OOZING : (See Moisture).

PAIN : agar, *aur,* **Bell,** *caps, cham,* **Hep,** *mag-p, merc.*

night : *aur,* **Merc.**

right : *merc.*

coughing, when : *caps.*

lying on affected side : *merc.*

spells, coming in : *cham.*

swallowing on : **Apis, Lach, Nit-ac, Nux-v.**

warm application, amel : **Hep,** *mag-p.*

PAIN, burning : *caust, sulph.*

sore : *caust, chin.*

behind : **Caps.**

stabbing : **Merc.**

right : merc.

tearing : cham, **Merc.**

night : merc.

POLYPUS : mar-v, *merc, teucr, thuj.*

easily bleeding : thuj.

pale red : thuj.

RED : *caust, sulph.*

STOPPED, sensation : **Asar,** tril-p.

SWELLING : agar.

behind : **Caps** (mastoid).

VEINS, distended : dig.

□□□

Ear-Hearing

ACUTE : **Bell, Coff,** *colch, graph,* **nux-m, Nux-v, Nat-c, Op.**
      music, to : *cham, coff.*
      noises, to : **Bell,** *chin, coff,* **Nit-ac,** nux-m.
      sounds of vehicles, to : nit-ac.

CONFUSION : (See Impaired).

IMPAIRED : **Bar-c, Carb-an, Graph,** *hep, kreos,* **Nit-ac.**
      catarrhal : **Kali-m, Merc-d.**
      confusion : **Carb-an.**
      direction of sound, cannot tell : *carb-an.*
      menses, before : *kreos.*
            during : *kreos.*
      noise, amel : **Graph.**
      old people : bar-c, *cic, petr.*
      quinine, after abuse of : *calc.*
      reverberation of sounds : caust (one's own).
      riding in a carriage or train, amel : *graph,* **Nit-ac,** *puls.*
      rumbling sound, amel : *graph,* **Nit-ac.**

LOST : bar-c, **Caust,** *graph,* **Hep,** kreos, **Lyc,** *merc-d,* nit-ac, plb, psor, stram.
      inflammation and closure of eustachian tube, from : *kali-m.*
      old age : *merc-d, kali-m, phos* (deafness to human voice).
      riding in a carriage, amel : *graph,* nit-ac.

❑❑❑

Expectoration

DAYTIME only : **Ars, Cham, Hep,** *stann,* **Sulph.**

MORNING : ambr, hyos.

   evening, without : ambr, hyos.

NIGHT : *caust.*

ACRID : sulph.

ALBUMINOUS : (See White).

AMELIORATES : Ant-t.

BALLS, in the shape of : **Stann.**

   bitter : med.

BLOODY, spitting of blood : **Acon,** *cact,* **Crot-h,** dulc, *dros, kreos, mill,* **Phos,** tril-p.

   bright red : **Acon, Bell,** mill.

   cough, during : mill.

   fall, after a : mill.

   haemorrhoidal flow, suppressed : mill.

   haemorrhoidal patient, in : mill.

   menses, before : **Zinc.**

     during : **Zinc.**

     suppressed, during : mill.

   phthisis, incipient, in : mill.

   ruptured blood vessels, from : mill.

CASTS (See Membranous) : *brom, kali-bi.*

   morning, on awakening : *kali-bi.*

COPIOUS : *bals-p,* **Coc-c,** *dros,* **Euphr,** kali-i, myos, nat-s, phel, **Phos,** ph-ac, **Stann,** tril-p.

   large quantity, expectorated, after, amel : **Coc-c, Dros.**

DIFFICULT : Caust, med.

   adhering to throat : **Kali-bi.**

   aged people : *am-c.*

   swallow, must : (See Swallow).

EASY : Arg-n.

FLIES, forcibly out of mouth : *bad*, *chel*, kali-c.

FOUL smelling : *borx*, *cop*, *guaj*, *phel*, ph-ac, **Sang.**

FROTHY : ars, kali-i, med.

GELATINOUS : Arg-met.

GRAYISH : cop.

GREENISH : benz-ac, cop, dros, **Kali-i**, *kali-s*, med, **Nat-s**, par, **Psor, Stann**, sulph.

        gray : *cop*.

HAWKED up, mucus : **Euphr, Rumx.**

        morning : euphr.

        voluntary : *euphr.*

HEAVY : stann.

LUMPY : **Calc-s**.

MEMBRANOUS : *brom*, *kali-bi*, **Spong.**

MUCOUS : *ant-t*, **Arg-met**, benz-ac, **Caust, Coc-c, Dros, Euphr, Hep, Kali-bi**, *nat-s*, **Psor**, sil, *squil*, *seneg.*

        seems much, nothing comes out : **Ant-t.**

        tenacious : (See Viscid).

PURULENT : bals-p, cop, *dros*, **Kali-c**, lyc, pix, ph-ac, psor, **Sil**, stann, tril-p.

ROPY : (See Viscid).

SCANTY : **Bry**, med, rumx.

STARCH, like : *arg-met*, *sel*.

STICKY : (See Viscid).

STRINGY : *bov*, hydr, **Kali-bi.**

SWALLOW, must, what has been loosened : *arn*, **Caust**, *kali-c.*

TASTE, bitter : **Puls.**

        bloody : rhus-t.

        herby : *borx*.

        musty : stann.

        putrid : *stann.*

        salty : kali-i, lyc, **Phos**, psor, **Sep**, *stann.*

        sour : stann.

        sweetish : **Calc, Phos, Stann.**

TENACIOUS : (See Viscid).

THICK : alum, ant-t, kali-i, lyc, *puls*, stann.

TOUGH : alum, *ant-t*, bov, *coc-c*, **Kali-bi.**

TRANSPARENT : Arg-met, *sel*, *stann.*

VISCID, tenacious : **Arg-met**, *bov*, canth, **Coc-c**, dros, **Hydr**, **Kali-bi**, *kali-c*, *med.*

WHITE : *med*, **Phos**, *stann.*
        albuminous : *stann.*

YELLOW : Calc, *dros*, **Hydr**, *kali-s*, lyc, *psor*, **Puls**, **Stann.**
        green : *kali-s*, nat-s, **Puls.**
        grey : lyc.

Extremities

ARTHRITIC, nodosities, gout stones : **Benz-ac**, berb, **Led**, **Lith-c**, **Lyc**, *rhod*, sabin, *staph*, *sars*.
        painful : **Led**.
        finger joints : **Benz-ac**, caul, **Caust**, *colch*, **Led**, **Lyc**, *staph*.
ATAXIA (See Inco-ordination) : *agar*, **Alum**, *arg-n*, *kali-br*.
AWAKWARDNESS : Agar, **Apis**, **Bov**, *nat-m*.
        hands : *agar*, *apis*, **Bov**.
          diverted or talking, when : **Hell**.
          drops things : **Apis**, **Bov**, *nat-m*.
            objects fall from powerless hands : *bov*.
            though careful : **Apis**.
        fingers : agar, *apis*, **Bov**.
        lower limbs : **Agar**.
          makes missteps when walking : *ph-ac*.
          stumbling when walking : **Agar**, ph-ac.
BITES, nails : (See Mind).
BLOOD, oozing from finger nails : **Crot-h**.
        rush of, to arms : **Sulph**.
          to legs : **Sulph**.
BRITTLE nails : ant-c, *dios*, **Graph**, *thuj*.
BUNIONS, foot : hyper.
        painful : hyper.
BURNING : (See Heat, Pain, Burning).
        hands and feet : **Lach**, **Med**, *sang*, **Sulph**.
          uncovers them : *lach*, **Med**, *sang*, **Sulph**.
        palm : sang, **Sulph**.
        soles of, at night, puts feet out of bed : **Calc**, cham, *med*,
          puls, *sang*, sanic, **Sulph**.
CHAPPED hands (See Roughness) : **Petr**.
        winter agg : **Petr**.

CHILBLAINS : abrot, **Agar**, **Petr**, pyrog, *zinc*.
    burning : *agar*.
    itching : *agar*.
    painful : *petr*, zinc.
    rubbing, agg : zinc.

CHOREA : **Agar**, caul, **Cic**, *cocc*, *croc*, **Tarent**.
    right arm and left leg: **Tarent**.
    left arm and right leg : **Agar**.

CLENCHING fingers : **Cupr**.
    thumb : *aeth*, **Cupr**.

CLUMSINESS : (See Awkwardness).

COLDNESS : **Calc**, **Carb-v**, chin, **Dig**, diph, ip, *kalm*, lil-t, *med*, *puls*, **Sec**,
   Stram, *tab*, **Verat**.
    night : carb-v.
    deficient capillary circulation, from : **Carb-v**.
    icy : *sec*.
    arm : carb-v (left).
      icy : *verat*.
    fore arm : *arn*, *brom*, med.
      icy or deathly cold : **Arn**, **Brom**, *verat*.
        diarrhoea, in : **Brom**.
    hands : *calc*, **Chin**, *dig*, **Ip**, **Meny**, med, **Puls**, **Sep**, *stram*, *tab*,
      Verat.
      hot face, with : **Arn**, **Stram**.
      icy : calc, carb-v, *meny*, sep, tab, **Verat**.
        body warm : tab.
      one cold, the other warm : *chin*, *dig*, *ip*, *puls*,
    knee : *apis*, **Carb-v**.
      night : *apis*, **Carb-v**.
    legs : **Calc**, carb-v (left), *med*, *meny*, *tab*, **Verat**.
      icy : **Calc**, *tab*, **Verat**.
    foot : **Bell**, **Calc**, *chel*, **Caust**, *med*, **Meny**, **Sep**, **Sil**, **Stram**,
      Sulph, *verat*.
      right : *chel*.
      daytime : sulph.
        with burning soles at night : **Sulph**.

bed, in : **Calc**.

headache, during : **Gels**, **Sep**, *sulph*.

hot face, with : **Stram**.

icy cold : **Calc**, *chel*, meny, **Sep**, **Verat**.

right icy cold, left neutral : *chel*, **Lyc**.

menses, before : **Calc**.

during : *calc* (as if cold damp stocking put on).

one cold, other hot : chin, dig, ip, **Lyc**.

CONCRETIONS : (See Arthritic Nodosities).

CONTRACTION of muscles and tendons : abrot, **Caust**, *guaj*, *nat- m*.

colic, from : abrot.

painful : abrot, am-m.

spasmodic : abrot.

flexors, of : **Caust**.

joints : *caust*.

upper limb, flexor tendons : *caust*.

upper arm, tendons : **Caust**.

elbow, bend of : *caust*.

flexors : *caust*.

forearm : *caust*.

wrist, shortening of tendons : *caust*.

hand, flexor : caust.

fingers : cann-s (after sprain), **Caust**.

lower limbs : **Am-m**, **Caust**, *guaj*, *nat-m*.

thigh, hamstring : *am-m*, **Caust**, *cimx*, **Guaj**, med, **Nat-m**.

walking while : am-m.

knee : *am-m*, **Caust**, *cimx*, **Guaj**, **Nat-m**.

leg : **Am-m**.

calf : *caust*.

ankle : med.

CONVULSIONS : *bell*, **Cic**, **Cina**, **Cupr**, **Hyos**.

clonic : cupr.

begining in fingers and toes and spreading over entire body : **Cupr**.

fingers : *cupr*.

toes : *cupr*.

CORNS : Ant-c.

       burning : *ran-b*, sal-ac.

       horny : *ant-c*.

       painful : *hyper*.

       sensitive : (See Sore).

       sore : *ran-b*.

       soles horny : **Ant-c**, *ran-b*.

CORRUGATED nails : fl-ac, **Sil**, *thuj*.

CRACKED skin, joints, bends of : **Graph**.

       hands : **Graph**, nat-m, **Nit-ac**, **Petr**, **Sars**.

         finger tips : **Graph**, **Petr**.

           nails, around : **Graph**, *nat-m*, *petr*.

         nails : **Ant-c**.

       feet : **Sars**.

       toes, between : *graph*.

       sides of fingers and toes : sars.

CRACKING, joints, in : *benz-ac*, *caust*, *cocc*, **Nit-ac**, *petr*.

       motion, on : *benz-ac*, *graph*, **Nit-ac**.

CRAMPS : Coloc, **Cupr**, mag-p.

         pregnancy, during : *mag-p*.

         upper limbs : **Coloc**.

       hands : *cupr*, verat.

         cholera, during : **Verat**.

         extending all over : **Verat**.

       fingers : *cupr*.

         cholera, with : **Cupr**, **Verat**.

         parturition, during : **Cupr**.

         playing piano or violin : *mag-p*.

         writer's : *mag-p*, **Stann**.

         extending all over : **Cupr**, **Verat**.

       lower limbs : **Cupr**.

       thigh : podo.

       legs : **Cupr**.

         labor, during : cupr.

         calf : **Cupr**, *med*, podo, **Sulph**, *verat*.

           night : **Sulph**.

           cholera, in : **Cupr**, **Verat**.

CRAMPS, foot : **Cupr**, podo, *sulph*, verat.

          cholera, in : **Cupr**, **Verat**.

          extending all over : **Cupr**, **Verat**.

          sole : med, **Sulph**.

              night : **Sulph**.

          toes : *cupr*.

CRIPPLED, nails : ant-c, **Graph**, **Sil**, *thuj*.

CRUMBLED, nails : **Graph**, *thuj*.

CRUSHED nails grow in splits like warts : **Ant-c**.

CURVED finger nails : *nit-ac*.

CURVATURE, long bones of : **Calc**.

DAMPNESS of feet, as if they had cold damp stocking : calc.

DEFORMED, bones : **Calc**.

        finger joints : *med*.

DEFORMED nails : (See Distorted).

DISCOLOURATION,

            joints, redness : *benz-ac*, *bry*, *kalm*.

            arm, red streaks up the arm : all-c.

            hand, palm, yellow : *chel*, **Sep**.

                  redness : **Agar**.

            feet, redness : agar.

            nails, finger, blue : carb-v.

DISLOCATION,

            patella, going up stairs, when : cann-s.

            ankle : nat-c.

DISTORTION, limbs, : **Cic**.

DISTORTED nails : **Ant-c**, *fl-ac*, **Graph**, *thuj*.

DRAWING up of limbs amel : thuj.

DROPSY : (See Swelling).

DRYNESS,

        hands : *nat-m*,

        fingers : nat-m.

           nails, about : nat-m.

EMACIATION : Plb, *sec*, *sil*, **Sulph**.

    diseased limb : **Led**, **Plb**, **Puls**, *sec*, sel.

    paralysed limb : *kali-p*, **Plb**, *sec*,

    hands : **Plb**, **Sel**.

    lower limbs : *abrot*, am-m, *arg-n*, sel (thighs).

    legs : *abrot*, acet-ac, **Iod**, **Sanic**, sel, **Tub**.

    foot : sel.

ENLARGEMENT, joints, finger : med.

    large and puffy : med.

ERUPTION : *graph*, kali-br.

    upper limb : kali-br.

    shoulder, pustules : kali-br.

    hands, between fingers : *graph*.

    palm, eczema of : **Ran-b**.

    lower limbs, knee, hollow of, herpes : **Graph**, hep, **Nat-m**.

        foot, between toes : *graph*.

EXTENSION of limbs, agg : thuj.

FALLING, closing eyes, when : **Alum**, arg-n, *gels*.

FANNED, wants hand and feet : lach, **Med**, sulph.

FELON (onychia, paronychia, panaritium, etc.),

    panaritium : *all-c*, **Am-c**, **Anthraci**, apis, **Dios**, **Sil**, **Tarent**.

        burning : **Anthraci**, **Ars**, **Tarent** (atrocious).

        deep-seated : *am-c*.

    periosteum : *am-c*, dios, **Sil**.

    painful, agonising : dios, *tarent*.

        making patient walk the floor for nights : **Tarent**.

    purple : *lach*, **Tarent**.

    sloughing, with : **Anthraci**, *ars*, carb-ac, *lach*.

    tendency to : dios, *hep*.

FIDGETY : (See Restlessness).

FISSURES : (See Cracks).

HANG nails : **Nat-m**.

HEAT : agar.

    joints : *kalm*, **Led**.

hands : **Agar, Chel, Lach, Led, Lyc, Med, Sep, Sulph**.
and feet are hot alternately : sep.

HEAT, palms : *calc*, **Lach**, *med*, *petr*, *puls*, **Phos**, *sang*, **Sulph**.
foot : agar, calc, **Cham**, lach, **Puls, Sulph**.
bed in *: calc*, sang, **Sulph**.
burning : calc, cham, **Med, Puls**, *sang*, **Sec, Sulph**.
uncovers them *:* cham, **Med, Puls**, *sang*, **Sulph**.
one foot, coldness of other : chel, chin, dig, ip, **Lyc**.
sole *: calc, cham, lach,* **Lyc**, *petr, phos, puls, sang, sep,* Sulph.
uncovers them : *calc*, **Cham, Puls**, *sang*, **Sulph**.

HEAVINESS, tired limbs : **Ars, Bry, Gels, Kali-p, Ph-ac**, pic-ac.
exertion, on : pic-ac.
lower limbs : *alum*, *med*.
walking, while : *med*.
legs : *med* (feels like lead).
walking, difficult : *alum, med*.

IMPRESSION, fingers, on, deep, from using blunt instruments : bov.

INCOORDINATION (See Ataxia) : *agar*, **Alum**, *aster*, caust, **Gels**, kali-br,
phos.
daytime, inability to walk except, in : alum.
children, in : *caust*.
muscles refuses to obey will : **Alum**, *aster*, *gels*, kali-br.
tottering and falling when closing eyes : *alum, arg-n, gels,*
stram.
when thinks unobserved : *arg-n*.
uncertainty in walking : **Agar**.

INFLAMMATION,
bones : **Fl-ac, Merc, Sil**.
joints : **Apis, Bell, Bry, Led**, *rhod*.
night : *rhod*.
rest, agg : *rhod*.
storm, during : kalm, *rhod*.
wandering : kalm, ṛhod.
wrist : abrot.
fingers : hep, staph.
ankle : abrot.
knee : stict.

INGROWING toe nails : **Graph, M-aush,** *nat-m, nit-ac.* **Sil,** teucr.

        touch, agg : nit-ac.

        ulceration, with : *nit-ac.*

INJURIES,

        hands, laceration : *calen, hyper.*

        fingers, nails : *hyper, led.*

        lacerations : **Hyper.**

ITCHING : abrot, **Agar.**

        bends of joints, in : psor.

        hands : **Agar.**

          between fingers : psor.

        ankel : **Led.**

          scratching : *led.*

          warmth agg : **Led,** puls, rhus-v.

        foot : *agar,* **Led, Sep, Sulph.**

          night : **Led.**

          bed, in : **Led.**

          scratching agg : *led.*

          warmth of bed agg : **Led,** puls, rhus-v.

LERKINGS : Cham, Cic, Cina, Hyos.

        arms : **Cic.**

        legs : cic.

LAMENESS : abrot, *dulc* (after damp cold), *rhus-t, ruta.*

        as from a blow or fall : **Arn,** *ruta.*

        sprain, after : *ruta.*

        joints : **Rhus-t, Ruta.**

          sprain after : **Rhus-t, Ruta.**

          wrist : **Ruta.**

LIGHTNESS, sensation of : *aster.*

LOCOMOTOR ataxia : (See Ataxia).

MOTION, constant : apoc.

        arm and leg, left : apoc, bry. hell.

MOTION, constant, one arm and leg : apoc.

          hands and fingers : *kali-br.*

          sleep during : **Caust.**

involuntary : **Agar,** *hell.*

one arm and one leg : *apoc, hell.*

hands, of : zinc.

one hand and head : apoc, bry, *hell*, zinc.

sleep, ceases during : agar.

voluntary, one arm and leg : apoc, **Hell.**

left : **Bry.**

NODOSITIES : (See Arthritic Nodosities).

NUMBNESS : *acon, cham,* cocc, graph, **Kalm,** plat, nat-m (fingers and toes).

heels, of : *alum.*

arm, left : cact.

ODOR of feet, offensive, without perspiration : *sil.*

OEDEMA : (See Swelling).

PAIN : *abrot,* **Agar,** *arn,* **Bell,** berb, **Bry,** cact, calc, calc-p, caps, *caul,* **Caust,** *cham, chin,* **Colch,** *dulc,* **Eup-per,** ham, **Kalm,** *kali-br,* led, **Med,** *ph-ac,* **Phyt, Puls, Rhod, Rhus-t,** *sang, sars,* thuj, **Verat.**

morning, on getting up : **Rhus-t.**

night : **Cham, Rhus-t,** *sars.*

autumn, agg : *calc-p.*

bed, drives out of : **Cham, Rhus-t.**

chill, before : **Eup-per.**

cold, applied, amel : **Led** (ice cold), **Puls, Sec.**

exposure in winter : *sars.*

diphtheria, after : phyt.

motion, on : **Bry, Colch,** *kalm, led.*

amel : **Kali-s, Puls, Rhus-t.**

continued, amel : **Rhus-t,** tub.

move, on begining to : **Ferr, Lyc, Puls, Rhus-t.**

neuralgic : *coloc,* kalm, *mag-p.*

stump of, after operation : **All-c,** *ph-ac.*

rheumatic : *abrot,* **Arn, Benz-ac, Calc-p,** *caul,* **Caust, Cham, Colch,** *dulc,* eup-per, *ham,* **Kalm,** led, lith-c, **Med,** nux-m, **Phyt, Puls,** *ran-b.* **Rhod, Rhus-t, Sang, Sars, Sulph,** *syph,* thuj, verat.

acute : **Acon, Bry, Colch,** *dulc, kalm, rhod,* verat.

cold, weather, of : **Calc-p,** *dulc, rhod.*

cold, wet clothes : *nux-m,* **Rhus-t.**

wet weather : *nux-m, rhod,* **Rhus-t,** *verat.*

colchicum, after abuse of : *led.*

damp weather : *dulc,* **Rhus-t.**

diarrhoea checked : *abrot.*

drive him out of bed : **Cham, Rhus-t.**

exposure to draft of air, after heated : acon, *bry,* nux-m.

getting feet wet : *nux-m.*

gonorrhoea, after suppressed : *clem,* daph, *sars,* **Thuj.**

hot weather, sudden changes, in : *bry, dulc.*

mercury, abuse of : *phyt,* **Sars.**

rest, agg : rhod, **Rhus-t.**

secretions cheched, from any : abrot.

spring, amel : *calc-p.*

sudden changes in hot weather : bry, dulc.

suppressed haemorrhoids : *abrot.*

syphilitic : *phyt.*

walking, amel : **Rhus-t,** *verat.*

continued, amel : *verat.*

wandering : *caul, kalm, kali-bi,* **Kali-s,** *mag-p,* **Puls,** *rhod, tub.*

warmth, agg : **Sec.**

amel : **Ars, Mag-p, Rhus-t.**

of bed, agg : *led,* **Merc,** *verat.*

wet weather : dulc, **Rhod, Rhus-t.**

PAIN, bones : chin, **Eup-per, Nit-ac, Ruta,** *sars,* **Still.**

damp weather, after : sars.

cold, after : sars.

joints : bar-c, **Bry,** *caust, chin, colch, kalm, kali-bi, lac-ac,* **Led,** *med,* sal-ac, *sang,* thuj, verat-v.

night, agg : *benz-ac,* led.

gouty : *abrot,* **Arn,** *benz-ac,* bar-c, *berb,* **Caust, Colch,** fl-ac, *kalm,* **Led** (especially after abuse of colch), *thuj.*

motion : *kalm,* **Led.**

amel : *rhod,* **Rhus-t.**

rheumatic : *arn, benz-ac, berb, bry,* caul, (women, small joints), cact, **Caust, Colch,** ham, *kalm, kali-s, led, lith-c,* **Sang,** thuj.

gonorrhoea, suppressed, after : **Med, Thuj.**
small joints : *caul, cimic.*
touch, agg : *colch.*
wandering : caul, *colch,* **Kali-bi,** *kalm,* kali-s, **Lac-c, Puls,** *tub.*
downwards : cact, **Kalm.**
upward : **Led.**
warmth, agg : **Led, Merc, Puls.**
amel : **Ars.**
PAIN, upper limbs : **Bry, Colch,** *caust,* **Eup-per,** *kalm.*
chill, before : *eup-per,*
heart symptoms, with : **Cact, Kalm.**
motion : **Bry.**
rheumatic : berb, **Bry, Colch,** *kalm,* med.
extend downwards : *kalm* (especially left).
shoulder : *caust,* **Chel, Ferr,** *led, med,* ran-b (especially women of
sedantery habits), **Sang.**
right : **Chel, Sang.**
left : *agar,* **Ferr, Led,** nux-v.
and right hip : **Led.**
night : **Sang.**
rheumatic : *caust,* **Med,** *sang,* syph.
right : *sang.*
left : *ferr.*
motion, agg : med.
extending to fingers : med.
upper arm, rheumatic : med, **Sang,** syph.
singing, when : stann.
biceps, after lifting : **Rhus-t,** syph.
deltoid region : ferr, **Sang,** *syph.*
elbow : *caust.*
wrist : abrot, *caul, eup-per, guaj,* hep, **Rhus-t, Sulph.**
dislocation, as if : *arn,* **Eup-per.**
paroxysmal : *caul.*
rheumatic : *caul.*
hands : caul, rhus-v, sang.
paroxysmal : caul.
rheumatic : **Caul,** sang.

back of : rhus-v, *sang.*

fingers : caust, **Caul,** cimic, **Rhod.**

joints : **Caul, Caust,** cimic.

    intermittent : caul.

    paroxysmal : caul.

    rheumatic : **Caul.**

    spasmodic : caul.

nails : *graph, nit-ac,* **Sil.**

    splinters, as from : hep, **Nit-ac.**

lower limbs : *caust, colch, mag-p.*

motion, from : **Bry.**

    amel : **Ferr, Lyc, Puls, Rhus-t.**

paroxysmal : *mag-p.*

rheumatic : *caust.*

sciatica : am-m, ars, *bell,* **Bry,** chel, **Coloc, Gnaph,** kali-c, *lyc,* **Mag-p,** phyt, *podo,* **Rhus-t,** *valer.*

    right : bell, bry, chel, *coloc, lyc,* **Mag-p.**

    left : coloc, rhus-t.

    lying on painful side, amel : **Bry,** coloc.

    pressure, amel : **Coloc,** *mag-p.*

    rest on floor, letting foot : bell, valer.

    rest, during, after previous exertion : valer.

    standing, agg : **Valer.**

    straightening leg, agg : *valer.*

    walking, amel : **Ferr, Lyc, Rhus-t.** *valer.*

    warmth, amel : **Mag-p.**

wandering : *caul.*

hip : *caust,* **Coloc, Colch, Led,** *med,* **Stram.**

right : *agar,* ant-t, **Led,** *stram.*

left : **Caust.**

coughing, on : **Caust.**

rheumatic : **Led,** *med.*

    alternating sides : *lac-c.*

    extending upwards : *led.*

walking, when : *med.*

extending downwards : *med.*

    running around : *med.*

    knees, to : *med.*

thigh, walking : *am-m*.

        hamstrings : *am-m*.

        feel painfully short : *am-m*.

knee : caps, **Caust, Led.**

        cold, amel : *led*.

        cough, when, : caps.

        rheumatic : *caust, led,* **Stict** (sudden acute attack).

leg : *caps, caust,* eup-per, *led,* mag-c, *rhus-v, sang.*

        cold, amel : *led*.

        cough, when : caps.

        rheumatic : *med*.

        walking, when : med.

    tibia : rhus-v, sang, **Still.**

    calf : cupr.

    ankle : abrot, *caul, caust,* **Led.**

        cold, amel : **Led.**

        gouty : **Led.**

        step, from a false : **Led.**

        warmth agg : **Led.**

    foot : am-m, *caul, caust, led,* mag-c.

        ascending : **Led.**

        cold water, putting feet in amel : **Led,** *sec.*

        gouty : bar-c, fl-ac.

        menses, during : am-m.

        paroxysmal : caul.

        rheumatic : caul, *caust,* **Hep, Led.**

        sole : *ant-c,* calc, **Caust,** cupr, **Led,** lyc, **Sil.**

        heel : agar, am-m, caust, cycl, **Led,** mang, phyt.

    toes : *benz-ac, caul, caust, colch,* **Rhod.**

        first : **Led,** *rhod.*

            joints : *benz-ac, colch,* **Led.**

                gouty : **Led,** *rhod.*

                    fibrous deposit, in : colch, **Led,** rhod.

                paroxysmal : *caul.*

                rheumatic : *caul, colch.*

PAIN, aching : **Agar, Eup-per, Nux-v, Rhus-t.**

     upper arm : **Rhus-t.**

        heart disease, with : **Rhus-t.**

     lower limb : **Eup-per, Gels,** *med,* **Rhus-t.**

        night : med.

     hip : aesc.

     legs : med.

   boring, neuralgia : ph-ac.

   broken sensation, as if : aesc, **Eup-per,** tril-p.

     wrist : **Eup-per.**

   burning, hands : **Agar,** *calc,* chel, *fl-ac,* **Med,** *petr, phos, puls, sang,* **Sulph.**

     evening : **Puls, Sulph.**

     palm : *calc, fl-ac,* lach, *petr, phos, sang, sep,* **Sulph.**

        uncovers them : **Med, Puls,** *sang,* **Sulph.**

     fingers, sides : sars.

     foot : agar, *calc, lach,* **Med,** *petr, phos, puls,* sang, *sep,* **Sulph.**

     sole : **Calc,** *cham,* fl-ac, *graph, lach,* **Lyc,** med, petr, *phos, puls, sang,* sep, sanic, **Sulph.**

        uncovers them : *calc,* **Cham,** fl-ac, **Puls,** sanic, *sang,* **Sulph.**

     heel : agar, *caust, cycl,* phyt, valer.

     toes, sides : sars.

   crampy, hip : **Coloc** (as though in a vice).

   digging : (See Boring).

   drawing : *chin,* med, ph-ac, **Nit-ac,** *rhod.*

     motion, amel : rhod, **Rhus-t.**

     neuralgic : ph-ac.

     rest, agg : *rhod,* **Rhus-t.**

     rheumatic : **Rhod, Rhus-t.**

     weather, windy : *rhod, rhus-t.*

     bones : *chin.*

     joints : chin

     arms : caust.

     hands : caust.

     thighs : caust.

     legs : caust.

PAIN, neuralgia, thigh (along sciatic nerve, alternating with numbness) :
  Gnaph.
    foot, menses, during : *am-m.*
  rawness, foot : all-c, *calc.*
    soles : *calc.*
      perspiration from : *calc, graph,* sanic.
      heel : all-c.
  screwing : coloc.
  shooting, lower limb : *coloc.*
    left : *coloc.*
    extending from hip to knee : coloc.
  sore, bruised, beaten : **Arn, Bapt, Chin, Cimic, Eup-per,** mag-c,
      merc, ph-ac.
    exertion, after : cimic, **Rhus-t.**
    bones : **Eup-per.**
    joints : **Chin.**
    upper limbs : **Eup-per.**
    upper arm : **Eup-per.**
    fore arm : **Eup-per.**
    wrist : **Eup-per.**
    fingers, nails as if ulcerated : graph.
    lower limb : **Cimic, Eup-per.**
      exertion, after : *cimic.*
    pelvic region, cannot walk erect : **Arn.**
    thigh : *am-c.*
      menses, during : *am-c.*
    leg : **Eup-per,** mag-c.
    calf : **Eup-per.**
    foot : all-c, *graph,* **Lyc,** mag-c, petr, **Sil.**
      rubbing, from : dios.
    sole : **Ant-c, Bar-c, Led, Med,** puls.
      stone pavement, agg : *ant-c.*
      walking, while : **Ant-c, Hep, Led, Lyc, Med, Ruta.**
    heel : agar, all-c, *caust, cycl,* **Led,** med, phyt, valer.
      standing, when : agar, cycl.
      walking, when : caust, *cycl,* **Led.**
    balls of feet : med.
    toes : **Nit-ac,** sanic.
      perspiration, from : bar-c, sanic.

PAIN, sprained, as if : rhod, **Rhus-t.**

PAIN, sprained : **Rhus-t,** *ruta.*

      chronic : *bov,* stront-c.

      joints : **Arn,** *carb-an,* **Led, Rhus-t,** *ruta.*

          exertion, by slight : *carb-an,* **Led.**

      wrist : **Rhus-t, Ruta.**

      ankles : carb-an, **Led,** nat-c, **Rhus-t, Ruta.**

    stitching : abrot, apis, benz-ac, *bry.*

      joints : *apis,* **Bry, Kali-c.**

      toes, joint, first : *benz-ac.*

  tearing : benz-ac, **Chin, Lach, Merc, Rhod, Rhus-t.**

      motion, amel : *rhod,* **Rhus-t.**

        rheumatic : *rhod,* **Rhus-t.**

      wandering : *puls,* rhod.

      weather, wet : *rhod, rhus-t.*

      joints : *chin.*

      lower limbs : **Caust, Coloc, Rhus-t.**

        stool, during : *rhus-t.*

      foot : *benz-ac.*

      toes, joint, first : *benz-ac.*

PANARITIUM : (See Felon).

PARALYSIS : **Caust, Cocc,** pic-ac, **Rhus-t,** *sec.*

      apoplexy, after : *caust.*

      appearing gradually : **Caust.**

      ascending : agar, *con, kali-c.*

      cold, after catching : dulc, rhod.

      descending : *bar-c.*

      exertion, after : *caust.*

      hemiplegia : **Caust.**

        right : **Caust.**

        left : **Apis, Lach, Nux-v.**

        anger, after : staph.

        mental excitement : stann.

          shock, after : apis.

        twitching of one side, the other is paralyzed : *apis, bell.*

        old people : *bar-c, con.*

post-diphtheritic : *caust, cocc.*

stiffness, with : caust.

suppressed eruptions : *caust.*

typhoid, in : caust,

wet, after getting : **Caust.**

upper limbs : **Caust,** *cocc.*

    right : *caust.*

    left : **Dig.**

    coldness, with : caust.

    diphtheria, after : *caust.*

    sensation, of : **Aesc.**

upper arm, sensation of : *aesc.*

hands : **Caust, Plb** (wrist-drop).

    right : **Caust, Plb.**

    left : bar-c.

lower limbs : *cocc.*

    painless : **Cocc.**

    parturition, after : *caust.*

    post-diphtheritic : *cocc.*

    sensation of : **Aesc.**

leg, sensation of : **Aesc.**

PARONYCHIA : (See Felon).

PERSPIRATION,

hands : **Calc, Nit-ac, Sep, Sil, Sulph, Thuj.**

    cold : *lil-t.*

fingers : staph.

knee : *calc,* sep.

foot : am-m, alum, **Bar-c, Calc,** *cupr,* **Graph,** *petr,* **Psor,**
sanic, **Sep, Sil, Sulph, Zinc.**

    cold : *lil-t.*

    offensive : am-m, **Bar-c, Calc, Graph,** *petr, psor, sanic,*
    Sil, *zinc.*

    suppressed, bad effects : *cupr,* graph, **Sil, Zinc.**

sole : bar-c, **Nit-ac,** sanic, **Sil.**

    as if stepped in cold water : sanic.

toes, between : sanic, **Sil,** zinc.

    offensive : sanic, **Sil,** *zinc.*

    rawness, causing, : **Bar-c, Zinc.**

RELAXATION : *carb-an.*

       ankles : *carb-an.*

         turn when walking : *carb-an.*

RESTLESSNESS : Ars, Chin, Ferr, graph, **Kali-br,** *med,* **Puls, Rhus-t. Tarent, Zinc.**

            sitting at work, while : graph, zinc.

            typhoid, in : **Rhus-t,** tarax, zinc.

       arms : *tarent.*

       hands : **Kali-br,** *phos,* **Tarent.**

       fingers : **Kali-br.**

       lower limbs : **Tarent, Zinc.**

       legs : **Ferr, Med,** *phos,* **Tarent, Zinc.**

       feet : **Med,** *puls, tarent,* **Zinc.**

         night : *zinc.*

         in bed for hours after retiring, even when asleep : **Zinc.**

         sitting, while : **Zinc.**

ROUGH, hands : *petr.*

         finger, tips : **Petr.**

         winter, in : **Petr.**

SENSITIVE, finger tips : tarent.

SHOCKS : Cic.

SHORTENING (See Contraction also) : *am-m,* **Caust, Cimx, Guaj, Nat-m.**

SLEEP, go to (See Tingling) : cocc (hands and feet), dig (fingers).

SPASM of limbs : (See Convulsions).

SPLIT, nails : **Ant-c, Sil.**

SPRAIN : (See Pain, Sprained).

STAND, late learning to : **Calc, Calc-p.**

     unable to : **Calc-p.**

STAGGERING : (See Ataxia and Vertigo).

STIFFNESS : abrot, **Caust, Cupr,** *med,* **Rhus-t.**

       morning on getting up : **Rhus-t.**

       cough, before : **Cina.**

         during : *cupr,* ip.

       motion, amel : **Rhus-t.**

continued, amel : **Rhus-t.**
move, on beginning to : **Rhus-t.**
rising, on : **Rhus-t.**
joints : abrot, *bry,* **Caust,** med, **Rhus-t.**
upper limbs : *caust.*
shoulder : caust.
fore arm : *caust.*
finger : *caul.*
lower limb,

> knee : **Caust.**
> ankle : **Caust,** med.
> foot : caust.

STUMBLING : (See Awkwardness).

SUBSULTUS tendinum : *agar,* **Hyos, Iod, Zinc.**

SUPPURATION, fingers : staph.

SWELLING : apis, led, **Merc-sul.**

dropsical : **Apis,** apoc, **Ars, Coll** (cardiac), led, merc-sul, sulph.

joints : *abrot, apis,* apoc, ars, benz-ac, bry, *kalm,* **Led,** med, *rhod.*

inflammatory : ars, rhod.
puffy like windgalls : med
wandering : rhod.
wrist, arthritic swelling : sabin.

hand : *agar,* **Apis,** cact (left).

finger, joints : med.

lower limbs : *led.*

dropsical : **Apis, Ars, Chin,** *led,* **Samb.**

knee : **Led.**

leg : cact (left), **Led, Samb.**

ankle : **Apis,** apoc, *led,* **Med,** samb.

feet : agar, **Apis, Led,** *samb.*

oedematous : **Apis,** apoc, **Samb.**

one foot only : cact (left), *kali-c.*

toe : Grpah, *led.*

ball of first : *led.*

F-6

TENDERNESS : (See Pain, Sore).

TENSION, joints : *am-m,* nat-m.

    as from shortening of muscles in : *am-m, caust, cimx.*

    arm : meny.

    hand : meny.

    finger : meny.

    thigh : **Am-m.**

        hamstrings : *am-m,* **Caust,** cimx.

THICK, nails : *ant-c,* **Graph.**

    finger : **Graph.**

    toe : *graph.*

TINGLING, prickling, asleep (See Numbness) : **Acon, Graph, Lyc, Phos, Puls, Rhus-t,** *sec.*

    fingers go to sleep : dig.

    fingers and toes in : nat-m.

TOTTERING (See Weakness) : **Alum,** arg-met, **Cocc** (while walking), *gels.*

TREMBLING : Arg-n, Cocc, Gels, Merc, tarax, zinc.

    arms : *cocc.*

        excitement, exertion of pain from : cocc.

    hands : ant-t, *gels,* **Merc,** *phyt,* **Zinc.**

        menses, during : *zinc.*

        writing, while : **Caust, Sulph,** *zinc.*

    lower limb : **Arg-met.**

    legs : *cocc,* gels.

        exertion, excitement of pain, from : cocc.

TWITCHING : *agar,* **Hyos, Ign.**

    fingers : **Cupr,** kali-bi.

ULCERS, lower limbs : *calc.*

    foot : **Ars.**

    sole : calc.

        blisters, from : calc.

WALK, late learning to : **Calc, Calc-p, Caust, Nat-m,** *sanic, sil.*

WALKING : (See Awkwardness).

    daytime : alum.

    inability, except with eyes open : alum, arg-met.

WARTS, hand : anac, **Caust, Dulc,** *nat-c, nat-m,* **Thuj.**
        fleshy : **Dulc.**
        large : dulc.
        smooth : dulc.
        sore : ruta.
        palm : *anac, nat-c, nat-m,* ruta.
            flat : ruta.
            sore to touch : *nat-c.*
        back of hands : *dulc.*
     fingers : *dulc.*
         sore : ruta.
WEAKNESS : bov, cocc, *cupr,* **Merc, Sil,** *zinc.*
        exertion, after least : **Ars,** *med.*
        loss of nervous force, from : med.
        joints : *bov, carb-an.*
        hand : **Med,** *zinc.*
            menses, during : zinc.
            writing, while : *zinc.*
        lower limb : **Alum,** am-c, **Arg-n, Cocc, Carb-an.**
            menses, during : cocc (scarcely able to stand).
        thigh : am-c,
            menses, during : am-c.
        knees : cocc (give out when walking), *dios.*
        legs : med (legs give way), **Ph-ac.**
        ankle : **Carb-an,** led, med, **Nat-c, Sil.**
            walking, while : carb-an, med, *nat-c,* nat-m.
               easily turns : med, *mat-c,* nat-m.
        foot : nat-c, *nat-m.*
            bends under : carb-an, nat-c.
WEARINESS : bov, *cupr,* **Merc.**
        hands : *bov.*
        feet : *bov.*
        legs : med (legs give way), pic-ac.
WOODEN sensation, lower limbs : thuj.
WRIST drop : **Plb.**

◻◻◻

Eye

AGGLUTINATED : Arg-n, Graph, thuj.

        morning : apis, **Arg-n,** *eup-per,* **Graph,** *merc,* **Rhus-t.**

        night : **Alum, Graph,** *syph,* thuj.

AMAUROSIS : (See Paralysis).

BLEEDING, from eyes : arn, **Crot-h.**

        in anterior chamber after iridectomy : *led.*

        conjunctival haemorrhage, from injury : **Arn.**

        cough, from : arn.

        retinal : **Arn,** ham, *led,* **Nux-v.**

           cough, from : *arn,* **Led,** ham, **Nux-v.**

BLINKING : (See Winking).

BLOATED lids : (See Swelling).

BLOOD shot : **Bell,** op, verat-v.

BOILS on lids : (See Pustules).

BRILLIANT : Bell, Camph, *coff, stram.*

CATARACT : Calc, Calc-fl, *calc-p,* **caust.**

CHALLAZAE : (See Tumors).

CHEMOSIS : Arg-n.

CLOSE, difficult to : **Nux-v.**

        half close : (See Open, Half).

        involuntary : **Caust,** *gels.*

        must, bathing, while : *lyss, phos.*

CLOSED (See Open, Unable to) : nux-m, op.

        constantly : nux-m.

        unconscious, during : *op.*

COLD, sensation as if cold wind blowing across eyes : **Croc.**

        agg : **Merc.**

        amel : *asar.*

COLOR, orange : lach.

CONDYLOMATA : *nit-ac,* **Thuj.**

        eye-lids : *caust,* **Thuj.**

CONESTION : (See Redness).

CONTORTED : (See Distorted).

CRACKS, canthi, in : **Graph.**

CRUSTY, margin, lids : (See Eruption).

DARK around eyes : (See Face).

DISCHARGE of mucus or pus : *arg-n,* **Calc, Calc-s, Graph,** kali-bi, kali-s, **Merc,** nat-s, **Puls.**

        acrid : euphr.

        bland : **All-c,** Puls.

        bloody : *crot-h, graph.*

        gonorrhoeal or sycotic : **Nat-s.**

        green : *nat-s.*

        profuse : **Arg-n, Euphr,** syph.

        purulent : **Arg-n, Merc, Puls.**

        sensation of, as if weeping : croc.

        sticky mucus on cornea : **Euphr.**

        thick : *kali-bi, puls.*

        touch : kali-bi.

        yellow : kali-s, nat-s, **Puls, Sil.**

           green : **Puls.**

DISTORTED : **Bell,** *cupr, stram.*

DROOPING of lids : (See Falling).

DRYNESS : **Alum,** bry, **Nux-m, Op,** thuj.

DULLNESS : diph.

ECCHYMOSIS : **Arn,** *ham,* **Led, Nux-v.**

ECZEMA : (See Eruption).

ENLARGEMENT, sensation : cimic, *com,* **Spig.**

ERUPTION about eyes : *graph.*

        lids, on : **Graph.**

           blisters : nat-s, thuj.

           crust : *graph.*

           eczema : **Graph.**

           moist : graph.

           scaly, margins on : **Graph.**

EVERSION of lids : **Arg-n.**

EXCORIATION of lids : **Arg-n.**

EXOPHTHALMUS : (See Protrusion).

EXTRAVASATION of blood into chambers of eye : *ham.*

　　　　　cough, from : *ham.*

EYE brow : (See Hair).

EYE lashes : (See Hair).

FALLING of lids : caul, *caust,* **Gels**, graph, sep, *syph.*

　　　　　upper : caul, *caust,* **Gels**, graph.

　　　　　both : sep.

FIRE, looking into, agg : *merc.*

FISSURE, canthi : (See Cracks).

FISTULA, cornea, of : **Sil.**

　　　　　lachrymalis : **Fl-ac, Sil.**

FIXED look : (See Staring).

GLASSY appearance : **Op.**

GLAUCOMA : *osm,* phos, *spig.*

GRANULAR lids : *arg-n, nat-s.*

HAIR, falling from brows : **Kali-c,** sel.

　　　　　eyelashes, agglutinated in the morning : *borx.*

　　　　　　　　loaded with dry gumy exudation : borx.

　　　　　　　　turn inward and inflame eye : *borx.*

　　　　　　　　wild hairs, tendency to : borx.

　　　　　eye brows, light : **Brom.**

HEAT in : **Bell, Kali-c,** *op,* **Ruta.**

　　　　　exertion, during : **Ruta.**

　　　　　using eyes : **Ruta.**

HEAVINESS : Aesc, aloe.

　　　　　lids : caul, **Caust, Con, Gels,** *graph.*

　　　　　　　upper : *caul,* **Gels.**

　　　　　　　　has to raise with fingers : *caul,* **Gels,** *sep.*

HOLLOW : (See Sunken).

INFANTS, eye complaints of : (See Inflammation).

INFLAMMATION : Acon, *arg-n,* **Arn, Ars, Bell,** *borx,* **Euphr,** *glon, ham, kali-bi,* **Merc, Puls, Rhus-t, Sulph,** *thuj.*

    burn, after : **Canth.**

    catarrhal, from cold : **Acon, Bell, Dulc, Euphr.**

    fire, agg : **Ant-c.**

    foreign body : **Acon.**

    gonorrhoeal : *merc,* **Nit-ac, Puls,** *thuj.*

    infants : **Arg-n.**

        ophthalmia neonatorum : **Arg-n,** *bell, merc,* **Puls, Rhus-t,** *sulph,* syph, thuj (sycotic or syphilitic).

    scrofulous : *bar-c.*

    vaccination, after : thuj.

    warm covering, amel : *hep,* thuj.

    conjunctiva : **Acon, Arg-n, Bell, Euphr,** *ham,* merc-d, **Rhus-t, Sulph,** *thuj.*

        acute : *arg-n.*

        granular : **Arg-n,** *thuj.*

        pustular (including cornea) : thuj.

        traumatic : *arn, ham.*

    cornea : *crot-h,* **Merc, Sulph.**

    iris : **Merc-c, Crot-h, Rhus-t.**

    lids : **Arg-n,** *psor.*

        margins : *arg-n,* graph, staph.

INJECTED : all-c.

INJURIES, from : *arn, led,* **Symph.**

INSENSIBILITY : hell.

INVERSION of lids : *borx.*

JERKINGS : (See Twitchings).

LIGHT, aversion to : **Con** (student's remedy for night work).

LACHRYMATION (See Tears) : **All-c,** *chel, crot-h,* **Euphr, Nat-m, Rhus-t,** *sabad,* squil.

    daytime only : **Alum,** euphr, ferr, nat-m.

    coryza, during : **All-c, Euphr, Carb-v, Nux-v,** squil.

    cough, with : **Euphr, Nat-m.**

        whooping cough, during : euphr, ferr, nat-m.

    water all the time : **Euphr,** chel (right eye, in right-sided headache), **Spig** (left eye, in left-sided headache).

MOVEMENTS, eye balls,

    constant : agar, *bell,* phys.

    convulsive : **Bell.**

    pendulum like, from side to side : **Agar.**

    quick : **Bell.**

    rolling : *bell, zinc.*

NYSTAGMUS : (See Movements).

OPACITY of cornea : **Arg-n, bar-c, Calc, Sulph.**

OPENING of lids difficult : **Caust, Gels.**

OPEN, lids : *stram.*

OPEN, half open : **Cupr, Op.**

    hard to keep open : caust, **Gels,** graph.

    unable to : **Nux-m,** *psor.*

    wide open : *hell,* **Op, Stram.**

OPENNESS, spasmodic : **Bell, Stram.**

PAIN : *arg-n,* asar, **Bell,** *chel, cimic,* eup-per, *hep,* **Nat-m,** *phys,* **Ran-b, Ruta, Seneg, Spig.**

    begins at sun rise, increases till noon and ceases at sunset : **Kalm,** *nat-m.*

    night : **Merc, Merc-c,** *syph.*

        2 to 5 a.m. : *syph.*

    air, cold, amel : asar.

    ascending stairs, agg : *cimic.*

    bathing eye in cold water, amel : *asar.*

    blow, from : **Arn, Symph.**

        obtuse body, ball, infant's fist, etc., from : **Symph.**

    cold water, amel : *asar,* syph.

    looking, when : **Nat-m,** *ruta.*

        intently : **Nat-m,** *ruta, seneg.*

    lying, amel : *cimic.*

    neuralgia : *chel,* **Cimic, Spig.**

        left : spig.

    periodic : chel (right), spig (left).

    reading : asar, **Nat-m,** phys, **Ruta.**

    sewing, while on fine work : nat-m, **Ruta.**

    short attack : **Bell.**

strained, as if : **Ruta.**

sudden, comes and ceases suddenly : **Bell, Mag-p.**

touch, agg : **Hep.**

turning side ways : **Kalm, Spig.**

work, while on fine : (See Sewing).

eyebrows : *chel.*

right : *chel.*

PAIN, aching : **Cimic, Eup-per, Puls,** *rhus-t, ruta.*

neuralgic : **Cimic.**

reading, while : **Ruta.**

PAIN, burning, smarting, biting : **Acon, All-c, Apis, Ars, Bell, Euphr,** *op, phos,* **Ran-b, Ruta,** sabad, **Sulph.**

rubbing, amel, : all-c.

smoke, as, from : *all-c.*

margins of lids : **Euphr,** sabad.

bursting : *gels.*

one sided : *sang, sil.*

cutting : spig.

darting : (See Shooting).

drawing : *hep.*

backward into head, the eye ball : hep, *olend,* **Par.**

neuralgia : cimic (ciliary), *spig* (ciliary),

pressing, pressure, etc. : asar, **Bry, Calc, Cham, Nat-m,** *phos,* **Ran-b,** sang, **Spig.**

false step, agg : *spig.*

headache, during : sang.

reading, while : asar.

turning eyes, agg : **Spig.**

shooting : (See Stitching).

smarting : (See Burning).

sore, bruised, tender : *arn,* arg-n, **Bry, Calen, Euphr, Ham, Hep,** led.

blow, from : **Symph.**

moving the lids : **Bry.**

eyes : *bapt,* **Bry.**

touch, agg : **Hep.**

lids : arg-n.

stabbing : (See Cutting).

stitching : *cimic, kalm*, **Spig.**

    right : *kalm.*

    left : *spig.*

    ascending stairs, from : cimic.

    cold, from : spig.

    lying down, amel : cimic.

    weather, rainy, from : rhus-t, spig.

    extending backwards : **Spig.**

        occiput : cimic.

        temples : cimic.

        vertex : cimic.

PARALYSIS of lids : **Sep.**

    upper : *caul,* **Caust, Gels,** *graph,* **Rhus-t, Sep,** *syph.*

        cold, from : **Caust,** rhus-t.

    superior oblique : *syph.*

PHOTOPHOBIA : *asar,* **Bell,** *coff,* colch, **Con,** euphr, *kali-bi,* **Nat-s,** nux-m, **Nux-v,** *psor.*

    night : con (student's remedy for night work).

    artificial light : *con.*

    daylight : asar, *con.*

    headache, during : kali-bi.

    intense : **Con,** psor.

    sunshine : asar.

    wind : asar.

PROMINENT : Stram.

PROTRUSION : Bell, iod, **Stram.**

    exophthalmus : **Ferr, Ferr-i, Iod, Sec.**

PTERYGIUM : *ars, calc, euphr, nux-m, sulph, zinc.*

PTOSIS : (See Paralysis of Eyelids).

PUFFY : (See Swollen).

PULLING sensation : (See Pain, Drawing).

PULSATION in eyes : **Bell.**

PUPILS, contracted : **Op, Thuj.**

    alternately contracted and dilated : *hell.*

    dilated : *aeth,* **Bell,** gels, *hell,* **Hyos,** *nat-c,* **Stram,** verat-v.

child reprimanded, when : stram.

epileptic fit, before : arg-n.

insensibility to light : **Bell, Cupr, Hyos, Op,** *stram.*

REDNESS : Arg-n, Bell, Euphr, Glon, Sulph.

raw beef, like : *arg-n.*

scarlet-red : *arg-n.*

lids : **Euphr,** *graph,* sabad.

edges : **Euphr, Graph.**

veins : dig.

ROLLING : (See Movements).

SCALY on the edges : thuj.

SENSITIVE to light : (See Photophobia).

touch : *spig.*

SPASM OF LIDS : agar, *bell, mag-p,* ruta.

lower lids : ruta.

STARING : aeth, **Bell,** hell, **Hyos,** mosch, ruta.

STRAINING (See also Vision, Dim) : arg-n, **Nat-m,** *ruta, seneg.*

air, open, amel : arg-n, *nat-m,* ruta.

fine work, from : **Nat-m, Ruta.**

sewing, from : arg-n, **Nat-m, Ruta.**

warm room, agg : arg-n, **Nat-m, Ruta.**

STIFFNESS of muscles about eyes : **Kalm.**

STRABISMUS : Bell, Cic, *tab.*

brain troubles, in : *tab.*

STYES : Con, Graph, Lyc, Puls, Sep, Staph, Sulph, *thuj.*

upper lids : **Puls,** staph.

eating fat, rich food or pork : **Puls.**

one after another : *staph.*

SUFFUSED : (See Lachrymation).

SUGGILATIONS : (See Ecchymosis).

SUNKEN, hollow : *berb,* **Chin,** *ph-ac, phos,* sil.

SWOLLEN : Apis, *kali-c.*

lids : **Apis, Arg-n, Euphr,** *kali-c.* **Nat-c,** *phos,* syph.

margin : **Euphr.**

oedematous : **Apis, Kali-c,** *phos.*

lower lids : **Apis.**
upper lids : **Kali-c.**
over the eyes : **Kali-c** (between eyebrows and upper
   eyelids).
under the eyes : **Apis.**

TEARS, acrid : **Ars, Euphr, Merc-c, Sulph.**
   bland : **All-c.**
   burning : **Euphr, Sulph.**
   gushing out : *chel,* rhus-t.

TENSION : Ruta.

THICKENING of cornea : *arg-n.*
   lids : **Arg-n.**

TUMORS on lids : *staph, thuj.*
   meibomian glands : **Staph,** *thuj.*
   nodules in lids : *con,* **Staph,** *thuj.*
   tarsal tumors : *thuj.*

TURNED (See Movements) : bell, **Spig,**
   down-wards : **Aeth.**
   upwards : *op.*

TWITCHING, lids : **Agar, Croc** (especially eyelids), **Phys.**
   muscles of : **Agar,** phys.

ULCERATION, cornea : *arg-n.*

VACANT : (See Face, Expression).

VEINS : (See Redness).

WARTS on lids : *caust.*

WATERY : (See Lachrymation).

WEAK : *kali-c.*
   abortion, after : kali-c.
   coition, after : **Kali-c.**
   emission, after : kali-c.
   measles, after : *kali-c.*

WILD look : **Bell.**

YELLOWNESS : *chel, chin,* **Crot-t,** *plb,* **Sep.**

❑❑❑

Eye-Vision

ACCOMMODATION defective : *arg-n,* nat-m, ruta, seneg.

ACUTE : Bell, *coff,* colch.

AMAUROSIS : (See Loss of Vision).

BLURRED : Gels, *phys,* **Nat-m,** *ruta.*

    headache, before : *gels, kali-bi,* lac-d.

        which returns as headache ceases : iris, kali-bi, lac-d, nat-m.

    headache, at beginning of : **Iris.**

COLOR before the eyes : *cycl.*

DAZZLING : nat-m.

DIM : Aur, *crot-h,* **Cycl, Gels,** phys, *psor,* **Ruta, Sulph,** tab, tril-p, *verat-v.*

    morning : cycl.

    blurr, from : phys.

    clears up, after keratitis or kerato-iritis : *crot-h.*

    exertion of eyes, after : *nat-m, ruta.*

        on fine work : *nat-m,* **Ruta.**

    film, from : phys.

    headache, before : *gels, kali-bi, psor.*

        during : **Cycl.**

    over use in bad light, from : *ruta.*

    reading : **Nat-m, Ruta, Seneg.**

    refraction, anomalies of from : *ruta.*

    sewing, from : *ruta.*

DISAPPEAR, letters : cic, cocc.

DIPLOPIA : Gels, glon, **Hyos,** syph, verat-v.

FIERY, sparks : *cycl.*

FLASHES : Phys.

FLICKERING : Bell, Cycl, Graph, Nat-m, Phos, *psor.*

    morning headache, with : **Cycl.**

    colours, various : **Cycl.**

    headache, before : *psor.*

FOGGY : caust, **Croc, Cycl,** *ran-b, ruta,* tab.

    sensation as if room filled with smoke : **Croc.**

GLITTERING objects : *cycl.*

     needles : **Cycl.**

HEMIOPIA : *aur,* gels, *glon,* verat-v.

     right half lost (sees left half) : **Lith-c,** *lyc.*

     left half lost (sees right half) : calc, cic.

     lower half lost (sees upper half) : *aur,* sulph.

     upper half lost (sees lower half) : **Aur,** *dig.*

LIGHTNING : nat-m.

LOSS of Vision (blindness) : **Acon,** *chin, gels, lac-d, psor,* stram, *tab.*

     daytime : ran-b.

     one eye : apoc.

     atrophy of retina or optic nerve, from : *tab.*

     headache, before : *gels,* kali-bi, lac-d, *psor.*

      during : *lac-d.*

      vision returns as headache increases : iris, kali-bi, lac-d, nat-m.

MIST : (See Foggy).

MOVING, letters up or down : cic, *cocc.*

RINGS, black, headache before : *psor.*

SMOKY : (See Foggy).

SPARKS : *cycl.*

SPOTS, black, floating : phys.

     headache, before : *psor.*

TURN, letters seem to : **Cic.**

VANISHING of sight : (See Loss of Vision).

VEIL, as though : (See Foggy).

                ❑❑❑

Face

ABSCESS : Hep, Merc, Sil.
        antrum : *merc,* **Sil.**
        parotid glands : **Ars,** lach, **Sil.**

BLEEDING, lips, : **Arum-t,** cund (with malignant tendency).

BLOATED (See Swelling, Congestion) : apis, **Ars,** bar-c, *chin,* ferr, *nat-m,*
        op, spig.

BLUSHING, acute or chronic : (See Flushing).

BURIED in pillow, lies with : psor.

CACHECTIC : (See Expression).

CHEWING motion of jaw (See Grinding Teeth) : **Bry,** *hell.*

CHLOROTIC : *acet-ac,* **Calc, Calc-p,** *chin,* **Ferr,** *helon,* **Kali-c, Nat-m,**
        Puls.

COBWEB, sensation of : *bar-c,* borx, *brom,* **Graph,** *ran-s.*

COLDNESS : *ant-t,* **Carb-v,** *iod,* **Verat.**
        icy coldness : *agar,* **Verat.**

COMPRESSION of jaw as in lock jaw : cic.

CONGESTION : Aml-ns, bar-c, **Bell, Glon, Meli, Stram.**

CONTRACTION of face : (See Distortion).

CRACKED lips : **Arum-t,** *ars,* **Bry,** *hell,* **Nat-m,** nit-ac.
        lower lip : *nit-ac,* **Sep.**
           middle of : *am-c, hep,* nat-m.
        upper lip : *kali-c, nat-m.*
           middle of : *hep, nat-m.*
        corners of mouth : ant-c, **Arum-t, Cund** (with malignant
           tendency), *hell,* **Graph,** *nat-m,* **Nit-ac.**

DANDRUFF in eyebrows, beard : sanic.

DISCOLOURATION, ashy : *plb,* pyrog, sec.
        bluish : ant-t, **Bapt, Camph,** *carb-an,* **Carb-v,** *cic, cina,* **Cupr,**
           Dig, *dros,* **Ip,** plb, *tab,* **Verat.**
        cheeks : *carb-an.*
        cholera, in : camph, **Cupr, Verat.**
        eyes, circles round : **Berb,** *bism, cina,* **Chin, Nat-c,** *ph-ac,*
           phos, **Sec.**
           lids : *dig.*

DISCOLOURATION,

bluish, lips : **Camph,** *carb-an ,* cina, *chin, dig, mosch.*
whooping cough : cupr, dros.

blushing : (See Redness).

changing colour : *ferr,* **Ign** (when at rest).

cyanotic : **Ars,** *cupr.*

dark (dusky) : **Bapt.**

dirty : **Lyc.**

earthy : *berb, lyc,*

grayish : *carb-v.*

greenish : **Carb-v.**

mottled : *ail, bapt, bell, crot-h, lach, rhus-t.*

pale : abrot, *acet-ac,* aml-ns (of affected side), alum, **Ant-t,**
Ars, Berb, bism, **Calc, Camph, Carb-v,** castm, *cham,*
Chin, Cina, *cycl,* **Dig, Ferr,** *iod, ip, kalm,* lach, **Lob,**
Lyc, Med, Nat-c, Op, Ph-ac, *plat,* **Plb,** psor, *puls, pyrog,*
rheum, samb, **Sec, Sep,** *sil, spig,* **Tab, Verat, Zinc.**
flushes easily : **Ferr.**
before, as well as, after a haemorrhage : **Carb-v.**

child, at birth : ant-t.

deathly pale : *bism,* **Dig,** plb, **Tab.**

lips : *dig,* **Ferr.**

menses, after : alum.

one side : *cham.*

one side pale and cold, other side red and hot : **Cham, Cina.**

rising up, on, red face becomes deathly pale : **Acon.**

red and pale alternately : **Acon** (in fever), **Ferr** (from emotion,
exertion and pain), zinc.

red : acet-ac, **Acon,** aeth, *agar, aml-ns, arn,* **Bapt, Bell, Bry,**
Calc, cact, **Chin,** cham, **Cic, Cina,** *coca,* erig, **Ferr,** *ign,*
Meli, mag-p, **Mez,** *nat-m,* **Nux-v, Op,** *sabad, spig,* **Stram,**
sulph, *verat.*

left : *acet-ac.*

bluish-red : *dig.*

chill, during : **Ferr,** *ign.*

circumscribed : **Chin, Ferr, Sang,** stram.
afternoon : **Sang.**
in bronchitis, pneumonia, phthisis : phos, **Sang.**

cough, during : **Bell.**

dark red : *arn,* **Bapt, Bell,** spig, *sulph.*

    cheek : *spig.*

dull : *gels.*

emotion, from : **Ferr.**

exertion, from : **Ferr.**

fever, during : **Acon, Bell.**

glowing red : *acon,* **Bell,** *cina* (pale around mouth), *ferr.*

headache, during : **Bell.**

inflammatory : *mez.*

lying, while : acon, verat.

    becomes pale on rising : *acon, verat.*

one red, the other pale : **Cham,** *cina.*

pain, when in : **Ferr.**

red and white alternate : **Ferr.**

spot : acet-ac.

    left cheek : *acet-ac.*

    straining at stool, when : caust.

    cheeks : *brom.*

    lips : *bell,* **Sulph,** *tub.*

        as if blood would burst through : **Sulph,** *tub.*

        red and white alternate : **Ferr.**

sallow : **Chel,** lyc.

sickly colour : *chin,* **Lyc,** *ph-ac,* psor.

spots, moth, forehead on : *caul, sep.*

white : (See Pale).

yellow : *carb-v,* caust, **Chel, Lyc, Plb, Sep.**

    saddle across cheeks and nose : **Sep.**

DISTORTION : bov, cic, **Hyos, Ign, Spig, Stram.**

    stammering, while : bov, ign, spig, **Stram.**

DRAWN : **Aeth, Ars, Lyc, Op, Sec.**

    linea nasalis, well marked : *aeth.*

DROPPING of jaw (See Mouth Open) : **Lach, Lyc, Mur-ac.**

DRYNESS (See Skin) : **Ars.**

    lips : *ars,* **Bry,** *helon, nat-m.*

EMACIATION (see Generalities) : *psor, sel,* tab.

    cheek of : tab.

F-7

ERUPTION : bell-p, **Calc,** *calc-p, cic,* **Dulc, Kali-br, Nat-m, Phos, Rhus-t, Sang,** syzyg.

   scanty menses of young women, during : bell-p, **Calc, Psor,** sang, syzyg.

   cheeks : *dulc.*

   chin : *dulc,* **Rhus-t.**

   forehead : dulc.

   lips : **Nat-m.**

   mouth : **Nat-m, Rhus-t.**

   temples : *dulc.*

ERUPTION, acne : calc-p, **Kali-br,** *psor.*

   coffee, from : psor.

   fat, from : psor.

   meat, from : psor.

   menses, during : psor.

   puberty, at : *calc-p.*

   sugar, from : psor.

   bluish-red : kali-br.

   indurata : kali-br.

   rosacea : kali-br, psor.

   scars unsightly, follows : *carb-an, kali-br.*

   young fleshy persons, in : *kali-br.*

   blisters, lips on : **Nat-m.**

   fever, during : **Nat-m.**

   pearl, like : **Nat-m.**

   boils, nose, inside : tub.

   painful : hep, tub.

   crusty : *cic,* **Dulc.**

   bleeds, when scratched : dulc.

   reddish borders, with : *dulc.*

   yellow : *cic,* **Dulc,**

      brownish : **Dulc.**

   chin : *cic,* **Dulc.**

   fore-head : *dulc.*

   temples : *dulc.*

   discharging, fetid : sec, tub.

   greenish : tub.

eczema : **Ars, Calc, Dulc, Graph.**
    moist : **Graph.**
    excoriating : **Graph.**
    fissures : **Calc, Graph.**
herpes : *dulc, graph,* **Nat-m, Rhus-t.**
    chin : *nat-m,* rhus-t.
    lips : **Nat-m.**
    mouth, around : **Nat-m,** *rhus-t.*
    nose : **Aeth.**
itching : *graph,* **Mez, Rhus-t,** *sars.*
    forehead : *sars.*
        menses, during : psor, *sang, sars,* syzyg.
moist : **Dulc, Graph, Mez.**
pimples : *led.*
    cheeks : led.
    forehead : *led.*
pustules : **Cic,** *kali-bi.*
    confluent : *cic.*
        yellow scabs with : *cic.*
red : *led.*
    stinging, painful : led.
tubercles, : *led.*
    cheeks : *led.*
    forehead : *led.*

ERYSIPELAS : Apis, Bell, *canth,* **Graph.**
    right : *bell.*
        to left : apis, **Graph.**
    left : lach, **Rhus-t.**
    oedematous : **Apis.**
    phlegmonous : *graph.*

EXCORIATED, lips : am-m, **Arum-t, Ars.**
    corners of mouth : *ars,* **Arum-t.**

EXOSTOSIS : *fl-ac, hecla.*

EXPRESSION, anxious : **Acon, Aeth,** *bapt, plb.*
    abashed : *staph.*
    besotted : apis, **Bapt,** diph, *gels.*
    drunken : *bapt.*
    frightened : **Acon** (life rendered miserable by fear), *aeth.*

EXPRESSION,

> guilty : *staph.*
>
> lively : *arn.*
>
> old looking : *abrot, ambr,* **Arg-n, Lyc,** *iod,* **Nat-m, Op,** *sanic, sars.*
>
> pinched : *aeth.*
>
> sickly : *chin,* **Cina, Lyc.**
>
> sleepy : **Cann-i, Op.**
>
>> dropping lids, from : *caust,* graph, *syph.*
>
> stupid : *bapt, hell, gels.*
>
> suffering : aeth, **Ars,** plb.
>
> 'tell tale face' of uterine ailments : **Sep.**
>
> vacant : *hell.*
>
> wild : (See Eyes),
>
> wrinkled : (See Old Looking).

FALLING of whiskers : nat-m, sel.

FLUSHING (See Discolouration) : **Aml-ns, Bell, Chin,** coca, crot-h, **Ferr, Meli.**

> emotion, on slightest : *aml-ns,* coca, **Ferr.**
>
> but parts below icy cold : *aml*-ns.
>
> prostration, followed by : *anl-ns.*
>
> sweating, followed by : **Aml-ns.**

FURROWS, on forehead : *lyc.*

GREASY : *nat-m, plb, psor,* sanic, thuj.

HAIR, growth of, on child's face : nat-m, ol-j, psor, sulph.

HANGING down of jaw : (See Dropping).

HEAT : *agar,* **Bell, Bry, Nux-v,** sabad, **Stram.**

> cold body, with : *arn.*
>
>> hands, with : **Arn.**
>
> flushes : **Graph, Lach, Sep.**

HIPPOCRATIC (See Sunken) : **Ant-t, Ars,** *camph,* **Carb-v,** chin, **Sec, Tab, Verat.**

INFLAMMATION,

> parotid gland : **Bell, Carb-v, Merc, Puls,** *sil.*
>
>> right : **Merc.**
>
>>> then left : **Lyc.**

left : **Brom,** *lach,* **Rhus-t.**

metastasis to mammae : **Puls.**

to testes : *carb-v,* **Puls.**

suppuration, with : **Ars, Brom, Calc, Hep, Merc, Rhus-t, Sil.**

submaxillary : **Merc, Rhus-t.**

ITCHING : *agar,* **Calc, Caust,** mez, **Rhus-t.**

night : mez.

child scratches face continually until bleeds : **Mez.**

LINES, premature : **Lyc.**

LOCKJAW : aeth, **Cic, Hyper** (also prevents).

splinters into flesh, from : **Cic, Hyper.**

NUMBNESS of lips : nat-m.

NECROSIS of lower jaw : **Phos.**

PAIN (aching, prosopalgia) : **Acon,** all-c, **Bell, Caust, Cedr, Coloc, Mag-p, Spig, Stann,** *sulph.*

right : **Bell, Chel,** *mag-p.*

left : **Spig.**

morning till sunset : *spig.*

cold air, agg : **Mag-p, Rhus-t.**

cold application, agg : **Mag-p, Rhus-t, Sil.**

gradually increasing and decreasing : *plat,* **Stann.**

and cease suddenly : puls, sul-ac.

intermittent : (See Paroxysmal).

neuralgic : all-c, **Coloc, Mag-p,** mez, *sang,* **Spig,** *stann.*

right : **Mag-p.**

left : *spig.*

kneeling down and pressing head against floor, amel : sang.

paroxysmal : caust, *mag-p.*

periodical : *mag-p,* **Spig.**

left side : spig.

pressure, amel : **Mag-p.**

quinine, after : **Nat-m.**

suddenly coming, suddenly going : **Bell,** *mag-p, spig.*

PAIN, tea agg : *spig.*

        warmth, amel : **Ars, Hep, Mag-p.**

        weather, during rainy : spig.

        wind, dry cold : **Acon, Hep, Mag-p.**

        extending from upper jaw to all directions : sang.

        eye, above (supra-orbital) : mag-p.

                right : *mag-p.*

        below (infra-orbital) : mag-p.

                right : *mag-p.*

        malar bone : *stann.*

           left : *spig.*

                menses, during : *stann.*

PAIN, burning : *agar,* **Ars, Rhus-t,** *spig,* **Sulph.**

        left : **Coloc,** *spig.*

        redness, without : *sulph.*

        cramp-like (See Drawing) : mag-p.

        cutting : *bell,* mag-p.

           right : **Bell,** *mag-p.*

           cold air, agg : **Mag-p.**

           heat external, amel : **Mag-p.**

           touch agg : *mag-p.*

PAIN, darting : (See Stitching).

    lancinating : **Mag-p.**

           right : *mag-p.*

    neuralgia : caust, kalm (right), *spig* (left).

    sore, bruised : *nat-m.*

        lips : nat-m.

    stitching : *mag-p.*

        right : *mag-p.*

        cold air, agg : **Mag-p.**

        heat, external, amel : **Mag-p.**

        pressure, amel : *mag-p.*

        touch agg : *mag-p.*

    tearing : **Bell,** caust, *chel,* **Coloc, Mag-p,** *spig.*

        right : **Chel.**

        left : **Coloc.**

        morning to sunset : *spig.*

        periodic : spig.

        cheek bones : *spig.*

PARALYSIS : Caust.
>> right : *caust.*
>> cold, from : **Caust.**
>> one sided : **Caust.**
>> riding in wind : *caust.*
>> wet, after getting : **Caust.**

PARCHED, lips : ars, **Bry.**

PERSPIRATION : ant-t, **Carb-v, Ign,** lob, med, *tab,* **Verat.**
>> cold : *ant-t,* cact, **Carb-v,** hell, **Lob,** med, *tab,* **Verat.**
>> eating, while : *ign.*
>> face, only : ign.
>>> small spot, on : ign.
>>> eating and drinking, after : cham.

PICKING, lips : **Arum-t, Bry,** *cina,* hell.
>> until they bleed : **Arum-t.**

PUFFED : (See Swelling).

REDNESS : (See Discolouration).

RISUS sardonicus : **Bell,** *stram.*

RUSH of blood : (See Congestion).

SHINY : Apis, *nat-m,* plb, sanic, thuj.
>> as if oily : *nat-m,* plb, thuj.

STICK, lips : helon.

STIFFNESS, cough during : *cupr,* **Ip.**
>> jaw : caust.

SUNKEN : Berb, Chin, *lach, ph-ac, plb,* **Sec,** sil, *staph, tab,* **Verat.**

SWELLING : agar, **Apis,** *bar-c,* **Ferr, Nat-m, Op,** *sep.*
>> lips : **Apis, Arum-t, Bell, Sep.**
>>> lower : *sep.*
>>> upper : bell, calc-c, nat-m.
>> parotid gland : **Arum-t,** *bapt,* **Brom,** diph, merc-i-f, **Merc, Rhus-t, Sil.**
>>> dark red : *bapt.*
>>> hard : **Brom.**
>> sub-maxillary : **Brom.**
>>> hard : **Brom.**

TRISMUS : (See Lockjaw).

TINGLING of lips : nat-m.

TWITCHING : Agar, *mygal*.

ULCERS : nat-m, *nit-ac*.

        lips : nat-m, nit-ac.

        mouth, around : *nit-ac*.

            corners of : *nat-m,* **Nit-ac, Rhus-t.**

VEINS, distended, lips : *dig*.

WARTS : Caust, Dulc, *thuj*.

        fleshy : *dulc*.

        large : *dulc*.

        smooth : *dulc*.

        chin : *lyc,* **Thuj.**

        lips : *caust*.

WAXY (See Shiny) : **Acet-ac,** *apis, ferr,* **Med.**

WHISKERS : (See Falling).

WRINKLED : *abrot,* ant-t, bar-c, hell, op.

◻◻◻

Fever

HEAT in general : **Acon, Ant-t, Apis, Arn, Ars**, *arum-t, bapt*, **Bell**, benz-ac, **Bry, Cact**, cadm, *caps, cham*, chel, *chin, chinin-s, cina, cocc, eup-per*, **Gels**, hyos, ign, **Ip, Lyc**, meny, **Nat-m, Nux-v**, *podo, samb*, **Verat**, *verat-v*.

MORNING : **Apis**, *cham*, eup-per, *nat-m*, nux-v, sulph.

FORENOON : **Cham**, *eup-per*, **Nat-m**, sulph.

> 9 a. m. : **Cham**.

AFTERNOON : **Apis**, *ars*, **Bell**, calc, *chel*, **Gels, Ign**, *nit-ac*,**Phos, Puls**, sulph.

> 1 p. m. : *ars*.
> 2 p. m. : **Puls**.
> 3 p. m. : *bell*.
> 4 to 8 p.m. : *hell, lyc*.

EVENING : **Acon, Bell, Chin**, hep, **Lyc, Puls, Rhus-t**, *sulph*.

NIGHT : **Bapt, Bell, Bry, Cina, Merc**, *nit-ac*, **Sulph**.

MIDNIGHT : **Ars**, *rhus-t*.

> midnight and noon : *ars*, sulph.
> > before : **Bry, Calad**, *graph*.
> > after : **Ars**, *kali-c*.

ANGER, paroxysm brought on by : **Cham**, nux-v, **Staph**.

ANNUAL : lach.

AUTUMNAL : lach, **Nat-m**.

BODY, upper part : **Agar**, *arn, puls*.

BURNING heat : **Acon, Apis, Ars, Bell**, *bry*, **Gels**, *nux-v*, **Tub**.

CEREBRO-SPINAL fever : **Apis, Bell, Gels**, hell, **Nat-s**.

CHILL, with : **Acon**, *apis*, **Bell**, *eup-per*, eup-pur, **Ign**, meny, **Nit-ac, Nux-v**.

> chill predominates : meny.
> 9 a.m. one day, noon the next day : eup-per.
> 11 a.m. : cact.
> 3 p. m. : **Apis**, ign, thuj.
> 11 p. m. : cact.
> 3 a. m. : thuj.

CHILLINESS with : **Apis, Calc, Puls**.
    wants to be covered in every stage of fever : **Nux-v**.

CONTINUED fever, typhoid, typhus : ant-c, **Ars, Arum-t, Bapt, Bry**, calad, **Carb-v, Crot-h, Gels, Hyos, Lach**, *lyc, mur-ac, nit-ac, ph-ac, phos, psor, pyrog*, **Rhus-t, Stram**.
    cerebral : *apis*, arn, *bapt*, bry, **Hyos**, *lach, lyc*, nux-m, *op, ph-ac, rhus-t*, **Stram**.
    exanthemic : **Apis, Bell, Rhus-t**.
    haemorrhagic : **Cror-h**.
    stupid-form : **Bapt, Hyos, Mur-ac, Op, Ph-ac**.

COVERED, wants to be in every stage of : **Nux-v**.

DRY heat : **Acon, Ars, Bell, Bry**, *cham*, **Nux-v**, *sulph*.

EXANTHEMATIC fevers,
    measles : **Acon, Bry**, *coff, dros*, **Euphr**, *gels*, **Puls**, *rhus-t*, **Sulph**, zinc.
    scarlatina : **Am-c**, *arum-t*, **Bell**, *bry, carb-ac*, hyos, mur-ac, *sulph*.
    malignant : **Am-c**.

GASTRIC fever : **Ant-c, Ars, Bry, Ip, Puls**, *sulph*.

HAY fever : (See Nose, Coryza, Annual).

HECTIC fever : *abrot, acet-ac*, **Ars, Ars-i**, eup-per, **Iod, Lyc, Phos, Sep, Sil**, *sulph*, **Tub**.
    in children : *abrot*.

INFLAMMATORY fever : *acon*, **Bell, Bry, Merc, Rhus-t**, *sulph*.

INFLUENZA, epidemic : *eup-per, lac-c*.

INSIDIOUS fever : cocc.

INTENSE heat : **Acon, Arn, Ars, Bell**, *bry*, **Gels, Pyrog, Rhus-t**.
    of head and face, body cold : **Arn**, *op*.

INTERMITTENT, chronic, : apis, **Ars**, *carb-v* (after quinine), **Chin, Chinin-s, Eup-per**, eup-pur, lyc, **Nat-m**, petros, verat.
    congestive or pernicious : camph, *verat*.
    gastric disturbance, from : *ip*.
    irregular cases : *ip*.
    old : *nat-m*.
    quinine, abuse or suppression, from : *carb-v*, **Ip, Nat-m**.
    spoiled cases : **Nat-m, Sep**.

NERVOUS : Cocc.

PAROXYSM,

> 7 a. m. : *podo.*
> 10 or 11 a.m. : **Nat-m**.
> 11 a.m. : cact.
> 11 p.m. : cact.
> every spring : *carb-v*, **Lach**, *sulph.*
> felt 2 or 3 hours before attack : chin.
> frequent sudden attack of high fever : **Cina**.

PERSPIRATION, absent : **Ars, Bell, Bry, Gels, Nux-m**, *rhus-t*.

> heat, with : **Caps, Con, Hell, Op, Psor, Puls, Pyrog**, *rhus-t*.

PERIODICITY : Ars, Cedr, Chin, Chinin-s, Ip, Nat-m, Sep, Sil.

> return every, other day : **Chin, Ars**.
>> seven days : *chin.*
>> fourteen days : *chin.*

PERPURAL fever : arn (prevents if given just after labor), **Echi, Lach, Puls, Pyrog, Rhus-t, Sulph**.

> suppressed lochia, from : **Sulph**.

SEPTIC fever (See Zymotic, Continued, Perpural) : **Anthraci** (rapid loss of strength, sinking pulse, delerium and fainting), **Ars** (see anthraci), **Arn, Crot-h, Pyrog** (see anthraci), *rhus-t*, **Sulph**.

SHIVERING, with : **Arn**, *bell*, *chinin-s*, eup-per, **Gels**, *hep*, **Nux-v**, *podo*, **Sulph**.

> uncovering, from : **Arn**, *chinin-s*, **Nux-v**, *rhus-t*, **Tub**.

SLEEP, heat, comes on during : ant-t, **Calad, Samb**.

>> after : *samb.*

> and wakes when it stops : **Calad**.

SUDDEN : Bell, *cina*.

UNCOVERING, amel : apis, *ars*, ign.

> aversion to : ars, **Bell**, *hep*, **Nux-v, Samb**.
> chilliness from uncovering : **Nux-v, Rhus-t**.
>> in any stage of paroxysm : **Nux-v, Rhus-t, Samb**.

ZYMOTIC fevers : **Arn, Ars, Bapt**, *cadm*, **Crot-h**.

> drunkards, in : *crot-h*.

Genitalia-Male

ATROPHY : iod, staph.

        penis : arg-met, **Lyc**.

        testes : *aur*.

           sexual excess, after : **Staph**.

COITION, aversion to : **Graph**.

        painful : *arg-n*.

COLDNESS : Agn, *dios*.

        penis : **Agn**, calad, **Lyc**, *sel*.

        testes : **Agn**.

CONDYLOMATA, warts : *cinnb*, **Nit-ac**, *staph*, **Thuj**.

        bleed easily : **Nit-ac**, *thuj*.

        sensitive : *staph*.

        penis : **Cinnb**, **Nit-ac**, *staph*, **Thuj**.

           bleeding : *cinnb*, **Nit-ac**, *thuj*.

           cauliflower-like : **Nit-ac**.

           fan shaped : **Cinnb**, *thuj*.

           oozing : *thuj*.

           glans : *cinnb*, *nit-ac*, **Thuj**.

           prepuce : **Cinnb** (preferable to thuj), *nit-ac*, **Psor**, **Thuj**.

           frenum : **Cinnb**.

        scrotum : **Thuj**.

DRAWN up, glans : berb, sel.

        down, glans : canth.

ENLARGED, testes : bar-c, *iod*.

        testicle, right : canth.

ERECTION,

        child, in a : *lach*, *merc*, *tub*.

        continued : *pic-ac*.

        delayed : **Bar-c**, *sel*.

        easy, too : *cinnb*, *coff*, lac-c, **Murx**, **Plat**.

        fails, when coition attempted : **Agn**, **Arg-n**, **Calad**, **Sel**.

        incomplete : **Agn**, arg-n, *calad*, **Lyc**, *sel*.

           penis becomes relaxed : *agn*, arg-n, calad, sel.

        long-lasting : (See Continued).

painful : **Canth**, *phos*, pic-ac, sel.

slow : (See Delayed).

troublesome : **Canth, Phos, Pic-ac.**

violent : **Phos, Pic-ac**.

wanting (impotency) : **Agn**, *arg-n*, **Calad**, ign, **Lyc**, nat-m, **Sel**, *thuj*.

    caresses, even after : *calad*.

    desire, with (See Sexual Passion) : *calad, ign, sel*.

    excitement, with : *calad*, **Lyc, Sel**.

    gonorrhoea, after frequent attacks : *agn*.

        bad effects, after suppressed : *agn*, **Med, Thuj**.

    onanism, from : *lyc*.

    penis relaxed when excited : **Calad, Lyc, Sel**.

    sexual excess, from : **Lyc**, nat-m.

    sudden : *chlor*.

ERUPTIONS : *crot-t*, **Petr, Rhus-t.**

    herpetic : **Petr**.

    itching : **Petr.**

    red : *petr*.

    sensitive : *crot-t*.

    vesicles : **Crot-t**.

    extending to perineum and thigh : *petr*.

FLACIDITY : **Agn**.

    penis : **Agn**.

HAIR, falling off : **Nat-m**, *sel*.

IMPOTENCY : (See Erections, Wanting).

INDURATION, testes : aur, *bar-c*, **Con** (stony hard), *iod*, **Med, Rhod**.

    gonorrhoea, after : *med, clem*, **Rhod**.

    epididymis : **Rhod, Spong**.

INFLAMMATION : apis, **Canth**, *rhus-t*.

    erysipelatous : **Rhus-t**.

    penis : merc.

        glans : *merc*.

        prepuce : **Merc-c**.

    testes : **Arn, Clem, Con, Ham, Puls, Rhod, Rhus-t, Spong**.

    gonorrhoea suppresed, from : ant-t (before puls), **Clem, Med, Puls**, *rhod, spong*.

epididymis : **Puls, Rhod, Spong**.

spermatic veins : **Ham**.

ITCHING : crot-t, **Rhus-t**, *sep*.

scratching does not amel : sep.

MASTURBATION, disposition : **Bufo, Orig**, *ph-ac*.

MOISTURE, scrotum : **Petr, Sulph**.

ORGASM, absent during embrace : *calad*, calc, **Sel**.

ODOR, stinking : *sars*.

PAIN, penis, root : *petros*.

spermatic cord : **Ham**, *spong*.

testes : **Arg-met**.

PAIN, crushing, testes : **Arg-met**, *aur*, cham, **Rhod**.

sore, penis : *cann-s*.

testes : **Rhod, Spong**.

prepuce : merc.

squeezing, testes : **Spong**.

PERSPIRATION : *calc*, **Fl-ac**, *petr*, **Thuj**.

sweetish : *thuj*.

scrotum : *calc, petr*, **Thuj**.

sweetish smeeling : *thuj*.

PHIMOSIS : Merc.

paraphimosis : *merc*.

PRIAPISM : (See Erection, Painful).

RELAXED, scrotum : **Agn, Staph**.

penis : **Agn**, *calad*, **Lyc**, *sel*, **Staph**.

RETRACTION, prepuce : **Nat-m**.

testes : **Clem**.

SMALL penis : *calad*, **Lyc**, *sel*.

SATYRIASIS : (See Sexual Passion, Violent)

SEMEN, dribbling : *sel*.

sleep, during : *sel*.

stool at : *sel*.

SEMINAL discharge,

bloody : *canth*, led, *merc, petr*, sars.

copious : *pic-ac*.

failing during coition : *calad*.

quick, too : **Lyc**, *sel*.
with long continued thrill : sel.

SEMINAL emission (nightly) : *arg-met*, **Canth**, **Dig**, **Dios**, **Nat-m**, **Ph-ac**, *sars*.

night, every : arg-met, **Nat-p**.
several in one: **Ph-ac**.
coition, after : **Nat-m**, *ph-ac*.
erection, without : arg-met.
frequent : arg-met, **Ph-ac**.
almost every night : *arg-met*.
onanism, after : arg-m.
premature : lyc.
profuse : **Ph-ac**.
stool, during : **Sel**.
unconscious : *sel*.
wanting (absent) : calad.

SENSITIVE : *mur-ac*, *murx*.

SEXUAL passion,

diminished : **Agn**, **Bar-c**, **Graph**, *ign*.
sexual abuse, from : *graph*.
increased : **Canth**, **Con**, *ign*, **Lyc**, *nat-m*, **Ph-ac**, *tarent*.
emission, after an : nat-m, *ph-ac*.
erection, without : **Calad**, **Con**, **Graph**, ign, **Lyc**, **Sel**.
excessive : *agar*, **Phos**, **Stram**, **Zinc**.
excitement, of easy : *cinnb*, coff, lac-c, **Murx**, plat.
suppressing the, complaints from : **Camph**, **Con**.
violent : **Canth**, **Phos**, **Pic-ac**.
wanting : **Agn**, calad, *ign*, **Kali-bi**, sel.
fleshy people, in : **Kali-bi**.

SWELLING : **Arn**, *ars*, **Rhus-t**.

dropsical : *apis*.
penis, oedematous : *apis*, merc, **Rhus-t**.
prepuce : **Merc**.
scrotum : dig, **Rhus-t**.
oedematous : **Apis**, **Ars**, **Rhus-t**.
spermatic cord : **Spong**.

testes : apis, *brom*, **Clem, Puls, Rhod, Spong**.

right : apis, **Clem, Rhod**.

gonorrhoea, after : **Clem, Rhod**, *spong*.

maltreated orchitis, after : **Spong**.

rheumatism, after : clem, *rhod*.

UNDEVELOPED testes : *aur*.

ULCERS, burning : **Ars**.

deep : *merc*.

gangrenous : *merc-c*.

spreading : **Ars, Merc-c**.

Penis : lac-c, **Merc**, *merc-i-f*.

bleeding : merc.

chancres, chancroids : cor-r, *lac-c*. **Merc, Merc-c**, *merc-i-f*.

elevated margins with or inverted : *merc*.

cheesy base : merc.

deep : merc.

discharge, fetid : merc.

yellow : merc.

elevated : *merc*.

hard (Hunterian) : **Merc, Merc-c, Merc-k-i, Merc-i-f**.

lardaceous base : **Merc**.

mercurio-syphilitic : **Hep, Nit-ac**.

painful : merc.

penetrating : merc.

red : cor-r.

round : merc.

shining, glazed : **Lac-c**.

sore : *merc*.

splinters, sticking pains, as from : arg-n, hep, **Nit-ac**.

ULCERS, penis, frenum destroying : *mer*.

glans : **Merc, Merc-c, Nit-ac**.

prepuce : **Merc, Merc-c**.

WARTS : (See Condylomata).

WEAKNESS : dig, **Sep, Staph**.

coition, after : *dig*.

retarded emission, with, during an embrace : *nat-m*.

❑❑❑

Genitalia-Female

ABORTION : **Apis**, *arn*, *canth*, *caul*, *cimic,* **Con**, *helon*, kali-br, plb, **Puls**, **Sabin, Sec, Sep,** vib.

        anaemia, from : helon.

        bad effects of : *helon, sabin.*

        cough, from : kali-br, **Con.**

        month-third : cimic, *sabin, sec.*

        tendency to : **Plb**, *sabin.*

            inability of uterus to expand, from : **Plb**.

        threatened : **Puls.**

        uterine debility, from : *alet, caul.*

AILMENTS during pregnancy, parturition, lactation : *caul.*

ATONY of uterus : *caul.*

CANCER, uterus : **Con**, *crot-h*, iod, *kreos*, lach, **Phos**, **Sep**, **Sil**, thlas, ust.

        ovary, left : lach.

COITION, aversion to : *graph*, **Nat-m, Sep.**

        enjoyment absent : **Sep.**

        painful : *arg-n.*

CONDYLOMATA (See Excrescences) : *calc*, **Nat-s, Nit-ac**, *sabin, staph,* **Thuj**.

        cauliflower-like : **Nit-ac.**

CONGESTION, ovaries : *lil-t*, sulph.

        uterus : **Bell, Lach, Puls, Sep.**

CONSCIOUS of a womb : *helon*, lyss, murx.

CONSTRICTION,

        os, spasmodic during labor : **Bell, Caul, Cimic.**

        uterus : *bell*, cact, cimic.

            hour-glass : **Bell**, *sec.*

            menses, during : *bell*, **Cact**, *puls.*

        vagina : *cact*, plat.

            touch, from : **Cact.**

CRACKS, labial commissure, of : ant-c, *graph.*

DESIRE, diminished : *agn*, **Caust**, *sep*.

       increased : aster, **Canth**, *lil-t*, *murx*, *sabin*, *tarent*.

          metrorrhagia, during : ambr, *sabin*.

      violent : **Murx**, **Orig**, **Plat** (especially in virgin), *zinc*.

          embrace, desiring for an : *murx*.

          least contact of parts, from : **Murx**.

          masturbation, driving her to : **Orig**, **Zinc**.

DISPLACEMENT of uterus : **Bell**, **Calc**, *helon*, lach, **Lil-t**, nat-m, **Sep**.

DROPSY : (See Swelling).

         ovaries : **Apis**, *lil-t*.

          right : **Apis**.

DRYNESS : *nat-m*, **Sep**.

         vagina : *lyc*, **Nat-m**.

          coition preventing : *lyc*, lyss, **Nat-m**.

ENLARGED, ovaries : **Apis**, **Con**, *iod*, lil-t.

         uterus : **Con**, *iod*, **Sep**.

EXCORIATION, *vulva* : *am-c*.

         leucorrhoea, from : am-c.

FEELS, lack of room for foetus, in uterus : plb.

FLATUS from vagina : **Brom**, *lac-c*, **Lyc**, *nux-m*, *sang*.

FOREIGN body in uterus : *canth*, sabin.

HAIR falling out : **Nat-m**, *sel*.

HAEMORRHAGE : (See Metrorrhagia).

HEAT flushes : sep.

         ascends from pelvic organs : sep.

HEAVINESS, in pelvis : helon, nat-c.

         motion, amel : nat-c.

         sitting agg : nat-c.

         ovaries : helon, lappa.

         uterus : **Chin**, **Sep**.

INDURATION,

         injuries, from : *con*.

         ovaries : **Con**, *iod*, lach, **Sabin**.

          right : *podo*.

abortion or labor after : *sabin*.
uterus : **Aur, Con,** *iod*, **Sabin**.
abortion or labor, after : *sabin*.

INFLAMMATION : *apis, bell*, **Merc**, med, **Rhus-t**.
ovaries : **Acon, Apis, Bell,** *lil-t*, **Lyc,** *med*, **Merc, Podo**.
right : *apis*, **Lyc, Podo**.
left : *lach, thuj*.
suppressed gonorrhoea, after : **Med**.
fallopian tubes : *med*.
uterus : **Bell, Sabin, Ter**.

INTOLERANCE of least contact or pressure : **Lach**.

IRRITATION : *apis, canth*.
uterus : lil-t.
ovaries : *apis*.

ITCHING : **Calad,** coll, *crot-t*, hydr, **Kreos,** *med*, **Merc, Plat, Rhus-t, Sep, Tarent**.
leucorrhoea, from : hydr, **Kreos**, merc.
pregnancy, during : calad, *coll*.
scratching does not amel : sep.
sensitive : crot-t.
voluptuous : *calad, kreos*.
vagina : **Calad, Kreos,** *med*.
pregnancy, during : *calad*.
thinking agg : *med*.
voluptuous : *calad*, **Kreos**.
vulva : **Calad,** coll, *merc*, plat, **Tarent**.
leucorrhoea, from : *merc*.
pregnancy, during : coll.
urine, from contact of, which must be washed off : *merc, sulph*.

LABOR, shortened when given during last months of pregnancy : cimic, **Caul,** cimic, puls.

LEUCORRHOEA : *aesc*, agn, **Alum,** ambr, *am-c, am-m, borx, bov,* **Calc, Carb-an, Carb-ac,** caul, **Con, Graph,** *hydr*, **Iod, Kreos,** *mag-m*, **Merc,** murx, *psor*, **Puls,** sang, sec, **Sep, Stann, Sulph,** syph.
day and night : **Graph**.
daytime only : *alum*.

night : ambr, *caust*, **Merc**, **Nit-ac**.

acrid, excoriating : aesc, **Alum**, *am-c*, carb-ac, caul, con,
    Graph, *iod*, **Kreos**, **Merc**, *sulph*.

    corrodes the linen : *iod*.

albuminous : **Borx**.

atony, from, in children : *calc*, mill.

black : croc, pyrog.

bland : *alum*, *caul*, **Puls**.

bloody : **Cocc**, con, thlas.

bluish-white : *ambr*.

    especially at night or only at night : ambr, **Caust**, **Merc**,
      Nit-ac.

brown : *am-m*, **Nit-ac**, *sec*.

burning : alum, *am-c*, **Borx**, **Calc**, **Calc-s**, *fl-ac*, merc.

carrion-like : (See Putrid).

children, in : **Calc**, kreos, merc, mill, **Sep**.

cold bathing, amel : *alum*.

copious : **Alum**, *am-c*, *borx*, *carb-ac*, *con*, iod, **Syph**.

    menses, during : iod.

    running down to heels : **Alum**, *syph*.

dark : aesc, thlas.

excoriating, corrosive : (See Acrid).

exercising, while : mag-m.

exhausting : caul.

girls, little : **Calc**, caul, **Sep**.

gonorrhoeal : *am-m*, cann-s.

greenish : *carb-ac*, **Carb-v**, **Merc**, **Nit-ac**, *sec*.

gushing : **Graph**.

intermittent : *con*.

lumpy : psor.

meat-washing, like : cocc.

menses, before : **Graph**, **Sep**, thlas.

      during : iod.

      after : *borx*, **Bov**, **Calc-p**, *eon*, graph, kreos, thlas.

        ten days after : *borx*, **Bov**, *con*.

        two weeks after : bar-c, *borx*, con, mag-m.

two weeks between : **Borx**, *bov*, con.

instead of : *cocc, nux-m*.

mental depression, agg : murx.

metrorrhagia, followed by : mag-m.

milky : *con*.

offensive : anthraci, **Carb-ac**, *kreos*, **Psor**, *pyrog*, *sec*, thlas.

decomposed foetus, from : *pyrog*.

fish brine : *sanic*.

LEUCORRHOEA, offensive, green corn-like : *kreos*.

putrid : **Psor**.

pregnancy, during : *cocc*.

painless : am-m.

stringy, tenacious : *bov*, **Hydr**, **Kali-bi**. ropy hanging from os in long string : **Hydr**, **Kali-bi**.

sensation as if warm water flowing down : borx.

serum, like : cocc.

sitting, agg : cycl.

slimy : am-m.

starch, boiled-like : **Borx**.

stiffens linen stiff like strach : *kreos*.

stool, after : mag-m.

thick : *ambr*, **Hydr**, *puls*.

thin, watery : am-c, con.

transparent : agn.

but stains linen yellow : agn.

urination, after every : *am-m*.

walking, amel : cycl.

watery : am-c.

white : *am-m*.

of egg like : am-m.

stains linen yellow : chel.

yellow : **Calc**, **Hydr**, **Kreos**, **Kali-s**, *puls*.

stains linen yellow : agn, **Kreos**.

green : *kali-s*, nat-s, **Puls**.

LOCHIA, acrid : **Kreos**, *pyrog*.

brown : *kreos*, pyrog.

dark : **Kreos**.

intermittent : *con*, *kreos*, rhus-t, *sulph*.

lumpy : **Kreos**.

offensive : **Kreos**, nit-ac, *pyrog*.

oozing for days from relaxed vessels : caul, **Sep**.

protracted : caul.

returning : con, *kreos*, sulph.

suppressed : **Pyrog**.

thin : *pyrog*.

MASTURBATION disposition : *calad*, **Orig**, zinc.

MENOPAUSE : aml-ns, *calc-ar*, *chin*, *crot-h*, kreos, **Lach**, **Mang**, *murx*, sang, **Sep**, **Sulph**.

MENOPAUSE, after lach and sulphur fail to relieve : sang.

MENSES, daytime only : cact, *caust*, lil-t, **Puls**.

     but ceases while lying : cact, caust, lil-t.

morning : carb-an.

night, ceases during : (See Daytime).

    only : **Bov**, cycl, **Mag-c**.

    more at : *am-m*, *bov*, **Mag-c**.

    on lying down : kreos.

     sleep, only during : mag-c.

absent, amenorrhoea : *acon*, *apoc*, *calc*, *cycl*, euphr, **Ferr**, lil-t, *phos*, **Puls**, **Sep**.

    in dropsical young girls : apoc.

    in plithoric young girls : **Acon**.

    fright, after : **Acon**.

acrid, excoriating : *am-c*, mag-c, *sulph*.

amel of all complaints during : *lach*, *zinc*.

appear as if it would : lil-t.

black : *croc*. **Cycl**, *ferr*, *mag-m*, **Puls**, ust.

bright-red : **Bell**, **Ip**, *lac-c*, lil-t, **Mill**, **Phos**, **Sabin**, tril-p.

    mingled with dark clots : **Bell**.

carrion-like : (See Offensive).

changeable in appearance : **Puls**.

clotted : bov, *croc*, **Cycl**, *ferr*, helon, mag-m, *med*, **Murx**, **Plat**, **Puls**, *ust*.

    dark : bov, *cycl*, *ferr*, *plat*, *puls*.

continuous up to next period : *sec*.

copious : *am-c*, **Calc**, **Calc-p**, **Chin**, *cimic*, **Cycl**, **Ferr**, *ham*, **Helon**, *kreos*, lac-c, *med*, **Mill**, **Murx**, **Nux-v**, **Plat**, *puls*, **Sabin**, **Sec**, *sep*, *stann*, *sulph*, thlas, tril-p, *tub*.

   night : *am-c*, *zinc*.

   alternate period more profuse : thlas.

   atony, from : *helon*.

   excitement, after : **Calc**, *sulph*, *tub*.

   exertion agg : **Calc**, **Calc-p**, tril-p.

   exhausting or faintness, with : *alum*, **Carb-an**, cocc.

   injury, after, : **Arn**, *ham*.

   menopause, during : *sabin*.

   miscarriage, after last : *sulph*.

   motion, from : *sabin*, tril-p.

      only during : lil-t.

   riding too long : tril-p.

   sitting, agg : am-c, zinc.

   walking, agg : *lil-t*.

   women who aborted previously : sabin.

dark : *bov*, **Croc**, *cycl*, *ferr*, **Ham**, helon, lil-t, *mag-c*, mag-p, *med*, **Puls**, **Sec**.

delayed : alum, cimic, con, **Graph**, lac-d.

   in girls, first menses : *ferr*, graph, **Puls**.

early, too : (See Frequent).

exhausting : *alum*, cocc, *ferr*.

fluid blood containing clots : **Bell**, *ferr*, **Sabin**, **Sec**.

flow agg : *cimic*, puls, **Thuj**.

   camel : cycl.

frequent, too early, too soon, : *am-c*, borx, **Bov**, **Calc**, *caust*, cycl, **Ferr**, *helon*, kreos, **Lac-c**, lil-t, mag-p, mill, murx, **Nux-v**, **Plat**, puls, **Sabin**, *sep*, *stann*, *sulph*, thlas, **Tril-p**, *tub*.

   every few days : bov.

   every two weeks : borx, bov, **Calc**, **Nux-v**, **Tril-p**.

gushing : **Ip**, lac-c.

intermittent : *cycl*, *ferr*, **Kreos** (at time almost ceases and then commences again), *lil-t*, *nux-v*, **Puls**, *sulph*.

   intermits two or three days and then returns : *ferr*.

irregular : *cimic*, cocc, cycl, ferr, graph, lil-t, *murx*, *nux-v*, puls, **Sec**, *sep*.

lactation, during : *calc-p*, *sil*.

  nursing the child, while : sil.

late : **Con**, cycl, euphr, *ferr*, **Graph**, **Puls**, **Sep**.

long lasting : (See Protracted).

lying down, flow, on : **Kreos**, *mag-c*.

  ceases while : bov, *cact*, *caust*, **Lil-t**.

membranous : **Borx**, *cycl*, **Lac-c**, puls.

  flow amel : cycl.

    agg : **Cimic**, **Puls**, **Thuj**.

mental excitement, agg : **Calc**, **Sulph**, tub.

mental symptoms agg, during : **Cimic**.

moving about : (See Walking).

new moon : rhus-t.

offensive : **Bell**, **Bry**, **Carb-v**, *croc*, helon, *lil-t*, *plat*, *psor*.

painful, dysmenorrhoea : bov, brom, *cham*, Cimic, cocc, coll, *croc*, *cycl*, euphr, ferr, *graph*, *lach*, *lac-c*, kreos, *lil-t*, mag-c, *med*, *plat*, *puls*, *sabin*, *sep*, thlas, *tub*, *verat*, *vib*.

  anger, following : **Cham**.

  cold drink amel : **Kreos**.

  congestion, from : coll.

  flow amel : **Lach**, mag-p, **Zinc**.

    agg : *cimic*, **Thuj**.

  feet wet, from getting : **Puls**, *rhus-t*.

  neuralgic : *cham*, caul, **Cimic**, **Mag-p**, *vib*.

  membranous : *brom*, *lac-c*.

  rheumatic : **Cimic**.

paroxysmal flow : *sabin*.

passive : helon.

pale : alum, **Ferr**, **Graph**, *puls*.

pitch-like : *mag-c*.

pregnancy, during : *nux-m*.

profuse : (See Copious).

protracted : **Calc**, cycl, **Ferr**, *kreos*, **Mill**, *murx*, **Nux-v**, **Plat**, **Puls**, **Sabin**, *sulph*, thlas (8, 10 even fifteen days), tril-p, *tub*.

  lasting a week or longer : **Calc**, **Calc-p**, **Tril-p**.

return after having ceased, the period : **Ambr**, *calc*.

accident, from (long walk, hard stool) : **Ambr**.

excitement, from : *calc*.

rheumatic : **Cimic**.

scanty : alum, *bar-c*, calc, *caust*, **cimic, Con, Cimic, Cycl**, euphr,
ferr, **Graph, Lach**, *lil-t*, **Puls, Sep**.

short duration : *con*, euphr, **Lach**.

only one day : bar-c, euphr.

only one hour : **Euphr**.

sitting, cease, while : *kreos*.

increased, while : cycl.

MENSES, slimy : puls.

stopped by taking cold : *con, dulc*.

by putting hands in cold water : *con, lac-d*.

stringy : *croc, lac-c*, mag-p, ust.

suppressed : ant-c, *bry, calc, cimic*, coloc, **Con, Cycl**, *ferr*, lac-
d, lil-t, mill, **Puls**, *stram*.

anger, from : *coloc*, cham, **Staph**.

bad effect of : *con*.

bathing, from : ant-c.

chagrin, from : **Coloc**.

colic pain, from : coloc.

cold, from : *cimic, con, dulc*.

by putting hands in cold water : *con, lac-d*.

drinking a glass of milk will suppress up to next period :
lac-d.

emotion, from : *cimic*.

fever, by : cimic.

girls, in young : podo, **Puls, Tub**.

plethoric women, in : *acon*.

water, working in : **Calc**.

wet, from becoming : *calc, dulc, rhus-t, sanic*.

putting hands in cold water : con, lac-d.

getting feet wet : **Puls, Rhus-t**.

tardy in starting : thlas, tub.

first day merely a show, second day colic, vomiting and
haemorrhage with large clots : thlas.

tenacious : **Croc**, lac-c.

thick : *lil-t*, **Puls**.

thin : **Ferr, Puls**.

vicarious : **Bry**, *crot-h*, *dig*, *ham*, **Phos**.

walking, only while : **Lit-t** (flow stops, while ceases to walk).

      cease while : am-m, kreos, mag-c.

      less while : cycl.

watery : **Ferr**.

wash off, difficult to : *mag-c*, *med*.

METRORRHAGIA : *acet-ac*, *apoc*, *arg-n*, *bov*, *canth*, **Chin**, **Croc**, **Crot-h**, *erig*, **Ferr**, **Ham**, **Ip**, mag-m, *med*, **Mill**, **Nit-ac**, **Phos**, **Plat**, **Puls**, **Sabin**, *sil*, thlas, **Tril-p**, ust.

    night : *bov*, *mag-m*.

    abortion, after : caul, **Lach**, mill, nit-ac, *sec*, thlas.

    active : *acon*, **Bell**, **Croc**, *ham*, **Ip**, **Sabin**, **Sec**, **Tril-p**, *ust*.

    between menstrual periods : *ambr*, *bov*, borx, **Sabin**.

    black : *anthr*, *croc*, **Crot-h**, *elaps*, nit-ac, **Plat**.

    bright : *nit-ac*, **Sabin**.

      clots with : **Sabin**.

    cancer, in : **Phos**.

    chlorosis, in : thlas.

    climacteric period : arg-met, arg-n, **Lach**, *med*, thlas, *Tril-p*.

    coagulated : *apoc*, *croc*, elaps, med, *plat*, Tril-p, thlas, ust.

    coition, after : **Arg-n**, **Nit-ac**.

    continuous : apoc, *sec*.

      for weeks : med.

    dark blood : *croc*, *crot-h*, med, sabin, Tril-p, thlas, ust.

      clots, mixed with : **Bell**, cham, *croc*, *crot-h*, *plat*, sabin.

    exertion, after : **Erig**, mill, *nit-ac*, *Tril-p*.

    faintness, with : **Tril-p**.

    flooding : (See Gushing).

    fluid : apoc, crot-h, plat.

    grumous : (See Clots, Dark).

    gushing : med, **Phos**, **Tril-p**.

      and then ceasing for a time : **Phos**.

    hard stool, from passing : **Ambr**.

    injuries : *arn*, ham.

    jolting, from, while riding over rough roads : *ham*.

    labor, during and after : caul (after hasty labor), **Erig**, **Ham**, **Ip**, mill, *nit-ac*, **Sabin**, thlas, Tril-p.

malignant disease of uterus in : med, *lap-a* (fibroids).

miscarriage, after : (See Abortion, Labor After).

motion agg : med, **Sabin**, **Sec**, Tril-p.

nursing the child when : *sil*.

offensive : crot-h, med.

oozing : anthraci, *crot-h*.

pale : sabin.

paroxysmal : apoc, sabin.

passive : caul, carb-v, **Erig**, *ham*, *sec*, thlas, **Ust**.

post-partum, prevents : **Arn**, (if given just after labor), mill.

profuse : **Bell**, calc, erig, iod, **Ip**, mill, med, nit-ac, **Phos**.

prolonged : *crot-h*.

rough riding, from : ham.

sterility, in : arg-n.

stool, during every : **Ambr**, lyc.

tarry : anthraci, crot-h, *plat*.

thick : anthraci, crot-h, plat.

tonicity, want of, for : caul.

traumatic : **Arn**, *ham*.

uterus, from displaced : Tril-p.

uterus, loss of tone of : sabin.

walk, from long : **Ambr**.

walking amel : *sabin*.

young widows : *arg-n*.

MISCARRIAGE : (See Abortion).

MOISTURE : petr.

MOLES : *canth*, sabin.

MOVEMENTS, sensation as if : (See Sensation).

MOVEMENTS like a foetus : (See Abdomen, Movements).

MUCUS discharge from vagina after embrace causing sterility : nat-c.

NUMBNESS : *plat*.

ovaries, right : *podo*.

NYMPHOMANIA : (See Mind).

ONANISM, pruritus vagina, from : *calad*, orig, zinc.

PAIN, ovaries : *arg-met*, **Bell**, **Coloc**, lil-t, **Lach**, **Lyc**.

right : **Bell**, lil-t, **Lyc**, *pall*, **Podo**.

        to left : **Lyc**.

        to thigh of right side : lil-t, *podo*.

     left : **Arg-met, Lach,** *lil-t*.

        to right : **Lach**.

PAIN, ovaries alternating sides : **Lac-c**.

        labor, after : **Lach**.

        menses, before : **Lach**.

        during : **Lach**, lil-t.

        extending downwards and forwards : arg-met.

    uterus ; **Bell**, *caul*, (needle like pricking pain in cervix), **Lach**, *lil-t,*
        plat.

        flow of blood, amel : **Lach**.

        jar, agg : **Bell**.

        menses, before : **Calc, Calc-p, Caul, Kali-c**, *lach*, **Sep**.

           at beginning : *calc, calc-p, kali-c, lach*.

           during : **Bell, Cact, Calc**, *calc-p*, castm, *kreos*, **kali-c**.
              lac-c, lil-t, **Nux-v, Puls**.

              amel : *lach, zinc*.

        motion, agg : **Bell, Bry, Cocc**.

        paroxysmal : **Bell, Cham, Plat, Puls, Sabin**.

        periodically, same time each day : cact.

        pressure, amel : *coloc, mag-p*.

        suddenly comes and goes : **Bell**.

        extending to back : *bell, gels*.

           back to groin : **Sabin**.

           back, from, go around and end with cramps in uterus :
              Vib.

           diagonally upwards : *murx*.

           downwards : *apis, graph, kreos*.

           down the thigh : apis, bufo, cact, *calc, kali-c*, kreos, *lac-c*.

           moves side to side : *cimic*.

           umbilicus, to : sep.

           upwards : **Lach**, *murx*.

    vagina, coition, during : **Arg-n, Nat-m, Sep**.

PAIN, after-pain : caul (after exhausing labor), cham, *cimic*, **Cupr, Sabin, Sec**.

        long-lasting : **Sec**.

        painful, to : cham, **Sec**.

spasmodic, across abdomen : caul.
extend into groin : caul.
 in the shin : carb-v, cocc.
groin, felt in : cimic.
bearing down, ovaries : *lil-t*.
 standing, while : **Lil-t**.
 walking, while : *lil-t*.

PAIN, bearing down, uterus and region of (See Labor-like Pains, also Pains in Abdomen) : **Agar**, **Bell**, bov, **Lil-t**, *lac-c*, **Murx**, *nat-c*, **Nat-m**, **Plat**, sanic, **Sec**, **Sep**.
 morning : **Nat-m**, **Sep**.
 come out as if every thing would : agar, **Bell**, **Kreos**, **Lil-t**, *murx*, *nat-c*, *nat-m*, sanic, **Sep**.
 crossing limbs, amel : **Lil-t**, murx, **Sep**.
 jar agg : sanic.
 lying, amel : sanic.
 menses, during : **Lil-t**, *sec*, **Sep**.
 mis-step, agg : sanic.
 pressing on vulva, amel : **Lil-t**. **Murx**, sanic, **Sep**.
 prolonged : **Sec**.
 rest, amel : sanic.
 sit down must to prevent prolapse : **Lil-t**, **Murx**, *nat-m*, **Sep**.
 standing, agg : **Sep**.
 urging to urinite, on : **Sep**.
 walking, agg : sanic, **Sep**.
 extending from back to abdomen : *sep*.
burning : kreos, thuj.
 ovaries : thuj.
  left : thuj.
  lying, amel, : croc, ust.
  menses, agg during : thuj.
  riding, while : thuj.
  sitting, amel : **Croc**, ust.
  walking, while : thuj.
 vagina : **Berb**, lyc.
  coition, during : *lyc*, *lyss*.
   after : *lyc*, *lyss*.

cramping, uterus : **Caul**, *coloc*, **Cham**, caust, *mag-m*, *mag-p*, *plat*, thlas.

> examination of parts, from : *plat*.
> leucorrhoea, followed by : *mag-m*.
> ovaries : *coloc*.

cutting, menses during : mag-c.

darting : (See Stitching).

labor-like : *act*, **Bell**, caul, **Cham**, *cimic,* **Kali-c**, mag-c, med, *sabin*, **Sec**, **Sep**.

> menses, before : mag-c.
> > during : med, *sec*.
> press feet against support, must : med.

labor pains : caul, cimic.

> ceasing : **Puls**, **Sec**.
> distressing : **Cham**, cimic, **Sep**.
> excessive : cham, cimic, **Sep**.
> fainting, causing : *cimic*, **Nux-v**, *puls*, *sec*.
> false : **Caul,** *cimic*.
> groin, felt in : cimic.
> ineffectual : **Kali-c**, **Puls**, sec.
> irregular : *caul*, **Puls**, sec.
> insufficient : **Kali-c**, *nux-v*,
> noise agg : cimic.
> prolonged : **Sec**.
> short : *caul*.
> spasmodic : **Caul**, **Cham**, *cimic*, *nux-v*, **Puls**.
> tearing down the legs : **Cham**.
> tormenting : *caul*, nux-v.
> useless in beginning of labor : caul, cimic.
> weak : caul (no progress), **Puls**, **Sec**.
> extending upwards : **Cham**.
> extending to rectum : **Nux-v**.
> back, begins in, and pass down innerside of thigh : cham.

lancinating, uterus : sep.

> extending upwards : sep.

lightening, ovaries : mag-p.

        right side : mag-p.

        bending double, amel : *mag-p.*

        heat amel : *mag-p.*

        uterus : mag-p.

pressing, uterus (See Bearing-down) : **Bell**, *sec*, *sep.*

        come out as if everything would : **Sep.**

        crossing limbs, amel : **Sep.**

        sit close, must, to prevent : **Sep.**

rawness : *merc.*

        leucorrhoea, from : *merc.*

shooting : (See Stitching).

sore, tenderness : arn, *caust*, helon, **Kreos**, **Plat**, **Staph**, *thuj.*

        labial commissures, of : ant-c.

        ovaries : helon.

        uterus : arg-n, **Arn**, caust, *conv*, *helon*, lappa, lach, lyss,

            Murx, nux-m, sanic.

           labor, after : **Arn**.

           splinter sensation when walking or riding : *arg-n.*

           wearing pessaries, from : nux-m.

           region of : conv.

        vagina : caust, **Kreos**, **Lyss**, *plat*, thuj.

           coition, during : *arg-n*, **Lyss**, **Plat**, *thuj.*

              preventing : coff, *plat*, *thuj.*

splinter, as if, uterus : **Arg-n**.

        riding, when : arg-n.

        walking, when : arg-n.

stinging : **Apis**, con, staph.

        ovaries : **Apis** (especially right).

stitching, ovaries : mag-p.

        right side : *mag-p*, *podo.*

        bending double, amel : *mag-p.*

        heat, amel : *mag-p.*

        uterus : *caul*, mag-p.

        side to side : **Cimic**.

        cervix : caul.

        vagina : *sep.*

        extending upwards : *sep.*

PERSPIRATION : *petr, thuj.*

PHYSOMETRA : (See Flatus).

PLACENTA, retained : **Canth,** *sabin.*

        atony of uterus, from : *sabin.*

POLYPUS, uterus : **Bell, Calc, Calc-p, Phos,** *sang,* **Teucr, Thuj.**

        vagina : **Calc,** teucr.

PROLAPSUS, uterus : *aesc,* agar, aloe, **Arg-met, Aur,** *helon, kali-bi,*
    lach, **Lit-t,** *lyss* (of years standing), *podo,* **Sep,** *stann.*

                atony, from : *helon, lit-t.*

                climacteric-post : agar.

                confinement, after : *podo.*

                constipation, from : *podo.*

                crossing legs, amel : lit-t, murx, **Sep.**

                hot weather, in : *kali-bi.*

                hypertrophy, from : *aur, con.*

                lifting, from : **Calc,** podo.

                menses, during : **Puls, Sep.**

                        after : agar.

                reaching up, from : *aur.*

                stool, during : **Podo,** *stann.*

                straining, from : *aur, podo,* **Rhus-t.**

                vagina : **Sep.**

PRURITUS vulva : (See Itching).

PUERPERAL complications : **Arn** (prevents if given just after labor).

REDNESS : *bell, sep, sulph.*

RELAXATION OF sphincter vaginae : *agn,* staph.

RIGIDITY of os during labor : **Caul,** cimic, **Gels.**

SENSITIVE : Bell, lach, *mur-ac, murx,* **Plat, Staph.**

           vagina : **Lyss, Plat,** *thuj.*

           coitus, to : **Plat,** *thuj.*

           vulva, touch of napkin, to : **Plat, Staph.**

           coitus, to : **Plat.**

SEXUAL passion : (See Desire).

SPASM in uterus : (See Pain, Cramping).

STERILITY : Aur, Borx, *caul,* **Nat-c, Sep.**

        leucorrhoea, from : *caul.*

        mucus discharge, from, during embrace : **Nat-c.**

SUBINVOLUTION : Cimic, *helon, lit-t,* **podo, Puls, Sep, Sulph.**

SWOLLEN : *apis.*

           ovaries : *apis.*

             right : *apis.*

TUMORS, ovaries : **Apis, Lach, Lyc.**

             right : **Lyc,** *podo.*

             left : **Lach.**

             cysts : *apis,* lach, *med.*

             uterus, fibroids : **Calc,** *lap-a, med.*

TWITCHING : plat.

VAGINISMUS : Cact, mag-p, plat.

ULCERATION of os : *sep.*

❑❑❑

Generalities

DAYTIME : *med*, nat-m, **Sulph**.

MORNING : *aloe*, **Bry**, **Calc**, **Cham**, **Chel**, chin, coc-c, *eup-per*, *hep*, **Kali-bi**, *kali-c*, **Kali-n**, **Lach**, **Nat-m**, **Nit-ac**, **Nux-v**, **Podo**, **Puls**, **Spig**, **Sulph**, *thuj*, *tub*.

    waking on : **Lach**, **Nux-v**.

    3 a.m. : *thuj*.

    4 a.m. : **Nux-v**.

    7 a.m. : *eup-per*.

    9 a.m. : *cham*.

    10 a.m. : **Nat-m**.

    11 a.m. : **Sulph**.

    sunset, to : *med*.

FORENOON : ars, **Nat-m**, **Sep**, **Sulph**, **Sul-ac**.

MOON : **Arg-met**, ars, sulph.

    eating, after, amel : **Chel**.

AFTERNOON : *apis*, *ars*, **Bell**, *bry*, *canth*, *chel*, **Lyc**, **Puls**, **Rhus-t**, **Sep**, *sulph*, **Thuj**, **Zinc**.

    1 p.m. : *ars*.

    3 p.m. : *apis*, ars, **Bell**, *thuj*.

    4 p.m. : *coloc*, **Lyc**.

    4 p.m. to 8 p.m. : *hell*, **Lyc**.

    4 to 9 p.m. : *coloc*, *mag-p*.

EVENING : *acon*, *all-c*, **Am-c**, **Ant-c**, **Ant-t**, **Bell**, **Bry**, **Calc**, **Carb-v**, **Caust**, **Cham**, coloc, **Cycl**, **Euphr**, **Hell**, **Hyos**, kali-s, **Lach**, **Lyc**, **Mag-c**, **Merc**, **Mez**, **Nit-ac**, *nux-v*, **Ph-ac**, **Phos**, **Puls**, *rhus-t*, **Sep**, **Sulph**, **Sul-ac**.

    amel : **Aur**, *med*, nux-v (while at rest), *sep*.

    twilight agg : **Puls**.

    9 p.m. : **Bry**.

    sunset till sunrise : *aur*, *colch*, *syph*.

NIGHT : **Acon**, **Ars**, *caust*, **Cham**, **Coff**, **Con**, *cupr*, **Ferr**, **Graph**, **Hep**, **Hyos**, *kali-br*, **Lach**, **Merc**, mez, **Nit-ac**, **Plb** (pain in limbs), *phyt*, *pic-ac*, **Rhus-t**, **Sulph**, *syph*, *thuj*.

midnight : **Ars**.

before : **Ars, Cham, Coff, Phos, Puls,** *rhus-t*.

after : **Ars, Dros,** nit-ac, **Podo, Rhus-t,** *Spong*.

uncovering, from : bell.

NIGHT, 12 to 2 a. m. : **Ars**.

3 a. m. : **Kali-c,** *thuj*,

ABSCESS : Anthraci, Hep, Lach, Merc, *sec*, **Sil, Tarent**.

boils all over : pic-ac, *sec*.

exertion, after physical : carb-ac.

slow to suppurate : *merc*.

vaccination, after : **Sil**.

bones : **Fl-ac, Hep, Merc, Sil**.

periosteum : *sil*.

glands : bar-c, **Hep, Merc, Sil**.

suppuration profuse : **Hep, Merc, Sil**.

ABSORPTION, power of, inflammatory process : **Bry, Kali-m, Sulph**.

ABUSE of argentum nitricum : **Nat-m**.

ACTIVITY, over activity of body : **Coff**.

AIR, open, aversion to : *bell*, **Calc,** *caps,* carb-an, **Cham,** *cycl, hep,* **Nat-c,** sel, **Sil, Sulph**.

cold open air goes right through her : **Calc**.

open, desire for : *aml-ns, arg-n, bry,* carb-an, **Carb-v, Kali-i,** *lach,* med, **Puls,** *sanic, sec,* **Sulph,** *tab, tub*.

child kicks off clothing even in coldest winter : acon, hep, sanic, **Sulph**.

fanned wants to be : **Carb-v** (quickly), *med* (slowly).

wants doors and windows open : *aml-ns, arg-n, lach,* **Sulph,** *tub*.

(when in a room), which inspires, benefits strengthens : **Calc,** *puls,* **Sulph**.

open, draft, agg : **Bell,** bry, **Calc,** *caust,* **Cham,** *chin, graph, hep,* mag-p, **Nux-v, Rhus-t,** *rumx,* **Sel, Sil**.

open, agg : *bell, bry, calc, caps, caust, cham, cycl,* euphr, **Hep** (imagines he can feel the air if a door in the next room is opened), *kali-bi,* **Kali-c,** *kreos, phos, rhus-t,* **Rumx, Sil**.

amel : acon, *all-c*, *aml-ns*, *ant-c*, *apis*, **Arg-n**, **Ars**, *bry*, **Iod**, **Kali-i**, *kali-s*, lyc, *lach*, **Mag-c**, **Mag-m**, *nat-m*, **Nat-s**, **Puls**, **Sabin**, *sanic*, *sec*, *sulph*, *tab*, tarent.

AIR, seashore : nat-s, *mag-m*, nat-m.

amel : med.

ALCOHOLIC stimulants : *agar*, alum, arn, **Ars**, **Asar**, **Bar-c**, *calc-ar*, *carb-v*, *coca*, cocc, colch, *con*, *crot-h*, *eup-per*, *hydr*, kali-bi, **Lach**, *led*, lob, *lyc*, mez, **Nux-v**, **Op**, **Ran-b**, **Sel**, **Sulph**, **Sul-ac**, verat, zinc.

hereditory tendency to alcoholism : **Asar**, psor, *sulph*, **Sul-ac**, *syph*, tub.

relapsing, continually : *psor*, *sulph*, tub.

stoppage, after : *calc-ar*.

brandy : ign, **Nux-v**, **Op**, **Sulph**, **Sul-ac**.

ANAEMIA : *acet-ac*, alum, **Calc-p**, **Chin**, *crot-h*, *cycl*, **Ferr**, ferr-p, *helon*, **Kali-c**, **Kali-p**, *nat-c*, **Nat-m**, *ph-ac*, **Phos**, *pic-ac*, **Plb**, psor, **Puls**, spig.

acute disease, after : carb-v.

haemorrhage, after : **Chin**, **Ferr**, helon.

pernicious : **Kali-p**, *pic-ac*.

ANALGESIA : bell, **Cocc**, **Op**, **Stram**.

ANIMAL matter, bad effects (See Wounds) by ingestion, inoculation, olfaction : **Ars**.

ANNUAL complaints : *ars*, **Carb-v**, **Lach**, **Sulph**, **Thuj**.

ANXIETY, general physical : **Arg-n**, **Ars**, **Camph**, **Cham**, *coff*, *lyc*, **Phos**, **Puls**, *sep*, **Sulph**.

APOPLEXY : **Acon**, *arn*, aster, bar-c, cact, *crot-h*, **Lach**, verat-v

congestive : verat-v.

controls haemorrhage in acute attacks and aids absorption : **Arn**.

drunkards, in : crot-h.

tendency, in old people : **Bar-c**.

ARSENIC poisoning : *merc*.

ASCENDING, agg : **Ars**, **Calc**, **Coca**.

high, agg (high places) : *coca*.

ASSIMILATION, imperfect : **Calc**, **Sil**.

ATTITUDE in bed, assumes strange : *plb*.

ATROPHY of, glands : *aur*, **Con**, **Iod**.

    muscles : *plb*.

      sclerosis of spine, from : **Plb**.

AUTUMN agg : calc-p, colch, ip, merc.

BALL, internally : **Ign**, **Sep**.

    lactation, during : *sep*.

    menses, durign : **Sep**.

    pregnancy, during : **Sep**.

BAND sensation of : (See Constriction or Seperate section Sensation).

BATHING, dread of : **Am-c**, **Ant-c**, **Psor**, **Rhus-t**, **Sulph**.

    agg : **Am-c**, **Ant-c**, *bar-c*, **Calc**, *caust*, **Rhus-t**, **Sulph**.

    amel : **Asar**, **Led**, **Puls**.

    cold, agg : **Ant-c**, cycl, *kreos*, **Mag-p**, mez, nux-m, **Rhus-t**.

     amel : apis, *arg-n*, *calc-s*, *fl-ac*, *nat-m*.

    face, amel : *asar*.

    sea, agg : *ars*, *rhus-t*.

    summer, too much, in, agg : **Rhus-t**.

BLOOD : (See Haemorrhage).

BLOOD vessels : aml-ns (rapidly dilates but later weakness and retards pulse).

BLACKNESS of external parts : agar, *anthraci*, arn, **Ars**, *carb-v*, *crot-h*, **Cupr**, *lach*, **Op**, **Sec**, **Verat**.

BLOOD poisoning : **Crot-h**, **Pyrog**.

BRUISE : (See Injuries).

BURNS : carb-ac (tends to ulceration and ichorous discharge), **Canth**, *caust*.

    never well since that burn : *caust*.

CAGED in wires, twisted tighter and tighter : **Cact**.

CALLOUS, promotes : **Calc-p**, *symph*.

CANCEROUS affections : *apis*, *aster*, **Brom**, **Carb-an**, **Con**, *hydr*, med.

    glands : **Carb-an**, **Con**.

    scirrhus : apis, **Carb-an**, **Con**, *hydr*, *med*.

CARIES of, bone : **Asaf**, *aur*, **Fl-ac**, *mez*, *ph-ac*, **Ther**.

    long bones : *calc-hp*, **Fl-ac**, *mez*.

    periosteum : **Ph-ac**.

CARTILAGES, affections of : **Arg-met**.

CATALEPSY : **Graph**, sabad.

CELIBACY : **Con**.

CHAMOMILE, abuse of : **Puls**.

CHANGE of symptoms, constant : **Puls, Tub**.

    begining suddenly and ceasing suddenly : *tub*.

    positions, agg : **Caps, Ferr, Puls**, nat-s, rhus-t.

        amel : *cham*, **Ign, Rhus-t**, *ruta*.

    temperature, agg : acon, *mag-c*, nit-ac, **Ran-b**.

    weather, agg : *calc-p*, *chel*, **Dulc**, meli, merc, nit-ac, **Nux-m**,
        Phos, Psor, Ran-b, Rhod, Rhus-t, *sulph*, tarent, **Tub**.

        cold to warm, agg : **Bry, Kali-s, Psor, Sulph, Tub**.

        spring, in : ant-t, **Kali-s**, nat-s.

CHLOROSIS : *acet-ac*, *alum*, **Calc**, *cycl*, **Ferr**, *nat-m*, **Phos**, phyt, **Puls**.

    winter, in : *ferr*.

    yet a fiery red face : **Ferr**.

CHOREA : *cimic*, **Agar** (of single muscle or of whole body), caul, caust,
    Cic, Cimic, *cocc*, *croc*, *mygal*, **Stram, Tarent**, *zinc*.

    left side : *cimic*.

    fright, from : *ign* (also from grief), *zinc*.

    puberty, at : caul.

    sleep, amel : **Agar**.

    suppressed eruptions, from : *caust*, **Sulph**, *zinc*.

    teething or worms : ign.

CIRCULATION, deficient, capillary : **Carb-v**.

    feeble : *carb-an*.

    imperfect oxidation : *arg-n*, *carb-v*.

    stagnated : *carb-an*.

    venous system, diseases : **Carb-v, Sulph**.

CLIMACTERIC, complaints during : **Lach**, murx, **Sep, Sulph**.

CLOTHING, intolerance : *aml-ns*, *bov*, **Calc**, *carb-v*, **Lach, Sulph**.

    loosening amel or must loosen it : *aml-ns*, *carb-v*.

CLOUDY weather agg : dulc, rhod, **Rhus-t**.

CLUMSY : *caps*.

COITION, after : **Agar**, **Calc**, **Kali-c**, **Kali-p**, *sel*, **Sep**, **Sil**.

COLD in general, agg : *acon*, agar, *alum*, *ambr*, *am-c*, *ant-c*, **Ars**, **Bar-c**, *bell*, *bry*, **Calc**, **Calc-p**, *camph*, **Caps**, *carb-an*, *carb-v*, **Caust**, *cham*, **Chin**, **Dulc**, **Graph**, *hell*, **Hep**, *ip*, *kali-bi*, **Kali-c**, *kreos*, *led*, **Lyc**, **Mag-p**, **Nit-ac**, **Nux-v**, **Phos**, **Psor**, **Pyrog**, **Rhus-t**, Sabad, **Sep**, **Sil**, *tub*.

    extremes of : *ant-c*, *lach*.

    head excepted : *arn*, *ars*, *hell*.

    single parts of : **Calc**, kali-bi.

  air, agg : *acon*, **Agar**, *alum*, *am-c*, arg-n, **Aur**, *bell*, *borx*, *bry*, **Calc**, **Calc-p**, **Caust**, *cham*, coff, cupr, **Dulc**, *graph*, **Hep**, **Kali-c**, **Lyc**, **Mag-p**, mez, **Nux-v**, *phos*, **Psor**, **Rhus-t**, **Rumx**, **Sep**, **Sil**, **Tub**.

    perspiration, during : acon.

    sensation, as if cold air blowing on her even when covered : *lac-d*.

        as if sheets were damp : lac-d.

  becoming : acon, *agar*, *am-c*, ant-c, **Ars**, **Aur**, **Bar-c**, *bry*, *calc*, *caust*, *cham*, **Hep**, **Kali-c**, *keros*, **Lyc**, **Nux-v**, *psor*, pyrog, **Rhus-t**, Sabad, **Sep**, **Sil**.

    amel : **all-c**, aloe, ant-t, *bry*, **Iod**. kali-m, *led*, *lach*, op, **Puls**, *sabin*, *sec*, verat.

  after : *acon*, agar, *am-c*, **Ars**, **Bar-c**, **Bell**, **Bry**, **Calc**, **Cham**, **Hep**, *kali-c*, **Nux-v**, *psor*, **Sep**, **Sil**.

    a part of body, agg : *bell*, **Hep**, **Sil**.

    feet : *bar-c*, *con*, *cupr*, **Sil**.

    hand out of bed, agg : **Hep**.

    head : **Bell**, **Hep**, **Sil**.

  damp : (See Wet Weather) : ant-t, borx, **Calc**, **Calc-p**, **Dulc**, **Rhus-t**.

COLD, dry weather, agg : **Acon**, *ars*, **Asar**, bell, *bry*, carb-an, **Caust**, **Hep**.

  heat and cold, extremes of : *ant-c*, colch, *lach*.

    less affected by : **Fl-ac**.

  place, entering a , agg : *hep*, **Sep**, tub.

    and stones, sitting on : **Nux-v**.

    often in search of, which, amel : **Op**.

  repugnace, to : **Nux-v**.

tendency to take : **Acon, Alum,** ambr, am-c, *ant-c,* **Bar-c,** *bell,* **Bry,** calc, **Calc-p,** camph, caust, **Cham,** *graph,* **Hep,** kali-bi, **Kali-c, Kali-p,** *led,* **Lyc, Nat-m, Nit-ac, Nux-v, Psor, Sep, Sil, Sulph, Tub.**

even when taking violent exercise : **led, Sep, Sil.**

extremely sensitive to cold : **Bar-c,** camph, **Hep,** *kali-m,* **Psor, Sep, Sil, Sulph, Tub.**

seems to take cold every time he takes a breath of fresh air : **Hep, Tub.**

COLD wet weather, agg : am-c, ant-t, *aran,* **Ars, Bad,** *bar-c,* borx, **Calc, Calc-p, Dulc, Med, Nat-s, Nux-m,** *phyt,* **Rhod, Rhus-t,** *thuj,* **Tub.**

lying in damp ground : **Rhus-t.**

living or working in cold damp basement or milk dairy : **Aran,** *ars,* **Dulc,** mag-p, nat-s, **Rhus-t.**

standing in cold water, while : **Calc,** *mag-p.*

swiming, from : *ant-c.*

COLD water, agg : **Calc,** cycl.

amel : aloe, pic-ac, sel.

swallow of : **Caust, Cupr.**

falling in : *ant-c,* **Rhus-t.**

workers and modellers in cold clay : **Calc,** *mag-p.*

COLDNESS, single parts : **Calc, Kali-bi.**

COLLAPSE : Am-c, *aml-ns,* **Ars, Camph, Carb-v,** *carb-ac, crot-h, diph, med, merc-cy, sec,* **Verat.**

diarrhoea or cholera, after : **Ars, Camph, Carb-v,** *sec,* **Sulph, Verat.**

haemorrhage, during : verat.

wants to be fanned : (See Respiration, Difficult).

CONGESTION of blood : **Acon Aesc,** *agar* (in indolent old people), *arn, aur,* **Bell, Cact, Chin, Ferr, Glon,** *ham,* **Meli, Phos, Puls, Sulph.**

haemorrhage, amel : *meli.*

single parts of (See Separate Section) : **Sulph.**

venous : ham, **Puls.**

CONSTIPATION, amel : **Calc.**

CONSTITUTION, Assimilation, defective : **Abrot, Calc, Calc-p,** *lac-d.*

averse to physical labor : (See Mind Indolence).

bilious : aesc, **Bell, Berb,** *bry, eup-per, mag-m,* **Nux-v, Podo,** tarax.

blonde : **Brom**, *chel*, *phos*, *sel*, *tub*.

brunette : *nit-ac*, tub.

complexion, dark : alum, *aur*, **Bry**, **Calc-p**, *chin*, coff, **Ign**, iod, *kreos*, lyc, *mag-p*, **Mur-ac**, **Nit-ac**, *thuj*.

fair : **Brom**, **Calc**, lob, *phos*, **Puls**, sabad, spong.

fine : **Bell**, *brom*, *calc*.

light : *calc*, chel, *hep*, petr, *sel*, sil, *tub*.

olive-brown : *aur*.

sallow : *caust*, lyc.

yellow : **Caust.**

diathesis, gouty and rheumatic : **Benz-ac**, **Bry**, **Colch**, **Led**, *lyc*, med, *phyt*, **Rhus-t**, **Sars**, spig.

gouty and rheumatic, engrafted on gonorrhoea or syphilitic patients : *benz-ac*, **Med**, **Sars**.

haemorrhagic : am-c, cact, *chin*, **Crot-h**, **Ferr**, **Ferr-p**, **Ip**, **Phos**, **Kreos**, **Lach**, **Sec**, **Sul-ac**, *ter*.

anaemic subjects, in : **Ferr**.

small wounds bleed profusely : **Crot**, *kreos*, **Lach**, **Phos**.

malignant : **Ars**, *aur*, **Brom**, **Carb-an**, **Con**, **Hydr**.

psoric : *bar-c*, **Calc**, **Caust**, *diph*, *fl-ac*, *graph*, hell, kali-bi, *kali-c*, kreos, *lyc*, merc-d, merc, **Psor**, **Sil**, **Sulph**.

To correct psoric diathesis of unborn : **Psor**.

scrofulous : **Apis**, **Bar-c** (expecially fat), **Brom**, **Calc-p**, **Con**, *crot-h*, *diph*, dulc, **Iod**, *kali-i*, kreos, *merc*, *nit-ac*, ruta, **Samb**, **Sil**, spig, **Sulph**, **Ther**.

children during first and second dention : **Calc-p**.

sycosis : **Arg-met**, **Arg-n**, *aster*, cinnb, **Kali-s**, **Med**, **Nat-s**, **Nit-ac**, ph-ac, sars, **Sep**, **Staph**, *sulph*, **Thuj**.

syphilitic : **Aur**, **Aur-m**, benz-ac, **Cinnb**, *fl-ac*, *kali-bi*, **Merc**, **Merc-c**, **Merc-i-r**, **Merc-i-f**, *mez*, **Nit-ac**, *ph-ac*, **Phyt**, **Sil**, **Syph**.

mercurial dyscrasia : *fl-ac*, **Nit-ac**.

tubercular : **Bar-c**, bell, chel, *diph*, *mag-c*, phos, rumx, *spong*, **Tub**.

dwarfishness : **Bar-c**, calc-p, *med*.

emaciation : **Abrot**, *acet-ac*, *alum*, *ambr*, *arg-met*, *arg-n*, **Ars**, **Bar-c**, *calc-p*, **carb-v**, **Graph**, *helon*, *hydr*, **Iod**, *kreos*, *lach*, **Lyc**, mag-c, mag-m, mag-p, myos, *nat-c*, **Nat-m**, **Nit-ac**, *op*, *ph-ac*, phos, phyt, **Plb**, *psor*, samb, sanic, *sec*, *sars*, **Sel**, staph, **Sulph**, syph, **Tub**, *verat*.

bilious or intermittent fever after : *eup-per*.

affected parts of : *ars*, **Graph**, **Led**, **Sec**, sel.

certain parts : (See Parts Affected),

of neck : **Nat-m**, sanic, sars.

upper parts emaciated, lower semi-dropsical : **Lyc.**

children (marasmus) : *abrot*, acet-ac, *arg-n*, **Ars**, bar-c, **Calc-p**, *carb-v*, **Iod**, *lyc* (head well-developed, body puny, sickly), *kreos*, *mag-c*, mag-m (puny), *med*, **Nat-m**, *op*, sanic, sars, **Sil**, sulph, ther, *tub*.

downwards spreads : lyc, nat-m, sars, sanic.

losing flesh, while living well : *abrot, calc*, con, **Iod**, **Nat-m**, **Tub**.

loss of animal fluid : **Chin**, **Lyc**, *nat-m*, **Sel**.

old people : *ambr*, **Bar-c**, eup-per, **Lyc**, *nit-ac*, *op*, *sec*.

old dried up, child looks : **Arg-n.**

pining boys : **Aur**, **Lyc**, *nat-m*, **Tub**.

upwards : abrot.

rapid : **Tub**.

eyes, blue : **Bell**, **Calc**, *caps*, lob, *puls*, tub.

light blue : **Brom**, cocc (children and women especially).

dark : **Acon**, *aur*, calc-p, *caust*, **Iod**, *lach*, mur-ac, *nit-ac*.

eye-lashes, delicate : *phos*.

eye brows, light : *brom*.

fat : (See Obesity).

flabby : *aster*, acet-ac, **Calc**, **Caps**, hep, puls.

fleshy : am-c, **Calc**, *calc-ar*, lob, *puls*, thuj.

florid : **Glon**.

grow rapidly : **Calc**, **Calc-p**, *kreos*, **Ph-ac**, **Phos**.

girls at puberty : **Calc**.

hair, dark : acon, *aur*, **Bry**, calc-p, caust, cina, *ign*, **Iod**, kali-c, *mur-ac*, *nit-ac*, **Nux-v**, *plat*, sars, **Sep**, *thuj*.

flaxen : **Brom**.

light : agar, *bell*, **Brom, Calc**, *caps*, coçc (women and
children especially), **Con**, *hep*, kali-bi, cob, *merc*,
mez, op, petr, sabad, spig, *spong*, sul-ac.

brown : cham.

red : lach, *phos*.

sandy : **Puls.**

soft : phos.

heat, lack of vital : **Alum**, *aur*, **Bar-c, Calc, Calc-p, Carb-an**,
carb-v, **Led**, *med*, *sep*, **Sil.**

acute disease, in : **Led.**

chronic disease, in : **Sep.**

hydrogenoid (of Grauvogl) : **Ant-t, Thuj.**

indolent, sluggish : **Aloe**, am-c, am-m, *ant-t*, cap, *hep*.

ill-developed, poorly nourished : *kreos.*

leucophlegmatic : **Calc**, *cycl*.

life, extremes of : ambr, *ant-c*, **Bar-c, Lyc**, verat.

children only : acon, **Aeth, Bell, Cham, Cina, Gels**, kali-
br, lyc, **Mag-c**, op, spong, **Samb.**

first and second childhood : **Bar-c**, cham, mill, op,
rhub.

old : **Bar-c**, *colch*, **Con**, dios, eup-per, *fl-ac*, **Kali-c, Lyc,
Op, Sul-ac.**

bachelor : *con.*

young people : *acon*, **Bell**, dios, *gels*, stram.

girls : *ambr*.

young people look old : **Fl-ac.**

lymphatic : *agn*, aster, *bapt*, *bell*, **Hep**, *thuj*.

muscle fibre, firm, rigid, : **Acon, Bry**, *caust*, **Con**, *nit-ac*, plat, *sep*.

lax: *acet-ac*, agar, kali-c, *mag-c*, merc, sabad, sec,
sil, spong.

nutrition, deficient : (See Emaciation, Marasmus).

old age, premature : **Agn, ambr, Arg-n**, *bar-c, fl-ac*, lyc.

abuse of sexual powers, from : *agn*.

people : (See also Life, Extremes of) : *agar, aloe*, **Ambr,
Aur, Bar-c**, *carb-an*, **Colch, Con**, eup-per, *fl-ac*, **Sec.**

old maid and bachelor : **Con, Kali-c.**

old looking : **Arg-n**, *kreos*, san   ic, sil.

nervous affections, with : *ambr*.

women of relaxed phlegmatic habit : aloe.

obesity, fat : *am-m*, *ant-c*, *aur*, bar-c, **Calc**, **Caps**, **Graph**, *kali-bi*, kali-br, *kali-c*, *lac-d*, op.

> body fat legs thin : *am-m*.

ossification, imperfect : **Calc**.

persons, children liable to brain trouble : **Bell**, **Calc**, **Hell**, **Tub.**

> chronic, disease, usually suffer from : alum.
>
> debilitated from exhausting disease, but once robust : **Carb-v**, **Chin**.
>
> intellectually keen but physically weak : **Lyc**.
>
> predisposed to, abdominal : *chel*, **Podo**, tarax.
>
>> gastric : aesc, **Ant-c**, **Hydr**, **Ip**, **Puls**, tarax.
>>
>> hepatic : **Calc**, **Chel**, **Hydr**, *lyc, phos*, **Podo**, **Sulph**.
>>
>> respiratory : **Caust**, **Calc**, **Lyc**, **Phos**, **Sulph**.
>>
>> urinary : **Caust**.
>
> smelling salts, always using : **Am-c**.
>
> venous : **Carb-v**, **Ham**, **Puls**, **Sulph**.
>
> varicose veins : **Ham**.
>
> women : aloe, **Am-c**, aml-ns, *apis*, bell, calc-ar, **Caul**, coca, con, *ferr*, gels, glon, graph, helon, **Ign**, **Mag-m**, **Nux-m**, op, **Plat**, **Puls**, **Sabin**, **Sec**, **Sep**, spong, sul-ac.
>
>> old maids : bar-c, bov, **Con**.
>>
>>> during and after climacteric : **Con**.
>>
>> unmarried and childless : cocc.
>>
>> widows : **Apis**, **Con**.
>>
>> worn-out women with exhausted nerves : mag-c.

plethora : *acon*, *am-c*, *amyl-ns*, arn, **Aur**, bar-c, **Bell**, *cact*, **Calc**, *caps*, *carb-an*, glon, kali-br, **Kali-bi**, *stram*, **Sulph**, verat-v.

phlegmatic, : aloe, ant-t, *caps*, **Dulc**.

rigid fibre : (See Muscle Fibre, Firm).

scrawny : (See Thin).

sedentary : **Acon**, aloe, am-c, anac, *arg-n*, bry, con, **Nux-v**.

short necked children : kali-bi.

skin, lax : merc.

> delicate : brom.

stooping : *coff*, **Sulph.**

stout : am-c, *caps*, *chin*, *colch.*

thin, lean : (See also Emaciation) : *acet-ac*, **Alum**, **Ambr**, *arg-n*, bry, **Calc-p**, *chel*, **Coff**, *kreos*, *lach*, mag-p, **Nit-ac**, **Nux-v**, **Phos**, **Plat**, **Sec**, spig, **Sulph**, **Tub.**

tall : *arg-met*, **Calc**, **Calc-p**, *coff*, **Kreos**, **Ph-ac**, **Phos**, **Tub.**

torpid : (See Indolent).

venous : **Aesc**, **Carb-an**, **Carb-v**, **Ham**, **Sulph.**

vitality defective : **Zinc.**

withered, dried up : **Abrot**, **Arg-n**, *iod*, *kreos*, *op*, **Nat-m**, **Sanic**, sars.

CONSTRICTION, worn-out : *eup-per.*

externally : *anac*, *cact*, carb-ac, gels.

as if caged with wires twisted tighter and tighter : **Cact**, med.

internally : **Cact**, *iod*, *mag-p*, med, *sulph.*

of orifices : **Cact.**

band sensation of (See also Sensation) : **Anac**, **Cact**, **Carb-ac**, **Sulph.**

CONTRACTIONS, spasmodic, of single sets of muscles : **Agar**, croc, *ign*, zinc.

CONTRADICTORY and alternating states : croc, **Ign**, nat-m, **Puls**, thuj.

CONVULSIONS : *acon*, *arg-n*, aster, **Bell**, **Calc**, **Calc-ar**, **Caust**, **Cham**, **Chin**, **Cic**, cimic, *crot-h*, **Cupr**, ferr, *hell*, **Hyos**, *kali-br*, *lyss*, mag-m, *mag-p*, **Nux-v**, **Op**, *phos*, **Plb**, sabad, *sil*, **Stram**, verat-v, zinc.

right side of body : bell, **Lyc.**

left paralysed : art-v.

left side of body : *calc-p*, *sulph.*

one side, of, the other paralysed : stram.

air, from current of : bell, *lyss.*

anger, from ; **Cham**, *kali-br*, **Nux-v.**

apoplectic : *bell*, *crot-h.*

begins in fingers and toes : *cupr.*

Bright's disease, from : kali-br.

bright light, from : bell, *lyss*, **Stram.**

cerebral selerosis, from : plb.

tumor, from : plb.

cataleptic : cic.

children : acon, **Bell**, *cic*, **Cina**, *cupr*, *hyos*, **Bell**, **Op**, *nux-v*, **Zinc.**

anger, fit of : **Cham.**

approach of strangers, from : op.

cerebral congestions, from : **Bell**, **Glon.**

crying, from : op.

dentition, during : **Acon** (skin dry, hot, fever high), **Bell**, *cic*, glon, meli, *zinc*.

fright, in mothers, after : hyos, **Op.**

meningitis : **Bell**, *glon*.

nursing, from, after a fit or anger in mother : **Cham**, **Nux-v.**

worms, from : **Cina**, *hyos*.

punishment, after : *cham*, **Ign.**

clonic : **Cic**, **Cupr**, hyos, **Plb**, nux-v, stry.

concussion, after : **Hyper.**

coition, during : *bufo*.

consciousness, with : **Cina**, *hell*, hyos, *nux-m*, *nux-v*, **Stram**, stry.

without : *bell*, **Cic**, **Hyos**, op.

dentition, during : *bell* (with fever), *caust*, *cic*, kali-bi, mag-p (without fever), *stann*.

distortion, with frightful, of limbs or whole body : **Cic.**

emotional causes, from : ign, kali-br, **Nux-v.**

epiceptic : *aeth*, *agar*, *aster*, **Bufo**, **Calc-ar**, caul, caust, *cic*, *cimic*, **Cupr**, **Hyos**, *kali-br*, *lach*, meli, **Plb.**

night : cic.

aura begins in knees and ascends : cupr.

congenital : kali-br.

distortion of limbs, with : **Cic.**

heart disease, from : **Calc-ar.**

loss of fluid, from : lach.

meals, after, child vomits, sudden shricks and then insensible : *hyos*.

menses, before : kali-br.

a day or two before : kali-br.

new moon : *cupr*, kali-br.

puberty, at : *caul, cimic.*

sleep, during : bufo, *cupr, lach.*

tubercular : kali-br.

syphilitic : kali-br.

twitching all over body , 4 or 5 days before attac : **Aster.**

epileptiform : *aeth*, **Agar, Bell, Cic, Cimic, Cupr, Hyos, Plb.**

suppressed eruptions, from : *agar*, **Psor, Sulph.**

eruptions fail to break out, when : *ant-t*, **Cupr, Zinc.**

eruptions, suppressed, from : ant-t, **Cupr, Zinc.**

exanthamata repelled or do not appear, when : *ant-t, bry, cupr*, **Zinc.**

excitement, from : cimic.

fever, with : *bell.*

without : mag-p.

fluids, from (even thinking of) : *bell*, **Lyss, Stram.**

fright : *cupr*, **Hyos**, ign, *kali-br.*

hysterical : *cimic*, hyos.

injuries : arn, *cic, cupr*, **Hyper.**

chronic effects from concussion of brain and spine : *cic, hyper.*

head, of : cupr, hyper.

jar, from : *cic.*

jealousy, after : lach.

labor, during : *hyos.*

light agg : *bell*, **Lyss, Stram.**

love, disappointed : hyos.

menses before : *bufo, cupr.*

during : *cimic, cupr.*

mirror : (See Shining Objects).

metastasis : *cupr*, zinc.

motion agg : *nux-v.*

new-born : *cupr.*

noise, from : *cic.*

onanism, after : *bufo, lach.*

onset, sudden : **Bell.**

opisthotonos : (See Back).

periodic : *cedr*, cupr.

pregnancy, during : *cupr*.

puerperal : aml-ns, **Cic**, **Cupr**, **Hyos**, kali-br, meli.

    continue after delivery : **Cic**.

    frequent suspension of breating for a few seconds as if
        dead : **Cic**.

    immediately after delivery : *aml-ns*, **Cic**.

    upper part of body most affected : **Cic**.

punishment, after : *cham*, **Ign**.

restlessness, preceded by : *arg-n*.

shining objects, from : bell, **Lyss**, **Stram**.

sleep, during : bufo, *cupr*, *ign*, *lach*.

    after loss of : **Cocc**.

small-pox fails to break out when : **Ant-t**.

suppressed eruptions, from : *agar*, *cupr*, **Psor**, **Sulph**.

        foot-sweat from : **Cupr**, **Sil**, zinc.

tetanic : **Cic**, **Hyper**, **Nux-v**, *phyt*, *stry*, verat-v.

    breath of passing person agg : *hyper*, lyss, nux-v, phys,
        stry.

    splinters into flesh, from : **Cic**, **Hyper**.

    traumatic injuries from : **Hyper**, phys.

threatened : **Bell**, verat-v.

tonic : **Cic**, plb.

touched, when : *bell*, **Cic**, *lyss*, *nux-v*, stram.

uterine trouble, from : *cimic*.

vaccination, after : **Sil**, thuj.

vexation, from : **Cupr**.

water, at sight of : *bell*, **Lyss**, **Stram**.

wet, getting : *cupr*.

whooping cough, during : kali-br.

worm, from : cic, **Cina**, *hyos*, psor, sabad.

CONVULSIVE movements : **Cic**.

COPPER poisoning : *merc*.

COVERED, cannot bear to be, surface though cold, throws of coverings:
    Camph, **Med**, **Sec**.

    wants to be : **Ars**, **Hep**, **Nux-v**, **Psor**.

CURVATURE of bones : **Calc.**

CYANOSIS : ant-t, **Camph**, carb-an, **Carb-v**, **Dig**, *ip*, *laur* (heart troubles).
　　　　infants, new-born : *ant-t*.

DAMP places, exposure to : *ant-t*, **Aran**, ars, ars-i, gels, merc, **Nat-s**, *ter*.
　　　　changes in weather : bar-c, sil.
　　　　weather, amel : **Caust**, *hep*, med, *nux-v*.

DARKNESS, agg : **Stram.**
　　　　amel : phos.

DECOMPOSITION of fluids, tendency to : **Bapt**, **Pyrog.**

DESCENDING, agg : **Borx**, stann.

DIABETIS : Helon, nat-m.

DIRTY : *caps*, **Psor**, **Sulph.**

DISCHARGES : (See Different Sections).
　　　　acrid : **Alum**, *am-c*, *am-m*, **Ars**, **Graph**, **Kreos**, **Merc**, *psor*,
　　　　　　　Sulph.
　　　　bland : *caul*, **Puls.**
　　　　sticky : **Graph.**
　　　　stringy : **Bov**, *kali-bi*.
　　　　suppressed, bad effects of : *asaf*, *bry*, *merc*, **Sulph.**
　　　　tenacious, viscid : **Bov**, *hydr*, **Kali-bi.**
　　　　transparent : **Graph.**
　　　　touch : (See Tenacious).
　　　　watery : **Graph.**

DISTENSION of, blood vessels : *aesc*, *lil-t*.
　　　　veins of lids, ears, lips, tongue : *dig*.

DRAWING up of limbs amel : thuj.

DRINKING, after : *aeth*, aloe, cocc, **Crot-t**, verat.
　　　　cold : (See Food, Cold Drink) : **Ars**, **Hep.**
　　　　　　amel : **Phos** (until it gets warm), **Puls**, **Caust.**
　　　　warm, amel : alum, **Ars**, **Lyc**, **Nux-v**, **Rhus-t.**

DROPSY : acet-ac, **Apis**, *apoc*, **Blatta-o** (after failure of apis, apoc and
　　　dig), **Ars**, **Chin**, **Colch** (after apis and ars), *coll*, conv, **Dig**, *dulc*,
　　　Hell, *kali-c*, *lach*, *samb*, *sulph*, **Ter.**
　　　　acute : apis, apoc.
　　　　acute diseases, resulting from : **Chin.**

F-10

Bright's disease, in : **Dig**, *lac-d*.

cirrhosis, after : apoc.

cold, from exposure to : *dulc*.

drunkards, of : sulph.

fever, with : hell.

    intermittent, after : lac-d.

heart disease, after, uncomplicated : *apoc*.

        complicated : *coll*, **Dig**, conv, *lac-d*.

inflammatory : *apis*, *apoc*.

liver complaints, from : lac-d.

loss of vital fluid, after : **Chin**, *ferr*.

quinine, after abuse of : *apoc*, carb-v, **Ferr.**

scarlatina, after : **Apis**, *colch*, **Dig**, *hell*, *lach*, *ter*.

suppressed, eruption, after : **Apis**, *dulc*, *hell*, **Zinc.**

    intermittent : **Carb-v**, **Chin**, *ferr*, hell.

    sweat, after : *dulc*.

DRUGS, after : **Nux-v.**

DRUNKARD : (See Alcoholic Stimulant).

DRY weather agg : *aloe*, **Asar**, **Caust**, **Hep**, ip, **Nux-v.**

    amel : am-c, **Calc**, **Nat-s**, **Nux-m.**

    warm, amel : *calc-p*, **Nux-m**, *sulph*.

DWARFISHNESS : (See Constitution).

EATING, before : **Iod, Phos.**

    while : **Sulph.**

        amel : alum, **Anac**, *iod*, *kali-p*, **Psor.**

    after : aeth, agar, aloe, *ant-c*, **arg-n**, **Ars**, **bar-c**, **Bry**, *cocc*, coloc,

        crot-t, **Kali-bi**, lyc, **Nux-v.**

    amel : *chel,* **Iod.**

EATS SELDOM but much : *ars*.

        over-eating : *ant-c*, **Nux-v**.

ELECTRICAL storm : (See Storm).

EMACIATION : (See Constitution).

EMISSIONS agg : **Kali-c**, **Kali-p**, **Nux-v**, **Sel**, **Sep**, *sulph*.

EMPTINESS in all parts : **Cocc.**

ERUCTATIONS : (See Stomach).

ERUPTIONS suppressed : *apis*, *ars*, **Caust**, **Cupr**, **Graph**, *hell*, **Psor**, **Sulph**,
Zinc.

EXERCISE, increased ability to : coca, *fl-ac*.

EXERTION, physical, agg : aml-ns, **Arn**, **Ars**, **Bry**, **Cocc**, mill, **Nat-c**.
    amel : rhod, **Rhus-t**, **Sep**.

EXHAUSTION : (See Weakness).

EXHAUSTING diseases, bad effects : **Carb-v**, *caust*, **Chin**, phos, psor.

EXOSTOSIS : **Aur**, **Calc-fl**, *mez*, *ruta*.

EXTENSION of limbs agg : thuj.

FAINTNESS : **Acon**, *alum*, anthraci, *ant-t*, apoc, **Ars**, asar, **Bry**, cact, **Caust**,
    Cham, **Chin**, colch, croc, **Crot-h**, **Dig**, lil-t, merc, **Mosch**, *nat-m*,
    Nux-m, **Nux-v**, **Plb**, **Puls**, sec, **Sep**, *sil*, spong, stann, **Sulph**, *tab*,
    Tarent, ter, **Tril-p**, **Verat**.
        morning : **Nux-v**.
        coition, during : *plat*.
        cold extremes of : sep.
        crowded room, on going into : *plb*.
        diarrhoea, after : ars, ter.
        eating, before : *ran-b*.
            after : **Nux-v**.
        exertion, on : *carb-v*, sulph, *verat*.
        frequent spells : **Ars**, **Sulph**.
        haemorrhage, during : chin, *tril-p*.
        heat, extremes of : sep.
            and then coldness with : **Sep**.
        kneeling in church, while : **Sep**
        labor pain, after : **Nux-v**.
        odor, from : **Nux-v**.
        odor of cooking food, from : **Colch**.
            of fish : *colch*.
        raising head from pillow, when : apoc.
        reading, while : *sep*.
        rising from bed, on : acon, **Bry**, **Phyt**.
        sit down, must : *alum*.
            up, from : **Bry**.
        stool, after : aloe.
        sudden : *sep*.
        upright position, when being raised to : *dig*.
        vomiting, from : ant-t.
        wet, after getting : *sep*.

FASTING, while : **Calc, Iod, Lach, Plat, Plb, Sep.**
        amel : cham.

FISTULA : Sil.
        offensive : sil.
        painful : sil.
        proud flesh, with : sil.
        spongy edges, with : sil.

FLUID, tendency to decomposition : **Bapt**, *pyrog*.
        loss of : (See Loss of Fluids).

FOGGY weather agg : **Rhus-t.**

FOOD, acids agg : **Ant-c**, lach, nat-m.
    beer agg : ars, ferr, *kali-bi*, lyc.
        sour : *ars*.
    bread agg : *ant-c*, lyc, *nat-m*.
    cake agg : puls.
    cheese agg : *ars*, coloc.
    coffee amel : coloc.
        agg : **Ign, Nux-v.**
    cold drinks agg : *ars*, *hep*, **Rhus-t**, spong.
        amel : **Bism, Bry, Caust, Phos** (until it gets warm), *puls*,
        Sep.
    cold food agg : *arg-n*, **Ars, Dulc**, *graph, nux-m*, **Nux-v, Rhus-t,**
        Sil.
        amel : **Phos, Puls.**
    craves things that make them sick : **Carb-v.**
    decayed vegetables, from : all-c, carb-an, carb-v.
        food or animal matter : *ars*.
    egg, agg : *ferr*.
    fat, agg : ant-c, **Carb-v, Cycl, Ferr, Puls.**
        bad : *carb-v*.
    fish, agg : plb.
    fish, spoiled fish agg : all-c, carb-an, *carb-v*.
    fruit, agg : *aloe, ant-t*, **Ars**, *crot-t*, samb.
        cold fruit, agg : **Ars.**
    ice-cream agg : arg-n, **Ars.**
    ice-water, agg : **Ars.**

lemonade agg : *sel.*

meat agg : *colch, ferr,* **kali-bi, puls.**

       bad, agg : **Ars**, *carb-v*, **puls.**

       fresh agg : *caust.*

milk agg : **Aeth, Calc, Lac-d**, *mag-c*, **Mag-m.**

onion, agg : **Lyc**

pastry, agg : ant-c, **Puls.**

pork, agg : **Carb-v, Cycl, Puls.**

       sight or though of, agg : **Puls.**

potatoes, agg : *alum.*

rich agg : **Carb-v, Puls.**

salt, agg : *alum, carb-v, mag-m*, nat-m, **Phos.**

       meat agg : *carb-v.*

sausage, bad, agg : **Ars**, puls.

seasoned food, agg : *nux-v.*

sight of, agg : *ars*, **Colch**, *sep.*

simplest, disagrees : *carb-v.*

smell of, agg : *ars*, **Colch**, sep.

soup, agg : alum.

sour : (See Acids).

spiced : (See Seasoned).

sugar agg : **Arg-n.**

sweets, agg : **Arg-n**, gamb, med, *merc, sulph.*

tea agg : ferr, **Sel**, thuj.

vegetables (green), agg : **Nat-s.**

       (decayed), agg : all-c, carb-an, *carb-v.*

vinegar, agg : **Ant-c.**

warm drink, agg : *stram.*

       amel : **Ars**, *lyc*, **Nux-v, Rhus-t.**

warm food, agg : **Bry, Lach, Phos, Puls.**

wine agg : ant-c, fl-ac, glon, *led, con*, **Sel, Zinc.**

       sour or bad, agg : *ant-c.*

FOREIGN body, promotes expulsion : **Sil.**

FOOT-SWEAT suppressed : *bar-c*, **Sil.**

FULL feeling : **Acon, Aesc**, lil-t.

GANGRENE : (See Inflammation, Blackness).

GONORRHOEA, suppressed (See Sycosis) or maltered : benz-ac, **Med**, **Thuj.**

HAEMORRHAGE : acet-ac, am-c, **Arn**, **Bell**, *bov*, *cact*, **Calc**, **Carb-v**, chin, *croc*, **Crot-h**, **Erig**, **Ferr**, **Ham** (venous), **Ip**, **Lach**, **Meli**, **Merc**, **Merc-c**, **Mill**, nux-m, **Nux-v**, **Phos**, **Sec**, **Sulph**, **Sul-ac**, *ter*, thlas, thuj, *tril-p.*

> flow and stop and flow again : **Puls.**
> broken down system, in : **Carb-v.**
> long continued : **Chin.**
> mucous membrane, from : **Carb-v**, **Chin**, **Phos.**
> oozing : **Carb-v**, *kreos.*
> orifices of body, from : acet-ac, arn, *chin*, *croc*, **Crot-h**, **Erig**, **Ham**, **Ip**, **Mill**, **Phos**, mur-ac, **Nit-ac**, ter, thlas.
> red face, preceded by : *meli*, **Phos.**
> pouring : **Phos.**
>> and then ceasing for a time : *phos.*
> traumatic : **Arn**, *ham*, *mill.*
> wounds, from : *bov*, *ham*, *mill.*
>> small wounds, bleed freely : **Crot**, *kreos*, **Lach**, **Phos**, *sec.*
> blood, black : carb-v, chin, *croc*, **Crot**, *kreos*, *lach*, *sec*, *sulph*, **Sul-ac**, thlas.
>> fluid : **Crot-h**, elaps, **Sul-ac.**
>> bright-red : **Acon**, **Erig**, ferr, ferr-p, **Ip**, *nit-ac*, **Phos**, *sabin*, *tril-p.*
>> coagulates : *croc*, ferr, ferr-p, *ip*, *phos*, thlas.
>> does not coagulate : am-c, **Crot**, **Lach**, **Nit-ac**, **Phos**, *sec.*
>> charred straw like : lach.
>> dark and clotted : chin.
>> fluid : **Carb-v**, **Crot**, *elaps*, *lach*, *phos*, **Sul-ac.**
>>> partly, and partly solid : ferr, *plat.*
>> hot : **Bell.**
>> hangs in strigs : **Croc**, *elaps.*
>> viscid : *croc.*
>> watery : sec.

HAIR : (See Constitution and Head).

HARD bed sensation of (See Pain, Sore) : **Arn**, *bapt*, bry, *pyrog.*

HARDNESS : (See Induration).

HEAT agg : (See Warm).

HEAT of upper part, cold lower part : **Arn.**

of face or head and face alone, and body cool : **Arn.**

extremes of heat : *ant-c*, *lach.*

flushes of : aml-ns, **Calc**, cham, crot-h, dig, *ferr*, **Glon**, **Lach**, *sang*, **Sep**, *sil*, **Sulph**, **Sul-ac.**

during day with weak faint spells, passing off with a little moisture : sulph.

climacteric, at : **Aml-ns**, *bell*, dig, **Glon**, **Lach**, *sang*, **Sep**, **Sulph**, **Sul-ac**, **Tub.**

menses, during : *ferr*, *glon*, **Sang.**

motion, from least : *sep.*

parts below are icy cold, with : aml-ns.

perspiration, with : *sep.*

upwards : **Glon**, **Sep.**

HEAT, sensation of : **Apis**, **Calc-s**, **Coff**, **Fl-ac**, **Iod**, **Kali-s**, **Nat-m**, **Nat-s**, **Puls**, **Sec**, **Sulph**, **Sul-ac.**

glands : med.

HEAT, vital lack of : (See Constitution).

HEATED, becoming (overheated) : **Ant-c**, bry, *carb-v*, *glon*, *sep*, *ip.*

fire, in : *ant-c.*

chilling after overheated : *bry.*

children getting sick by sitting or sleeping before open fire : *glon.*

HEAVINESS, externally : **Aesc**, **Con**, **Gels**, pic-ac.

HIGH places : (See Ascending, Vertigo).

HOT bed feels : **Op.**

HOT weather (See Warm Weather) : **Ant-c.**

HUNGER from : **Cina**, **Iod**, **Sulph.**

HYSTERIA : (See Mind).

INCOORDINATION : (See Extremities).

INDURATION : **Carb-an**, **Con**, *hydr*, *iod.*

glands : apis, bar-c (especially cervical and inguinal), **Carb-an**, **Con** (stony hard), **Calc-fl** (stony hardness), **Iod**, **Merc**, *sil*, **Spong.**

INFLAMMATION : *acon*, *apis*, **Ars**, bell, cann-s, **Canth**, **Echi**, *ham*, kali-m, *merc*, **Sil**, *verat-v*.

        blue : **Lach**, puls, tarent.

        gangrenous : **Ars**, **Canth**, **Lach**, **Sec**, **Sil**, sul-ac.

           after mechanical injuries : sul-ac.

        painful : verat-v.

        septic from absorption of pus or other deleterious substance
           with burning and prostration : **Anthraci**, **Ars**, **Pyrog**.

        blood vessels : **Arn**, **Ars**, *ham*.

           veins (phlebitis) : all-c.

               puerperal : all-c.

           long bones : **Fl-ac**, *mez*.

           periosteum : **Fl-ac**, **Mez**, **Ph-ac**, *ruta*, *sil*.

               suppressed gonorrhoea from : *thuj*.

        cartilages : **Arg-met**.

        bones : **Fl-ac**, **Mez**, **Ph-ac**, **Sil**.

        joints : (See Extremities).

        nerves : **Acon**, **Bell**.

           traumatic : all-c.

        veins : all-c, **Ham**.

           delivery, after forceps : all-c.

           puerperal : all-c.

INJURIES : (See also Traumatic Affections) : **Arn**, *carb-v* (bad effect of long ago injury), *cic*, **Con**, euphr, glon, ham, **Hyper**, mill, *ruta*, *staph*, **Sul-ac**, symph.

        blow, after : *con*, nat-s.

        blunt instruments, with : **Arn**, *sul-ac*, **Symph**.

        chronic effects of : **Arn**, **Con**, *glon*, ham, **Sul-ac**.

        extravasation with blood : **Arn**, **Sul-ac**.

        fall, from : **Arn**, ham, nat-s.

        sharp cutting instruments, from : **Staph**.

        bone : **Arn** (compound fracture with suppuration), calen, calc-p, **Ruta** (fracture), symph.

           frature : **Ruta**, *symph*.

           dislocation : ruta, symph.

        glands : aster, **Con**.

        nerves : **Hyper**.

           parts, full of sentient nerves : **Hyper**.

periosteum : *ruta*.

soft parts (muscles) : **Arn, Con.**

spinal cord : **Hyper.**

INOCULATION with animal poison : (See Wound).

INTOXICATION, after : **Nux-v, Op.**

IRON, after abuse of ; *puls.*

IRRITABILITY excessive : **Arn, Bell,** bry, **Coff, Nux-v, Staph.**

physical : **Apis, Arn, Coff, Med, Nit-ac.**

when too much medicine has produced an oversensitive state and remedies fail to act : *ph-ac*, **Teucr.**

lack of : **Caps, Carb-v, Gels, Laur, Op, Ph-ac, Psor.**

IRREGULARLY developed bones : **Calc.**

JAR : Arn, Bell, berb, **Bry, Cic, Con,** glon, **Lach,** sep, **Ther.**

JAUNDICE : (See Skin).

JERKING : *acon,* agar, cina.

convulsions, as in : acon, *cic, ign,* verat-v.

muscles of : acon, *agar,* ign, *tarent,* **Zinc.**

single limb or whole body : **Agar,** *ign.*

shock, from : *cic.*

sleep, on going to : *ign.*

KICKS off, child kicks off clothing at night even in winter : acon, hep, sanic, **Sulph.**

LASSITUDE : Am-c, *ant-t, benz-ac, caps, cocc* (requires exertion to stand firmly), **Con, Nux-v,** *plb,* **Puls,** *sulph.*

morning on waking : puls.

consumptive : med.

LEAD poisoning : *alum.*

LEAN : (See Constitution).

LIE down, inclination to : **Alum, Ars, Calad,** *caps,* **Nux-v, Sel, Sil.**

and sleep : caps.

eating, after : lach, *sel.*

wants to, in different position, lengthwise, crosswise, in a bundle, etc : stram.

LIFTING, straining of muscles and tendons, from : **Arn, Calc, Carb-v, Carb-an,** *mill,* **Rhus-t.**

LOSS of fat : phyt-b.

LOSS of fluid : agn, **Carb-v**, **Caust**, **Chin**, **Chinin-s**, ham, *kali-c*, **Ph-ac**,
    phos, psor, **Staph.**

LYING agg : arn, **Aur**, *bell*, caust, **Con**, dios, **Hyos**, *kali-br*, kreos, **Meny**,
    nat-m, **Nat-s**, **Rumx**, sil, **Tarax.**

        amel : **Caps**, **Nux-v.**

        after, agg : caust, *con.*

        on abdomen, amel, : *acet-ac*, am-c, med, podo.

            during early months of pregnancy : acet-ac, podo.

        desire to lie down : pic-ac, psor.

        with head low : ars.

        with head low, cannot lie : **Spong.**

        with head high, amel : **Bell.**

        on side, amel : *coloc.*

           right agg : **Merc**, *stann.*

                amel : ant-t, nat-m, **Phos**, *sulph*, tab.

                    with head high : ars, calc, spig, spong.

           left agg : **Phos**, **Puls.**

           painful side agg : *acon*, *ars*, **Bar-c**, **Hep**, **Iod**, *kali-c*,
             Nux-m, *nux-v*, *phos.*

                amel : am-c, **Bry**, *calc*, ign, ptel, puls,

           painless side, agg : **Bry**, **Cham**, **Puls.**

MALARIAL origin, complaints : **Chin.**

MEASLES after : **Camph.**

MENSES, before : *am-c*, **Bov**, **Lach**, **Verat**, **Zinc.**

        at commencement of : *am-c*, **Bov**, **Verat.**

        during : am-c, *cimic, cocc*, **Graph**, *ham*, **Hyos**, **Nux-v**, **Mag-c**,
        Puls, **Sep**, *sil*, *verat.*

           amel : **Lach** (by the flow), **Zinc.**

        after : **Lach**, **Nux-v**, **Graph**, *zinc.*

        suppressed, bad effects : *con.*

MENTAL labor, agg : sep.

MERCURY, abuse of : *arg-met*, **Aur**, **Carb-v**, *fl-ac*, graph, **Hep**, **Kali-i**, *lach*,
    mez, **Nit-ac**, *ph-ac*, podo, *puls*, **Sulph.**

METASTASIS : Abrot.

MOON, full : *alum*, *calc*, psor (involuntary urination), sabad.

    new : *alum*, *caust*, **Sil**, sabad.

    decrease of moon, during, amel : clem.

    increase of moon, during, agg : clem.

MOONLIGHT agg : *ant-c*.

MOTION, agg : aesc, ant-c, **Bell**, berb, **Bry**, **Colch**, *crot-h*, *dig*, *ip*, lob, *mag-p*, *med*, mez, **Nux-v**, *phyt*, pic-ac, **Ran-b**, **Sabin**, **Samb**, *sec*, spig, verat.

    amel : arn, chin, *dios*, **Dulc**, **Ferr**, iod, *kreos*, **Lyc**, *mag-c*, *meny*, nat-s, **Puls**, **Rhus-t**, *ruta*, *sep*, **Sulph**, **Tarax**, **Tarent**, *zinc*,

    at begining of : **Ferr**, **Lyc**, **Rhus-t**, **Puls**.

    aversion to : **Bell**, **Bry**, *gels*, **Nux-v**.

    continued, amel : **Ferr**, **Puls**, **Rhus-t**, sep.

    must keep in motion, though walking agg : *tarent*.

MUCOUS secretions increased : **All-c**, *alum*, am-c, **am-m**, **ant-c**, **Dulc**, **Hydr** (viscid), **Kali-bi** (viscid, stringy), kreos (corrosive, fetid, ichorous), mag-c, **Merc**, **Puls**, **Sulph**.

NARCOTICS, agg : **Cham**, **Coff**, **Nux-v**, verat, thuj.

NECROSIS bones : **Fl-ac** (especially long bones), *phos*, ther.

NEUROMA, idiopathic : calen.

NIGHT watching, bad effects : *cocc*.

NOISE agg : (See Mind Sensitive).

NUMBNESS : *acon*, *cham*, kali-br, kalm, **Op**, phos, *plat*, *rhus-t*, sec.

    whole body : **Kali-br**.

    parts lain on : *ambr*, **Puls**, **Rhus-t**.

    suffering parts or affected parts : *acon*, **Cham**, kalm, **Plat**.

OBESITY : (See Constitution).

ODOR, bad effects from inhalation of putrid : *anthraci*, **Pyrog**.

OLD age, premature : (See Constitution).

ONANISM, from : *arg-met*, calad, **Cocc**, dios, **Gels**, *kali-p*, **Orig**, **Ph-ac**, plat, **Staph**, **Zinc**.

OPUM eating : (See Narcotics).

ORGASM of blood, absent during an embrace : *calad*, **Sel**.

OSSIFICATION imperfet : **Calc.**

PAIN, appear gradually and disappear gradually : **Plat, Stann,** syph.

appear gradually and disappear suddenly : *ign*, **Puls**, *sul-ac.*

appears suddenly and disappear suddenly : **Bell**, *carb-ac*, eup-per, ign, **Kali-bi**, mag-p, **Nit-ac**, petr.

appear suddenly and disappear gradually : *coloc, puls.*

appear at sunrise increases till noon and ceases at sunset : **Kalm,** *nat-m*, *spig.*

afternoon 4 p. m. : *coloc*, **Lyc.**

evening : cham.

night (sunset to sunrise) : **Merc,** mez, **Nit-ac,** phyt, *syph.*

change of position amel : apis.

changing place : (See Wandering).

change of weather or temperature, agg : *nit-ac.*

chilliness, with : **Puls.**

coughing amel : apis.

delirium, with : **Verat.**

directions, downwards : cact, **Kalm.**

upwards : **Led.**

distant parts, on coughing : caps.

driving patient to crazy : **Acon, Cham**, *mag-p.*

fainting, with : **Hep.**

heat agg : cham.

light and superficial in warm weather, affects bone and deeper tissues when air is cold : **Colch.**

PAIN, micturition, with frequent : **Thuj.**

motion agg : **Bry**, *phyt.*

yet there is constant desire to move : lac-c, merc, *phyt.*

first motion, on : puls, **Rhus-t.**

amel : **Rhus-t.**

pressure amel : castm.

paroxysmal : mag-p.

side to side : (See Generalities, Side) : **Cimic.**

sleep, during : *nit-ac.*,

touch, light agg, but hard pressure amel : *caps*, **Chin**, plb.

thinking agg : ox-ac (as soon as he thinks about it).

amel : *camph, hell.*

unbearable, driving to despair : (See Sensitiveness to Pain): **Cham.**
> to delirium : verat.

walking amel : apis.

weather warm, pain superficial : colch.
> cold, pain deeper : colch.
>
> bones : bry, *chin*, colch, **Eup-per**, eup-pur, **Ip**, med, **Merc**, **Kali-i**, mez, ph-ac, ran-b, *sars*, ther, **Still.**
>> night : **Kali-i**, **Merc**, mez, *sars*.
>>
>> chill, before : **Eup-per**, *eup-pur*, caps,
>>> during : **Eup-per.**
>>
>> extending from above downward : mez.

gland : *carb-an*, con.

muscles : *bry*, sal-ac, *verat-v.*

periosteum : colch, *kali-i*, mez (of long bones), *merc*, *phyt*, sars, symph, **Still.**
> night, in bed : mez.
>
> damp weather : mez, merc, phyt.
>
> mercury, from : sars.
>
> suppressed gonorrhoea, from : sars.
>
> touch agg : mez.
>
> wounds, after healed : symph.

small spots : fl-ac, ign, **Kali-bi**, lil-t.

PAIN aching : *bapt*, cimic, *gels*, lyc, *mag-c*, nux-v.
> bones : med.

benumbing : acon, **Cham**, kalm, **Plat.**

broken, as if bones : *eup-per*, ther.

burning : **Acon**, *agar*, all-c, **Anthraci**, **Apis**, **Ars** (burns like fire), bell, *canth*, *caps*, carb-an, *con*, helon, *mez*, **Ph-ac**, **Phos**, *ran-b*, **Sec** (as if sparks of fire falling), spig, *staph*, **Sulph.**
> heat amel : **Ars.**
>
> hot drink, amel : *ars.*
>
> glands : *con.*
>
> small spots : agar, phos, ran-b, *sulph.*
>> circumscribed : ign.

constricting : **Cact**, iod, *mag-p*, sulph.

cramping : caust.

cutting : carb-an, cimic, **Con**, hydr, *mag-p*, spig.

       glands : con.

darting : **Bry**, cact, *cimic,* gels, con, kali-c, *kalm.*

drawing : caust, chin, colch, cycl (when bones lie near surface), lyc, puls.

       bones : chin, cycl.

          cold agg : colch.

gnawing : nit-ac.

gripping, ending in vice-like grip : *cact.*

jerking : podo.

lancinating : *carb-an, cimic,* **Con**, phyt.

lightening : cact, fl-ac, mag-c, *mag-p*, phyt.

       left side : coloc.

migrating : (See Wandering).

neuralgic : cact, caust, *chinin-s, cimic,* kali-bi, *kalm, mag-c*, **Magp**, med, *mez, phyt,* spig.

       cold air agg : **Mag-p.**

       diphtheria, after : phyt.

       gonorrhoea, after : phyt.

       heat, amel : **Mag-p.**

       mercury, after : *phyt.*

       periodical, daily at same hour : *cedr, chinin-s,* kali-bi.

       psoric origin : caust.

       pressure amel : *coloc, mag-p.*

       syphilis : *phyt.*

       touch, agg : mag-p.

       zona, after : *mez.*

pressing : *colch, cycl,* kalm, lyc, **Sulph,** sul-ac.

       bones : colch, *cycl* (when bones lie near surface).

          cold agg : colch.

raw : canth.

scraped, as if : ph-ac, *rhus-t.*

       periosteum : **Rhus-t.**

       bones : **Rhus-t.**

    shooting : cimic, kalm, *mag-p,* phyt.

    smarting : (See Burning).

    sprained, as if : psor, *rhus-t.*

    sore, bruised : abrot, apis, **Arn, Bapt,** *bel-p,* canth, **Chin,**

Cimic, Eup-per, Ham. mag-c, med, *nux-m, phyt,* Pyrog, Rhus-t, Ruta, *spig, sul-ac, thuj.*

cannot bear pain, whole body over-sensitive : **Arn, Cham, Coff, Ign.**

motion, amel : *chin, pyrog, rhus-t.*

parts lain on : **Arn, Bapt,** *nux-m,* **Pyrog, Ruta.**

glands : **Con,** *med.*

joints : *chim.*

bone and periosteum : **Ruta.**

springing : cact.

splinters, sensation : **Aesc, Agar,** *alum,* **Arg-n, Hep, Nit-ac.**

stabbing : *mag-p.*

stitching : **Bry, Bell,** *cimic,* **Kali-c,** *kalm,* **Led,** mag-p, **Nit-ac,** *nux-v,* ptel, **Puls, Spig, Staph,** symph.

night : *bry.*

cough agg : **Bry.**

inspiration : **Bry.**

lying on painful side, amel : **Bry.**

agg : *kali-c.*

rest amel : **Bry.**

agg : *kali-c.*

touch agg : nux-v.

stinging : all-c, **Apis,** con, nit-ac, *staph.*

strained as if, periosteum : **Chin.**

sympathetic : **Cimic.**

tearing : **Bry, Chin, Colch,** cycl, **Kali-c, Led,** ph-ac, ptel, **Puls, Rhus-t, Spig,** valer.

night : *bry.*

coughing agg : **Bry.**

inspiration agg : *bry.*

lying on painful side, amel : **Bry,** ptel, *puls.*

motion agg : **Bry.**

rest amel : **Bry.**

bones : **Chin,** colch, *cycl, ip* (as if torn to pieces).

cold agg : colch.

muscles : *colch,* rhus-t.

tendons : rhus-t.

tingling : acon, nux-v.

motion agg ; nux-v.

touch agg : nux-v.

wandering : apis, **Kali-bi, Kali-s, Lac-c,** lil-t, *mag-p, mang-act,* **Puls,** *phyt* (like electric shocks), syph.

PAINLESSNESS of complaints, usually painful : *hell,* **Op, Stram.**

PARALYSIS, agitans : **Merc,** *plb,* **Rhus-t, Zinc.**

apoplexy, after : lach, **Phos.**

cold wind or draft, exposure to : **Caust.**

coldness of paralysed parts, with : plb.

complete : **Op,** *phos.*

exertion, after : rhus-t.

gradually appearing : **Caust.**

from below upwards : con.

hysterical : ign.

internally : *cocc,* **Gels,** plb.

lead poisoning, from : **Caust.**

lying on damp ground, from : *rhus-t.*

motor : *gels,* kali-br, **Op,** phys.

one-sided : arn, **Caust,** *kali-c,* plb.

right : **Caust.**

left : *arn,* lach.

organs : *caust, plb.*

painless : **Plb.**

partial : **Op, Plb.**

parturition, after : rhus-t.

post-diphtheritic : *caust,* diph, gels, *plb.*

sexual excess, after : *nat-m,* rhus-t.

side, right : caust.

left : lach.

single parts : **Caust.**

sycotic : *med.*

typhoid, typhus, after : *caust,* rhus-t.

wet, from getting : *rhus-t.*

PERIODICITY : Ars, *carb-v,* **Chin, Chinin-s,** cupr, **Ip,** *lach, mag-c, sulph,* tarent.

complaints return every year : ars, carb-v, lach, *sulph,* thuj.

at same hours : cedr, ign, ip.

every other day : alum, **Chin,** ip.

every three weeks : mag-c.

neuralgia every day at same hour : **Kali-bi.**

PERSPIRATION gives no relief : **Ars, Caust, Cham,** hep, **Merc,** *nit-ac,* tilia, **Verat.**

amel : ars, **Bry, Nat-m, Psor,** *verat.*

suppression of ; **Bell,** *bry,* **Calc, Colch, Dulc.**

PHLEBITIS : (See Inflammation).

PLUG, sensation of : **Aloe,** *anac,* hep, **Ign,** plb.

POLYPUS : Calc, Calc-p, Con, *hep,* **Phos, Staph, Teucr.**

PREGNANCY, during : *cocc.*

PRESSURE, agg : **Agar, Apis,** arn, **Bar-c,** *bry,* **Hep, Lach, Lil-t, Lyc, Sil.**

amel : *am-c, apis, borx,* **Bry, Chin, Coloc, Con,** ign, **Mag-p, Meny,** *nat-s,* **Plb, Puls, Sil,** stann.

hard : **Chin, Coloc,** ign, *plb, stann.*

on painless side, agg : **Bry, Ign, Puls.**

PROSTRATION, sudden and complete, of vital force : **Camph.**

PULSATION : Acon, aesc, **Calc, Ferr, Glon,** iod, led, lil-t. **Nat-m.**

full and distended as if blood would burst : *aesc,* lit-t.

PULSE, abnormal : **Acon, Bell, Ars.**

bounding : **Bell.**

contracted : *sec.*

feeble : (See Weak).

frequent, accelerated, elevated, exalted, fast, rapid quick, etc.: *acon, aeth,* ant-c, aster, aur, coll, diph, lil-t, **Pyrog** (140-170), **Sec,** *tab,* **Verat-v.**

motion agg : *apoc.*

out of proportion to temperature : lil-t, pyrog.

full : *acon, arn,* aster, **Bell, Dig,** *tab, verat-v.*

globular, like buck shot, striking finger : **Bell.**

hard : *acon,* aeth, ant-c, aster, verat-v.

iron, as : verat-v.

imperceptible : *camph,* **Carb-v,** crot-h, tab, verat.

almost : **Camph,** crot-h, kalm, *tab.*

increase suddenly and decrease gradually below normal : verat-v.

intermittent : **Carb-v, Dig,** kali-c, mur-ac, nat-m, **Sec,** *tab,* verat-v.

every third, fifth, seventh beat : **Dig.**

every third : *mur-ac.*

irregular : *aur,* **Dig,** kali-c, lil-t, *naja* (in force but regular in rhythm), *tab,* **Verat-v.**

rapid : (See Frequent).

sinking : anthraci.

slow : **Dig, Gels** (of old age), kalm (35 to 40), *tab, verat-v.*

small : aeth, *aur,* **Camph,** pyrog, **Sec,** tab.

soft : verat-v.

strong : arn.

weak : **Aur, Camph,** coll, **Crot-h, Dig,** *diph,* kali-c, *laur,* mur-ac, *tab, verat-v.*

moved, when : apoc.

wiry : *carb-v,* pyrog.

PURPURA haemorrhagica : (See Diathesis, Haemorrhagic).

QUININE, abuse of : apoc (in dropsy), **Carb-v, Ferr, Ip,** *lach,* meny, **Nat-m, Puls.**

RACHITIS : *ph-ac.*

REACTION, lack of : **Ambr, Caps, Carb-v,** caust, *diph,* **Laur, Med, Op, Psor,** pyrog, **Sulph,** *verat, valer.*

acute disease, in : **Sulph.**

convalescence, during : **Psor.**

chronic : **Psor.**

carefully selected remedies fail to produce favourable results,

in acute : **Sulph.**

in chronic : **Psor.**

easily exhausted, in : *caps.*

fat people, in : **Caps.**

nervous affections, in : **Ambr,** *valer.*

patient improves for a while and then comes to a stand-still: *caust,* **Psor, Sulph.**

Sulphur fails, when : **Psor.**

REDNESS of all orifices : **Sulph.**

RELAPSING, complaints : **Sulph.**

RELAXATION of muscles : **Caps, Calc, Gels.**

REST : (See Motion, Aversion to).

RIDING in a carriage or rail-road : arg-met, berb, **Cocc,** *nux-m,* **Petr,** sanic.
    amel : **Nit-ac.**
    boat : *aml-ns,* **Cocc, Petr,** sanic.
    amel on deck in fresh cold air : **Tab.**

RISING agg : **Acon.**

RUBBING amel : **Phos, Plb,** sec, *tarent, thuj.*

SEASHORE : (See Air).

SEDENTARY : (See Lassitude).

SENSITIVENESS, external : aml-ns, **Arn,** *asar,* asaf, **Bell,** bov, camph, *canth,* **Cham,** chin, *coff, colch,* **Chin,** *hep,* **Ign, Lach,** *nux-m,* **Nux-v, Phos, Sil, Spig.**
        scratching of linen or silk : **Asar.**
        internal : *asar,* **Canth,** chin, colch, **Hep.**
    pain, to : **Arn,** asaf, *asar,* **Cham,** *chin,* **Coff,** *colch,* **Hep, Ign, Nux-v, Mag-p.**
        intolerance, driven to despair : **Acon, Cham, Coff, Mag-p.**
        tossing about in anguish : coff.

SEPTICAEMIA : *arn,* **Ars,** *bapt,* **Carb-v, Crot-h, Lach, Pyrog.**
    prevents : **Arn.**

SEWER gas infection : **Pyrog.**

SEXUAL excess after : **Agar,** *agn, chin,* cocc, **Con,** graph, **Kali-p, Lyc,** lyss, **Ph-ac,** samb, **Staph, Sep.**
    desire, suppression of agg : **Con.**
    excitement agg : **Lil-t.**

SHIVERS, cold, emotion from : *asar.*

SHOCKS from injury : **Arn, Camph, Hyper.**
    electric-like ; **Arg-met, arg-n.**

SHUDDERING, nervous : kali-c, **Nux-v,** *spig.*
    touch, from : kali-c, *spig.*

SIDE, symptoms on one side : *agar,* **Anac,** ant-c, bell, **Bry,** colch, kali-c, **Lach, Lyc,** rhus-t, thuj.
        alternating sides : ant-c, **Lac-c,**
        crosswise, left upper and right lower : **Agar,** ant-t, stram.
            left lower and right upper : **Ambr,** brom, med, **Phos, Sul-ac.**

right : **Apis, Bell, Bry, Chel,** crot-h, kali-c, **Lyc,** mag-p, *podo, rhus-t.*

then left : anac, **Lyc**

left : *colch,* coloc, **Lach,** lil-t, mag-c,rhus-t, *thuj.*

then right : *colch,* **Lach.**

SILICA, abuse of, after : ang, **Fl-ac.**

SILVER nitrate, after abuse of : **Nat-m.**

SITTING, while : alum, **Bry,** dig, dios, tarax.

upright amel : ant-t, apis, **Bell,** nat-s (cough), samb.

SLEEP at begining of, agg : **Lach.**

during, agg : **Arn, Ars, Bell, Bry, Cham, Hyos,** *lach,* **Merc, Op.**

after, agg : apis, *cocc,* **Lach** (especially mental symptoms), *op,* sep, **Spong, Stram.**

long agg : **Lach.**

amel : phos.

loss of, from or night watching : *caust,* **Cocc,** *colch, ign,* lac-d, **Nux-v,** *nit-ac.*

SLOW, bones slow to develop : **Calc, Calc-p,** *symph.*

repair of broken bones : **Calc, Calc-p,** *symph.*

SLIDES down in bed : **Mur-ac.**

SLUGGISHNESS of body : ph-ac, phos.

SOFTENING of bones : **Calc, Calc-p.**

SNOW air, agg : **Calc,** *calc-p,* ph-ac.

SPRING, in : **Lach,** *nat-s,*

STANDING, agg : *aloe,* sep, **Sulph.**

amel : **Bell.**

STOOL, after : aeth.

during : *verat.*

after, amel : aloe.

STOOP, inclined to : **Phos.**

shouldered : **Sulph,** tub.

sitting, while : **Sulph.**

walking, while : **Sulph.**

like old men : **Sulph.**

STORM, approach of : meli, nat-c, petr, *phos,* **Psor,** *ran-b,* **Rhod,** *rhus-t,*
    sep.

       during : am-c, *psor.*

       thunderstrom : *med, nat-c,* petr, *phos,* **Psor.**

         before : agar, nat-c, gels, phos, **Psor, Rhod,** sil.

STRAINING : (See Lifting).

STRETCHING : *aml-ns, calc,* **Nux-v,** plb, **Rhus-t.**

       constant, for hours : *aml-ns*

       sensation, in abdomen, from : aml-ns, plb.

       would seize the bed and call for help to stretch : *aml-ns.*

SULPHUR, abuse of : **Puls.**

SUMMER in : *aeth, ant-c, bell,* crot-t, **Fl-ac** (less affected by excessive
    heat), gels, **Kali-bi,** *lach,* **Nat-c,** *nat-m.*

       children, in, during dentition : *aeth.*

       mild, amel : alum, aur.

       amel : *calc-p,* ferr, *psor.*

SUN, from exposure : **Ant-c,** *bell,* gels, **Glon,** *lach, lyss,* **Nat-c, Nat-m,** *sel,*
    verat-v.

       ailments, sunburn, from : *ant-c.*

       exertion in : **Ant-c, Lach, Nat-m.**

SUPPURATION : (See Abscess).

       benign, change into ichorous or malignant : *carb-an.*

       prevents : **Arn.**

       profuse : *calc-s,* **Hep, Merc, Sil.**

       slightest injury, from : *calen,* **Borx, Graph, Hep,** *merc,* **Sil.**

       seems inevitable : **Hep.**

SWELLING in general : **Apis, Ars,** *bar-c,* **Bell, Bry,** *hep,* iod, lach, **Merc,**
    mez, samb.

       cold, from : dulc, merc.

       inflammatory : **Ars, Bell, Merc,** *sil.*

       bones : **Asaf, Calc,** *mez,* **Sil.**

         periosteum : *sil.*

       cartilages : **Arg-met.**

       glands : apis, **Bar-c** (especially cervical and inguinal), **Brom,**
         Carb-an, Con, Dulc (after repeated cold), **Hep, Iod,** kali-
         i, med, **Merc, Sil, Spong.**

inflammatory : **Bell, Con, Merc, Sil.**
painful : *carb-an.*
stony hard : *brom.*
tuberculous or scrofulous : **Brom.**
joints : *colch.*

SYCOSIS : (See Constitution, Diathesis).

SYPHILIS : (See Constitution, Diathesis).

TEA, drinking, abuse of : lob, **Puls.**

TISSUES fibrous affections of : *rhod,* **Rhus-t.**
serous, affections of : **Bry.**

TOBACCO agg : arg-n, **Ars,** cic, coca, *cocc, gels,* **Ign,** lob, *lyc,* **Nux-v, Staph,** verat.
chewing agg : **Ars,** lyc, nux-v, *verat.*
smoking, removes craving : **Calad.**

TONICS, abuse of : **Nux-v, Puls.**

TOUCH agg : **Apis,** arg-met, **Bell, Bry,** *cact,* camph, *caps,* **Chin,** cic, **Coff, Colch** (especially of affected parts), euphr, graph, **Hep,** ign, **Kali-c,** Lach, lob, **Mag-p,** *mez,* **Nit-ac,** Nux-v, **Ran-b,** spig, **Staph, Tarent.**
slight, agg : **Apis, Bell,** *camph,* **Chin, Hep, Lach.**
amel : arn.

TRAUMATIC affections : (See also Injury, Wounds).
disfiguring scars, prevents : **Calen.**
neuritis from lacerated wound : *calen,* **Hyper.**
neuroma : **All-c,** calen.
prevent suppuration : **Calen.**
promotes healthy granulation : **Calen.**
rupture of muscle and tendons : *calen.*
secures union by first intention : **Calen.**
sloughing of soft parts : *calen, carb-ac.*
surgical cuts (specific) : **Calen.**
wounds lacerated : **Calen,** *carb-ac,* ham, *hyper.*
penetrating articulations : *calen.*
bones, crushed, injured : *calen, carb-ac.*

TREMBLING, external : *agar, caust,* chin, **Gels, Lach,** med, **Merc,** mygal, *nat-m, ph-ac, phos,* phys, spig, staph, **Stram, Zinc.**
anger, from : *staph.*

children, in : cina, verat-v.

exertion, after least : *merc,* phys.

heart's pulsation, from : *nat-m,* spig.

internal : ant-t, caul, *caust,* **Sul-ac.**

drunkards, of : **Sul-ac**.

mental exertion, from : phys.

TWITCHING : acon, **Agar,** aster, caust, cimic, cina, croc, **Hyos, Ign,** nux-v, **Stram, Zinc.**

single muscle or groups of muscles : acon, **Agar,** croc, *ign,* stram, tarent, *zinc.*

single limb or whole body : ign.

sleep, on going : *ign.*

subsultus tendinum : **Hyos.**

upper part of body especially: stram.

TUMORS, cystic : (See Exostosis, Polypus) : **Bar-c, Graph.**

fibroid : **Calc-fl,** mez.

soften from within out : mez.

TURNING over in bed : **Con.**

ULCERS : Ars, *hep.*

canerous : **Ars,** *hep.*

UNCOVERING, agg : *arg-n,* **Ars,** *bell, graph,* **Hep, Mag-p, Nux-m, Nux-v, Psor, Zinc.**

cannot cover to warmly, but warmth does not amel : *caust.*

wants to be covered even in summer : **Psor.**

single parts, agg : **Hep.**

amel : acon, *aml-ns, lach,* lyc, **Op, Sulph.**

perspiration during : *zinc.*

UNWIELDY : Calc.

VACCINATION, after : *ant-t, ars,* crot-h, **Sil, Sulph, Thuj.**

Thuj fails, when, and Sil, not indicated : ant-t.

VERICOSE veins : **Arn, Calc, Carb-v, Fl-ac, Ham,** pyrog.

inflamed : *ham.*

VITALITY defective : **Zinc.**

too weak to develop exanthamata : **Cupr, Sulph,** *tub,* **Zinc.**

VOMITING, after : aeth.

WAKING, on : **Caust, Hep, Hyos, Lach, Nit-ac, Nux-v, Sulph.**

WALKING, agg : aloe, *berb,* **Bell, Bry,** ign, **Nit-ac, Nux-v, Sep,** *tarent.*
        amel : *dios,* **Ferr** (although weakness compels patient to lie
            down), *mag-c,* op, **Rhus-t,** *ruta.*
        constant : op.
        rapidly : lob (chest pains).
        slowly : **Ferr, Puls.**

WANDERING symptoms : *ant-c,* lac-c, **Puls.**

WARM, agg : acon, **Apis, Ars-i,** *bry,* cham, euphr, **Iod,** ip, kali-m, **Led,** med,
        Puls, Sec.
        amel : **Ars, Hep,** *ign,* kreos, **Mag-p,** podo, rhod, **Rumx,** *sep,* **Sil,**
            stram.
        air, agg : *bry.*
            amel : caust, *mag-c.*
            moist, agg : *ham.*
        bath, amel : ant-c.
        bed, agg : **Apis,** *bry, euphr,* **Led, Merc** (but amel, by rest in bed),
            mag-c, **Sulph,** *thuj.*
            amel : **Ars** (but agg by rest in bed), **Bry, Nux-v,** *sep.*
        days and cold damp night : merc.
        damp : *carb-v.*
        room, agg : **Acon,** *all-c,* ant-t, **Apis,** *bry,* euphr, lyc, *kali-s,* **Puls,**
            Sabin.
                coming from air into : *bry, caust.*
                amel : *cycl,* nux-m.
        stove, agg : apis, **Glon,** nat-m.
            amel : **Ars, Ign, Mag-p, Nux-v.**
        weather complaints : *aloe, ant-c,* **Bry** (especially. after cold days),
            kali-bi.
        wet weather, agg : **Carb-v, Nat-s.**
            amel : cham.
        wraps agg : **Apis,** *bry,* **Iod,** kali-m, **Led, Puls.**
            amel : (See Uncovering).

WASHERWOMEN'S remedy : **Sep.**

WASHING : (See Bathing).

WEAKNESS (Prostration, Exhaustion, Debility, etc.) : abrot, *acet-ac, aesc,*
        aeth, agar, *agn,* aloe, *alum, ambr,* **Am-c,** anac, anthraci, *ant-c,*

Ant-t, Apis, apoc, **Arg-met, Arn, Ars,** *aur,* **Bapt, Bar-c,** *benz-ac,*
bism, **Calc,** calen, *camph, canth, carb-an, carb-v,* **Carb-ac,** *castm,*
caust, **Chin,** *coca, cocc,* **Con,** *crot-h, cupr, cycl* (easily fatigued),
Dig, *diph,* eup-per, **Ferr,** ferr-p, fl-ac, **Gels, Graph,** ham, hell,
helon, *hydr, hyos, hyper,* ign, **Iod,** kali-br, **Kali-c, Kali-p,** *kreos,*
Lach, lac-d (whether does anything or not), **Lob,** mag-c, **Med,**
Merc, Merc-cy, mosch, **Mur-ac,** *nat-c,* nat-m, **Nit-ac,** *nux-m, nux-*
v, **Ph-ac, Phos,** *phys, phyt,* **Pic-ac, Plb, Psor, Rhus-t,** *sabad, sang,*
sanic, **Sec, Sel, Sep, Sil, Spig, Stann** (so weak she drops into
chair, instead of sitting), **Staph, Sulph, Sul-ac, Tab,** tarax, **Ter,**
thlas, **Tub, Verat,** *zinc.*

   morning : **Ars, Lach,** *nux-v, stann, sulph,* tub.
        dressing, while : *stann.*
        waking, on : **Nux-v.**
   acute disease, after : ph-ac, **Psor.**
   anaesthetic, after : *acet-ac.*
   ascending stairs, from : **Calc, Iod.**
   cares, after : *ph-ac.*
   children, in : *abrot, aeth.*
        cannot stand : **Aeth.**
        unable to hold up head : abrot, *aeth.*
   coition, after : **Sel.**
   cold, from : lach.
   convulsion after : aeth.
   debauchery, after : **Sel.**
   descending stairs : stann.
   diarrhoea, from : **Ars,** *carb-an,* acet-ac, ter, **Verat.**
   dying, as if feels : *dig.*
   emission, after : **Ph-ac, Staph.**
   epistaxis, from : ail, *apis,* carb-ac, diph.
   exertion, from slight or least : **Ars,** caps, *merc,* **Nit-ac,** nux-m,
        Sel.
   exhausted vital force : **Crot-h.**
   extremes of heat and cold : lach.
   fever, following prolonged : **Sel.**
   grief, from : **Ign,** *ph-ac.*
   heat, from : *lach, nat-c.*
        of the sun : **Nat-c, Sel.**

of the summer : *lach,* **Nat-c, Sel.**

haemorrhage, after : *ham* (piles), *kreos* (typhoid).

indolence, by : helon.

inebriety, from : eup-per.

injuries, after : *acet-ac,* **Sul-ac.**

leucorrhoea, from : **Ars,** *carb-an.*

lifting, from : **Carb-an.**

loss of blood, from ; *calen,* **Chin,** *ham,* **Ph-ac, Phos.**

    out of proportion to amount of blood lost : *ham,* hydr.

loss of animal fluid, from : **Chin,** *psor, nat-m.*

loss of sleep, from : **Cocc,** cupr, **Nux-v.**

love, after disappointed : *ph-ac.*

luxury, by : helon.

lying amel : ars.

menses, from : **Ferr,** thlas.

    scarcely recovers from one period before another begins : thlas.

    before : **Kali-c,** *mag-c.*

    during : *alum, am-c, ars,* calc, **Carb-an,** *cocc, graph, iod, verat*

        stand, can scarcely : alum, *carb-an,* cocc, verat.

        talk, can scarcely : *carb-an, cocc, stann.*

mental exertion, from ; *coca,* cocc, **Cupr,** fl-ac, helon, **Lach,** *lyc,* **Nat-c, Sel.**

mortification, after : ign, *ph-ac.*

motion, from : **Ars.**

nervous : *agn,* ambr, *coca,* dig, fl-ac, kali-br, **Kali-p, Nat-c, Pic-ac, Sil, Staph,** zinc.

    close confinement, from : sil.

    hard work, from : sil.

    following wound or surgical operation : *hyper.*

        sexual excess, after : agar.

    unmarried persons, in : *agn, con.*

nursing the sick, from : **Cocc,** *nit-ac.*

old people : *ambr,* **Bar-c,** *con, nux-m.*

over-exertion of mind and body, from : cupr.

perspiration, from : aloe, *stann.*

pain excessive, from : *calen.*
paralytic : **Gels, Mur-ac.**
    sliding down in bed : **Mur-ac.**
physical exertion, from : helon.
profund : **Camph.**
prostration of vital force : crot-h, diph.
rapid : *anthraci,* **Ars, Verat.**
sexual excess, after : *cocc,* nat-m, ph-ac.
senses, of all : *anac.*
sleep, from loss of : **Cocc,** *nit-ac.*
spasm, after : *aeth.*
standing imposible : merc-cy.
stool after : aeth, *aloe.*
sudden : **Ars,** *sel,* **Sep.**
surgical shock, after : **Acet-ac,** hyper.
sunheat, from : **Lach,** *ant-c, gels,* **Glon, Nat-c,** *nat-m.*
talking, from : **Alum,** *cocc* (feels too weak to talk loudly).
vomiting, from : *aeth, alum,* **Ant-t,** *verat.*
walking, from : aesc, *lac-d,* **Mur-ac,** *nat-c,* sep.
warm weather agg : **Ant-c,** lach.

WEAR out under physical strain : *aloe, ambr,* **Cocc,** *helon.*
    hard work from, mental and physical : *helon.*

WEARINESS (See Weakness) : aesc, **Alum, Arn, Benz-ac,** *bry,* calc, *con,* cycl, *hep,* helon, *mag-c, mag-p,* **Nux-v, Ph-ac, Phos, Pic-ac,** *plat,* op, **Sil,** *tab,* **Sulph.**
    morning : mag-c, **Nux-v,** *sulph.*
        more in morning than when retiring : bry, con, hep, *mag-c,* op, *sulph.*
        waking on : **Nux-v.**
    consumptive : med.
    cannot sleep so tired : helon.
    eating after : nat-m.
    loss of vital fluid, from : **Chin, Ph-ac, Phos.**
    sit down, must : *alum.*
    walking, when : aesc, calc, lac-d.
    weather, hot from : lach.
    women with exhausted nerves : mag-c.

WET, application : am-c, **Calc,** *merc,* **Rhus-t,** (especially, after being overheated)
  exposure in damp basement or cellers from : ant-t, **Ars, Aran,** ter.
  getting : apis, **Calc, Caust, Rhus-t.**
  weather, agg : **Am-c,** *aran,* **Calc, Dulc,** *merc,* **Nat-s, Nux-m, Rhod,** *ran-b,* **Rhus-t,** *phyt,* pic-ac, *sep, thuj,*
    amel : alum, *asar,* **Caust,** hep, *nux-v.*

WIND : *acon,* **Cham, Nux-v,** ph-ac, **Rhod.**
    cold : *acon,* **Bell,** *bry,* cupr, **Hep,** *mag-p.*
    east : calc-p, sep.
    north or west : *acon.*
    south : euphr, ip.
    snowy : ph-ac.

WINDY and stormy weather : **Bad, Nux-m, Rhod.**

WINE : alum, *arn, con,* **Nux-v, Op, Ran-b, Zinc.**

WINTER, in : *alum,* **Aur,** *ferr,* **Fl-ac,** ip, *merc, psor, petr.*

WORK, aversion to physical : (See Mind, Indolence) : *aloe,* chin, cycl.
    increased ability to : *coca, fl-ac.*

WOUNDS : *apis, arn,* **Calen,** con, **Led,** *staph, sul-ac.*
    anthrax poison : *ars.*
    bad effects of poison : *lach.*
    bites of poisonous animals : *apis, ars,* echi, hyper, **Led** (rat), merc.
    bleeding freely : *arn, ham,* **Lach,** mill, **Phos.**
      after a fall : **Arn, Hăm,** *mill.*
    bluish : *lach, lyss.*
    constitutional effects of : arn, con, **Led,** *sul-ac.*
    contused : **Arn,** *calen, ham,* sul-ac.
    crushed and lacerated : **Arn,** calen, carb-ac, ham, hyper, *led,* sul-ac.
      finger ends : **Hyper.**
      preserves integrity of lacerated parts when almost seperated from body : **Calen,** *hyper.*
    cuts : *arn,* **Staph.**
    dissecting : *anthraci, ars, crot-h, lach, pyrog.*
      gangrenous tendency to : anthraci.

incised : **Arn,** *calen, ham,* hyper.

old neglected : *calen.*

nails, needles, pins : **Hyper, Led.**

painful : *calen.*

penetrating : **Apis,** calen, *hyper,* **Led.**

post mortem : *lach.*

post surgical : *staph.*

rat bites : **Led.**

sloughing, modifies and sometimes arrests : **Calen,** carb-ac, *hyper.*

splinters from : *apis,* **Cic, Hyper,** led.

WOUNDS, stings of insects (venomous) : anthraci, *ars, crot-h,* led (mosquito).

red streaks radiate from site of sting : *anthraci,* lach, pyrog.

surgical : (See Dissecting).

tendency to erysipelas : calen, **Psor.**

Head

AIR, sensitive to a draft : **Bell, Sil.**

BALL, sensation of a, forehead in : *staph.*

BAND : (See Constriction).

BALDNESS : (See Hair).

BEATS head with hands : *hell.*

BORES head into pillow : **Apis, Bell,** *hell,* **Podo.**

BRAIN affections from suppressed eruptions : **Cic, Cupr,** *zinc.*

      symptoms, during dentition : **Bell,** *hell,* **Podo,** zinc.

BRITTLE cranial bones : *calc-p.*

CARIES : Aur.

           mastoid process : (See Ear).

COLD air, head sensitive to : **Bar-c, Hep, Nux-v, Sil.**

      amel : **Ars, Phos.**

COLDNESS : **Calc,** *sep,* valer, verat.

      vertex : sep, **Verat.**

CONCUSSION of brain : **Arn, Cic, Hyper,** sul-ac.

      chronic effects of : *cic,* **Hyper.**

CONGESTION, hyperaemia : *aml-ns, arg-n,* aster, *aur,* **Bell,** *calc-ar,* **Cact,** *chin,* erig, **Glon,** *hyos,* **Lach, Meli,** *nat-m, nat-s,* phos, *stram,* **Sulph,** verat-v.

      alcohol, after : *lach.*

      alternating with congestion to heart : *glon.*

      apoplectic, almost : verat-v.

      climaxis, at : **Lach.**

      exertion, after : aur.

      menses, delayed : *glon,*

          suppressed : **Glon, Lach,** verat-v.

      mental emotion : lach.

      brain, base of : **Verat-v.**

      spine, come up the : *phos.*

CONSTRICTION, tension (See also Drawing, Pressing) : carb-ac, **Gels,** med, nat-c, **Nit-ac,** *spig,* **Sulph.**

    band or hoop : anac, cact, **Carb-ac, Gels, Nit-ac,** *spig,* **Sulph.**

    string, as if by a : nit-ac.

    extending down length of spine : med.

    forehead : *carb-ac,* gels, *sulph.*

        band as from : **Carb-ac,** *gels.*

    nape : nat-c.

    occiput : nat-c.

        menses, before : nat-c.

DRAWN backward : **Cic,** med, verat-v.

DANDRUFF : *lyc,* **Nat-m, Phos,** sanic, **Sulph,** *thuj.*

    falls out in clouds : lyc, *phos.*

    white : **Nat-m, Thuj.**

ELONGATED sensation : *hyper.*

EMPTY, sensation, hollow : *cocc,* ign, **Phos.**

ENLARGED sensation : **Glon,** nat-c.

ERUPTION : **Ars, Calc,** cic, dulc, **Graph, Mez,** *psor.*

    crusts, scabs : *cic,* **Dulc, Mez.**

        brown : **Dulc.**

        thick : dulc, mez.

        vermin, with : *mez.*

        white : *mez.*

            with thick white pus beneath : **Mez.**

        yellow : cic, dulc.

        temples : *dulc.*

    dry : *mez.* **Psor, Sulph.**

    eczema : *cic* (without itching), *petr,* staph, *viol-o* (exudes and wets the hair).

    hair, at margin of : **Nat-m.**

    ichorous : mez.

    moist : **Graph, Hep,** *mez,* **Psor.**

        and glutinous : **Graph,** *mez.*

    offensive : *mez, psor.*

    pustules : *cic.*

        confluent with yellow scabs : *cic.*

scales : psor.

scurfy : **Graph,** *psor*.

suppuratng : *psor,* **Sulph.**

EXPANDED sensation : *arg-n*.

FONTANELES : (See Open).

FOREHEAD projected : apoc.

FULLNESS (See Enlarged) : am-c, *arg-n, bell,* **Glon,** verat-v.

blood seems to be pumped upwards : *glon*.

burst as if would : **Glon.**

HAIR, baldness : **Bar-c,** *fl-ac, graph, phos.*

patches, in : *phos.*

cut, bad effects of : acon, **Bell, Glon.**

combed, cannot be, easily : borx, fl-ac, lyc, psor, tub.

dryness : *psor,* **Thuj.**

falling : **Aur, Nat-m, Phos,** *sel,* **Sep, Syph, Thuj.**

climacteric, at : sep.

headache, after chronic : sep.

handfulls, in : **Phos.**

mercurial affections, in : **Aur.**

parturition, after : *nat-m, sep.*

pregnancy, during : **Lach.**

spots, in : **Fl-ac,** *phos.*

syphilis, in : **Aur.**

touched, when : *nat-m,* sep.

frowsy : *borx.*

gray, becomes : **Lyc,** *ph-ac.*

lustreless : *psor.*

plica polonica : bar-c, *psor,* sars, tub.

splits : *borx.*

sticks together : borx, lyc, **Mez,** *psor, tub.*

at ends : *borx,*

tangles easily ; *borx, fl-ac,* lyc, *psor, tub.*

HEAT, touch of, agg : *glon.*

HEAT : aster, **Bell,** *bry,* **Calc,** cic, **Graph,** *podo, sep, sulph,* verat-v.

air, surrounded by hot, as if : aster.

coldness of body, with : **Arn,** *hell.*

heat of face, and, but body cold : **Arn,** *hell, phyt.*

vertex : *calc,* **Graph, Lach,** *sep,* **Sulph.**

headache, during : **Sulph.**

menopause, during : **Lach.**

spine, come up the : *phos.*

HEAT flushes of : **Aml-ns, Bell,** cic, **Glon.**

forehead : **Bell.**

HEAVINESS (See Pressing) : *arg-n,* am-c, **Gels, Lach,** med.

occiput : *lach.*

lead, as if : *lach.*

vertex : (See Pressing).

HEMICRANIA : (See Pain).

HOLLOW : (See Empty).

HYDROCEPHALUS : **Apis,** apoc, *arn* (deathly coldness in forearm of children), *bry,* dig, *hell,* kali-br (first stage), *kali-m, sulph,* tub, zinc.

after Bry and Kali-m : sulph.

post-scarlatinal : *apis, hell,* **Sulph,** tub, **Zinc.**

tubercular : apis, hell, **Sulph, Tub.**

INFLAMMATION of brain : *acon,* apis, **Bell,** *hell,* hyos, verat-v.

meningitis : *apis, arn,* **Bell, Hell.**

after Apis, Hell and Sulph fail : tub.

injury, after : **Arn.**

basilar : *tub,* **Verat-v.**

tubercular : *calc,* hell, *sulph, tub.*

INJURIES of head, after : **Arn, Nat-s.**

JERKING of the head : *agar,* hyos, stram, verat-v.

LARGE (See Enlarged) : **Bar-c, Calc,** nat-c, *sil.*

brain feels : *glon.*

LOOSENESS of brain, sensation : bell, bry, **Chin,** *rhus-t,* **Spig,** sul-ac.

shaking the head : *rhus-t.*

stepping, on : **Rhus-t.**

falling from side to side, as if : bell, bry, rhus-t, *spig,* sul-ac.

forehead : *sul-ac.*

LUMP, sensation, of, vertex, ice on : sep, verat.

MOTION of the head : bell, *calc-p,* tarent.

        involuntary : zinc.

           and one hand : apoc, bry, *hell,* zinc.

        nodding of : *verat-v.*

        rolling head : **Bell,** *cina, hell, podo,* zinc.

        rub against something : **Tarent.**

NAEVUS of children, right temple : fl-ac.

NODDING : (See Motion).

NUMBNESS, sensation : *petr, plat.*

        brain : *plat.*

        forehead : **Plat.**

        vertex : *plat.*

OPEN, fontanells and sutures : apoc, **Calc, Calc-p, Sil.**

        close and reopen : *calc-p.*

PAIN, headache in general : agar, all-c, aloe, *am-c,* anac, *ant-c,* **Arg-n, Ars,** *aur,* bar-c, **Bell,** bism, **Bry,** *cact, calc-p,* carb-an, **Chin,** cocc, *coff,* croc, cycl, eup-per, *ferr,* **Gels, Glon,** hyper, *ign, kali-bi, kalm, kreos, lac-d,* **Lach,** lil-t, lob, lyss, *mag-m,* **Mag-p,** *med, meny, mez, nat-c,* **Nat-m,** *nat-s,* **Nit-ac, Nux-v,** *petr,* ph-ac, *podo,* phyt, pic-ac, plat, **Psor,** *rhus-t,* sabad, sang, sars, sel, **Sep, Sil,** *spig,* stann, **Sulph,** *syph,* tab, tarent, *ther, thuj,* **Tub.**

        morning : **Agar,** *bry,* cycl, lac-d, **Nux-v.**

          ceases towards evening : *bry.*

          increases and decreases with sun ; **Glon,** *kalm, nat-m, sang, spig,* tab.

          increases until noon, and then gradually decreases : *nat-m, spig,* tab.

          rising, on : **Bry, Cycl,** lac-d.

          amel by daylight : *syph.*

        forenoon, 10 a.m. : **Nat-m.**

        10 to 11 a. m. : mag-p.

        11 a. m. : sulph.

        afternoon ; **Bell, Lyc, Sel,** syph.

        4 to 5 p. m. : mag-p.

        until midnight : lob.

        4 p. m. : **Lyc,** syph.

worse from 10 to 11 p. m., ceasing at day-break :
   syph.
      ceases at 11 or 12 p. m. : **Lyc.**
evening : **All-c, Bell, Sulph.**
   amel, 10 to 11 p. m. : **Lyc.**
night : **Merc, Nit-ac, Syph.**
acids, from : ant-c.
air, draft of, from : **Sil.**
   open : coff, *mag-m, nux-v.*
alcohol, from : **Agar,** *ant-c.* **Lach,** lob, **Nux-v,** *sel.*
alternating with lumbago : aloe.
anger, from : *plat,* nux-v, rhus-t.
ascending steps, on : **Bell, Bry, Calc,** meny.
attention or application, too close : *arg-n,* sabad.
bandage, tight (See Pressure) amel : apis, *arg-n,* **Bell,** lac-d,
   puls.
bathing river, after : **Ant-c.**
   cold, after : **Ant-c.**
beer, from : *rhus-t.*
blindness precedes attack or vision blurred : gels, **Iris,** *kali-
   bi,* lac-d, d, **Nat-m.**
bright light, from : bell, **Lyc, Stram.**
businessmen, overworked, of : **Pic-ac.**
catarrhal : *all-c.*
chagrin, from : *plat.*
chill, during : **Nat-m.**
choriec persons, in : *agar.*
chronic : *lyss,* psor, sil, *thuj,* **Tub.**
   since some severe disease of youth : *psor, sil.*
   sycotic : thuj.
   syphilitic : thuj.
   tubercular : **Tub.**
climaxis, durig : cact, croc, glon, **Lach,** *sang.*
cold amel : **Aloe,** *ars* (temporary), spig.
cold, from becoming : **Bell, Bry,** ign (cold wind), **Mag-p.**
   from taking ; nat-c, rhus-t.
constipation, from : aloe, aur, **Bry,** *coll,* op, **Nux-v.**

coughing, on : **Bry, Caps,** nux-v.

    as if head would fly to pieces : **Bry, Caps.**

dancing, from : *arg-n.*

darkness, amel : *sang.*

debauchery, after : sel.

delirious (in fever or pain) persons, in : agar.

diarrhoea with : calc-p.

    alternating with headache : aloe, **Podo.**

dog-bite, rabid or not, from : *lyss.*

eating, after : **Nux-v.**

    overeating, after : **Nux-v.**

    amel : *anac, kali-p,* psor.

eat, if he does not : *lyc.*

emotion, from depressing : *pic-ac.*

epileptic attacks, after : kali-bi.

epistaxis amel : bufo, ferr-p, ham, mag-s, *meli, psor.*

exertion of body, from : **Bell,** epig, mag-p

excitement of emotion, after : kali-p, *lyss, pic-ac.*

    depressing emotion : *pic-ac.*

eye-strain, from : *calc-p, nat-m, ph-ac,* **Tub.**

    when glasses fail to relieve : **Tub.**

fall upon occiput, after, as if being lifted high up into air,
    great anxiety lest she fall from that height : **Hyper.**

fat food, from : ant-c.

fruit, from : ant-c.

gaslight, from : **Glon,** *lach,* **Nat-c.**

gastric : *anac,* **Ant-c,** arg-n, **Bry,** iris, lob, **Nux-v,** tarax.

    sedentary persons in : *anac, arg-n,* bry, **Nux-v.**

gastralgia alternating or attending with : arg-n.

grief, from : *pic-ac,* **Ph-ac.**

haemorrhage, after : **Chin,** glon (after uterine).

haemorrhoids, from : **Nux-v.**

hammering : **Bell, Ferr, Nat-m,** tab (right sided).

hat, from pressure of : calc-p, **Carb-v,** Nat-m, **Nit-ac.**

    heat, during : **Nat-m.**

    amel : **Mag-p, Sil.**

heated, from becoming : aloe, **Ant-c, Bell,** *thuj,*

by fire or stove : **Ant-c, Glon.**

hemicrania : arg-n, aml-ns (when afflicted side is pale).

beginning at nape and extend overhead : **Sang,** sil.

nail driven into, as if : **Coff, Ign, Nux-v, Thuj,**

women, in : sep.

right-sided : cact, *mez,* **Sang, Sil,** *tab.*

as if struck by hammer or club : tab.

left-sided : nat-m, **Spig.**

hepatic trouble : iris, nux-v.

hysterical : ign, mag-m, *nat-m, plat, sep.*

increases gradually and decrease gradually : plat, **Stann.**

intoxication : (See Alcohol From).

iron hoop around head, as if : *anac,* sulph, *tub.*

ironing, from : **Bry, Sep.**

jar, from : **Bell,** med.

lemonade, from : *sel.*

lie down, must : **Ferr,** kali-bi.

light in general, from : **Bell,** *bry, gels,* kali-bi, *lac-d,* nux-v, *sil,*
Tab, *tarent.*

artificial, from : *glon.*

bright, from : **Lyss.**

gas : (See Gas Light).

literary men, of : arg-n.

lumbago alternating with : aloe.

and : *phyt.*

lying, from : **Bell, Chin** (must walk), **Bry, Gels. Lach,** ph-ac,
rhus-t, *sil,* ther.

on back of head, by : *cocc.*

in cold, from : rhus-t.

with head low : gels.

amel : anac, *bry,* gels, mag-m, *ph-ac, sil.*

on affected side : **Ign.**

lying down in bed at night, amel : anac.

on painful side, amel : coff, ign, nux-v, thuj.

masturbation, from : **Nux-v.**

menses, before : *croc, lach,* lil-t, nat-c (with tension in nape
or occiput), *nat-m,* sep.

amel when flow begins and return when stops : all-c, **Lach, Zinc.**

menses, during : croc, **Kreos,** *lac-d, lach,* lil-t, *nat-c,* **Nat-m,** sep.

    amel : all-c, **Bell, Lach, Zinc.**

    return when flow stops : all-c, **Lach, Zinc.**

    after : chin, *croc, lach,* lil-t, *nat-m, sep.*

    in place of : **Glon.**

    suppressed : **Psor.**

mental emotion, from : *arg-met,* aur, lyss (chronic), mag-p, *pic-ac.*

    exertion, from : *arg-n,* coff, gels, epig, *kali-p,* lyss (chronic), mag-p, **Nat-c,** nux-v, **Pic-ac,** sep, **Tub.**

mercury, from : **Hep, Nit-ac,** *sars.*

motion, from : *anac,* **Bell, Bry,** lac-d, **Lach,** mag-m, *mag-p.* ph-ac, *phyt,* sep, *sil.*

    amel : indg, **Rhus-t,** sep.

move, on begining to : *sep,* ther.

moving head, from : **Bell, Bry, Gels,** ther.

music, from : *ph-ac.*

nervous : anac, **Arg-n,** bry, cocc, croc, ign, meli, mag-m, **Nux-v, Op,** verat-v.

nerves, exhausted, from : **Ph-ac.**

neuralgic : all-c, bell, spig, syph, tarent.

noise, from : **Bell,** kali-bi, *lac-d, lyss,* mag-m, nux-v, ph-ac, *sil,* tab, tarent.

    falling or running water, of : **Lyss.**

old people, of : *bar-c.*

overheating : (See Heated).

pain in the neck, with : **Gels.**

    in nape of : **Cocc, Gels, Ph-ac.**

paroxysmal : *mag-p,* tab.

periodic : *cact,* **Cedr, Chin, Chinin-s, Nat-m, Nit-ac, Sang,** *spig,* tab.

    morning : spig.

    every afternoon : *sel.*

    every two, three or four days : ferr.

    every seventh day : sabad, *sang, sil, sulph.*

eighth day : iris.

week : sulph.

every two or three weeks : ferr, sulph.

six weeks : *mag-m*.

perspiration, amel : *nat-m*.

pressure, from : **Lach.**

amel : apis, *arg-n,* **Bell, Bry,** cact, gels, ign, indg, lac-d, **Mag-m, Mag-p,** meny, puls, sep, *sil,* **stront-c.**

pulsating : **Bell, Chin, Ferr, Glon,** *lac-d,* **Nat-m,** petr.

rest agg : (See Motion).

amel : sang.

riding train, carriage or boat from : **Cocc.**

rubbing, amel : indg.

against pillow, amel : tarent.

school girls : **Calc-p,** mag-p, *nat-m,* **Ph-ac,** psor, **Tub.**

sexual excess, after : **Agar,** *chin,* **Sep, Sil,** *thuj.*

shaking head : *rhus-t.*

sick headache, chronic, after some serious illness of youth : **Psor, Sil.**

every week or every two weeks : **Sulph.**

lasting one or two days : tab.

coming each morning, intolerable at noon, deathly nausea : *tab.*

paroxysmal : tab.

sitting, by : chin, *rhus-t.*

erect, amel : **Bell.**

sit up and hold it together, has to : carb-ac.

skull would burst, as if : **Chin.**

sleep, after : **Lach** (dreads to go to sleep, because awakes with headaches).

falling asleep, on amel : anac.

smoking, from : *gels, ign, lob.*

spinal, affection from : *agar.*

spine, begining in cervical : **Gels.**

extending to : cocc.

down : med.

stepping : (See Walking).

stool insufficient, after : *aloe.*

stoopping, from : **Bell, Bry,** ign, lach, nux-v, **Sep.**

straining eyes, from : **Nat-m.**

students growing too fast : **Ph-ac,** pic-ac.

study, after hard : mag-p, pic-ac, *tub.*

summer : *ant-c,* **Glon, Nat-c.**

sun, from exposure to : **Ant-c, Bry,** *gels,* **Glon, Lach. Nat-c,** nux-v.

sun increases and decreases, every day, with : **Glon,** kalm, **Nat-c,** *nat-m,* **Spig,** tab.

suppressed eruption, from : *ant-c, psor.*

        gonorrhoea, from : *sars.*

sycotic : **Thuj.**

syphilis, from : *sars,* **Thuj.**

talking, from : coff.

tea, after : sel, thuj.

teachers, of : pic-ac.

terrific shocks, in : *sep.*

thinking, from : coff, **Sabad.**

tightly tying, amel : arg-n, *puls.*

tobacco smoking, from : (See Smoking).

tightly bound by a cord, as if with : cocc.

touch : **Mez,** tarent.

tubercular : *tub.*

urination, profuse, amel : acon, **Gels,** *ign, sil,* verat.

uterine haemorrhage, after : *glon.*

uterine irritation or displacement, with : lil-t, plat.

uncovering head : *sil.*

vexation, after : **Mez.**

violent pain : **Bell, Bry, Glon, Lach, Meli, Sil,** ther.

vision blurred, preceds the attack : kali-bi.

      with zig-zag dazzling, like lightening in eyes : nat-m.

      returns as headache increases : kali-bi, iris, lac-d, nat-m.

walking while : **Bell, Bry, Glon,** *rhus-t.*

      from others walking on the floor : ther.

wandering pains : mag-p.

warmth amel : ign, rhus-t.

water, noise of running, from : **Lyss.**

weight, pressing like a heavy, on vertex : *cact,* **Glon,** *lach meny.*

> crushing, on vertex from grief or exhausted nerves : **Ph-ac.**

wine, from : *sel,* zinc.

winter, returning every : **Bism, Podo.**

winter headache and summer diarrhoea : **Podo.**

work, from : anac, epip (after a hard day's work).

worms, from : *sabad.*

wrapping up head : **Iod, Lyc, Puls.**

> amel : **Bell,** *mag-m, mag-p,* **Rhus-t, Sil,** *stront-c.*

extending to eye : spig.

> left : spig.
>
> right : *sang,* sil.
>
> temple : spig.
>
>> left : *spig.*
>>
>> right : *sang,* sil.

PAIN, brain : plat.

> brain, deep in : gels (base), *spig,* ther.
>
> forehead : **Acon,** *aloe,* **Am-c,** *arg-n,* **Bell, Bry, Glon,** *lac-d, mag-m,* **Puls,** *sep.*
>
>> morning, rising, on : bry, lac-d.
>>
>> air open : *mag-m.*
>>
>> bandaging tight, amel : arg-n, lac-d, puls.
>>
>> foot steps : aloe, **Bell,** *bry,* **Nux-v, Sil.**
>>
>> menses, during : lac-d, sep.
>>
>> motion, on : *lac-d,* mag-m.
>>
>> noise, from : lac-d.
>>
>> periodic, every six week : mag-m.
>>
>> pressure from : arg-n.
>>
>>> amel : *lac-d.*
>>
>> extending to occiput : *lac-d.*
>>
>>> eyes around : mag-m.
>>>
>>>> above (supra-orbital) : mag-p.
>>>>
>>>>> right side : *mag-p.*

occiput : **Bell, Bry, Chin, Cocc, Gels, Glon,** *kali-bi, med,*
nat-m, **Petr, Ph-ac,** sil.

grief, after : **Ph-ac.**

load, as from : *petr.*

menses, before : nat-c.

motion : ph-ac.

music : *ph-ac.*

nerves, from exhausted : **Ph-ac.**

noise : *ph-ac.*

pulsating : ph-ac.

extending, eyes to, right : **Sang, Sil.**

left : **Spig.**

forehead, to : *kali-bi, ph-ac.*

suppressed nasal discharge from : *kali-bi.*

forward : ph-ac.

head, to : **Chin, Gels,** *mag-p,* ph-ac, sang, *sil.*

neck, to : **Cocc.**

spine, to : *cocc.*

nape : **Cocc,** ph-ac, **Pic-ac,** nat-m, sil.

temple, pressure in : arg-n.

screwing in : arg-n.

vertex : *calc,* plat.

anaemic girls : *calc-p.*

periodic from above downwards : meny.

PAIN, blown as if : (See Torn as if).

burning : graph, med.

brain : med.

occiput : med.

extending down the spine : med.

vertex : **Calc, Graph,** *lach,* **Sulph.**

menopause, during : **Lach, Sang, Sulph.**

menses, during : *lach.*

spots, in ; **Calc,** graph, **Sulph.**

cold spot : *sep,* verat.

bursting : am-c, **Bell, Bry, Calc,** caps, **Chin, Glon, Lach,** mag-m,
nat-c, **Nat-m** *sang,* **Sep,** sulph.

left : *nat-m.*

coughing, when : *bry, caps.*

ironing, when : *bry.*

lochia, suppressed when : *bry.*

mental exertion, from : sep.

motion, from : *bry,* sep.

    continued hard motion amel : sep.

pressure, amel : sep.

sleep, amel : *sang.*

stooping, while : *bry,* sep.

brain would burst out through forehead, as if : *bry.*

forehead : am-c, *bell, gels, glon, mag-m.*

    one sided : *sang, sil.*

temples : *lach.*

    lying, after : lach.

    motion : *lach.*

    pressure : lach.

    sleep, after : *lach.*

    stooping, on : lach.

    eyes around : mag-m.

vertex : **Calc, Graph, Sulph.**

    menopause, during : **Lach.**

crushed as if : **Arg-met,** ph-ac.

vertex : ph-ac.

    exhausted nerve and long lasting grief : ph-ac.

cutting : tub.

forehead, extending from about right eye to occiput :
    tub.

drawing : **Chin, Merc,** nat-c.

occiput : nat-c.

dull : *all-c,* **Nux-v, Puls.**

forehead : **Carb-ac.**

    as if a rubber band stretched over : **Carb-ac,** gels,
        plat, sulph.

temples : **Carb-ac.**

    from temple to temple : carb-ac, gels, *plat,*
        sulph.

nail, as from a : **Coff,** *ign, nux-v,* **Thuj.**

      sides : *coff, ign,* nux-v, **Thuj.**

pressing : *arg-n,* **Bell, Chin,** cimic, **Glon, Lach,** *meny,* nat-c, *petr, ph-ac, sep,* ther, *thuj.*

      as if top of head would fly off : cimic.

      button, convex, being pressed as from : *thuj.*

      mental exertion, from : **Pic-ac,** *sep.*

      motion, from : **Bell, Bry,** *sep.*

         continued motion amel : *sep.*

      pressure amel : *meny,* sep.

      stooping, on : sep.

      forehead : **Acon,** *arg-n,* **Bell, Bry, Nux-v,** petr, *stict, ther.*

         behind eyes : ther.

         extending into eyes : *cimic.*

    occiput : nat-c, **Petr,** ph-ac.

      lead, as from : petr.

      menses, before : nat-c.

      music : ph-ac.

      motion : ph-ac.

      noise : ph-ac.

      extending forward : ph-ac.

                down the back : *cimic.*

    temples : **Glon, Lach.**

      lying, after : lach.

      motion, on : **Lach.**

      pressure, from : *lach.*

      sleep, after : *lach.*

      stooping, on : *lach.*

    vertex : **Acon, Bell, Cact, Glon, Lach,** *meny,* **Ph-ac,** *sep, sulph.*

      ascending steps : *calc,* **Meny.**

      grief, after : *ph-ac.*

      nerves, from exhausted : *ph-ac.*

      pressure, amel : *alum,* **Cact,** *meny, verat.*

      weight, heavy, pressing upon head at every step : *cact, glon, lach, meny.*

      extendng downwards : **Meny.**

pulled, sensation as if hair were : **Chin,** mag-c, kali-n, *phos.*

screwing, forehead : *arg-n.*

temple : *arg-n.*

sore, bruised : caust, *eup-per,* **Gels,** ip, mag-c, *petr, phyt,* plat.

brain, in : **Gels.**

occiput : **Eup-per, Gels.**

vertex : kali-n, *mag-c,* phos.

as if hair were pulled : kali-n, *mag-c,* phos.

stinging : **Apis,** *nit-ac, sulph.*

stitching : *bry,* tarent.

torn, as if : **Carb-an,** *coff, rhus-t,* verat.

brain as if torn to pieces : verat.

has to sit up at night and hold it together : *carb-an.*

PARALYSIS of brain : am-c, hell, *zinc.*

threatened : am-c, tub, *zinc.*

PERSPIRATION, scalp : **Calc,** *mag-m,* **Merc, Rheum,** sanic, **Sil** (lower than calc).

fever, during : cham.

sleep, during : **Calc,** sanic, *sil.*

wetting pillow far around : **Calc,** sanic. *sil.*

sour : *hep,* rheum, **Sil.**

warm : cham (wetting the hair).

forehead : *carb-v,* croc, *stann,* **Verat.**

cold : **Carb-v,** croc, **Op, Verat.**

cold, with large drops on : **Carb-v,** *croc.*

occiput, back of head : **Calc,** *sil.*

PROJECTED, forehead : apoc.

PULSATING, beating, throbbing : aur, **Bell, Chin,** *croc,* **Ferr, Glon** (must hold with hand), *lac-d,* nat-m, *petr,* spig, *verat-v.*

jar, from any : **Bell,** glon.

lie down, must : ferr.

lying, while : glon.

pulse, at every : *glon.*

step, at every : *glon.*

brain : *bell,* meli.

forehead : **Bell, Glon, Lac-d.**

sides : aur.

temples : aur, **Bell, Glon.**

RETRACTION : (See Drawn, Backward).

ROLLING of the : (See Motion).

RUSH of blood : (See Congestion).

              pregnant women, in : **Glon.**

SENSITIVENESS of brain : **Bell, Chin, Gels, Glon.**

              brushing hair, from : **Arn, Sil.**

              jar, to the least : **Bell,** *glon,* **Nit-ac.**

              stepping, to : **Bell, Glon.**

SHOCKS, blows, jerks, etc. : *cic, glon.*

              pulse, at each beat of : **Glon.**

SUNSTROKE : Glon.

SURGING of blood : **Aml-ns, Bell, Glon.**

SWASHING sensation : rhus-t.

TENSION : (See Constriction).

THIN cranial bones : *calc-p.*

THROBBING : (See Pulsating).

TREMBLING : ant-t.

TIGHṬNESS : (See Constriction).

UNCOVERING head agg : **Bell, Hep,** *psor,* rhod, sanic, **Sil.**

              due to hair cut : **Bell, Glon,** *sil.*

WARM covering on head, agg : **Ars, Iod, Lyc.**

WATER, sensation, dripping on head, as of : cann-s.

WEAKNESS : phos, zinc.

              brain : *phos,* **Zinc.**

              feeling in head : cocc.

WEIGHT : (See Heaviness, Pressing).

◻◻◻

Kidneys

BUBBLING, sensation in region of : *berb, med.*

CALCULI : (See Urine, Sediment).

CONTRACTED : plb.

HAEMORRHAGE : (See Urine, Bloody).

INFLAMMATION : Apis, Benz-ac, Canth, *merc-c,* plb, **Ter.**

LAMENESS, region of, painful pressure, with : *berb.*

NUMBNESS, region of : **Berb.**

PAIN : Benz-ac, Berb, Canth, cann-s, *lyc, med, plb,* **Sars,** tab, *ter.*
    colic, left side : **Berb,** *tab.*
        either side with urging and strangury : **Canth.**
        right side : *lyc,* sars.
    fatigue, from : berb.
    jar, from : berb.
    lying, when : *berb.*
    sitting, when : *berb.*
    urination, amel : **Lyc,** *med.*
    extending downwards : berb, *sars.*
        right side : *lyc, sars.*
    ureters, right side : berb, **Lyc,** tab.
        left side : **Berb,** lyc, *tab.*
        radiatng, from renal region : **Berb,** med.
            into urethra : **Berb.**

PAIN, aching : *lyc, oci*
    urination, amel : **Lyc.**
   burning : *berb, cann-s, canth,* **Ter.**
   cramping : tab.
   cutting : *berb,* **Canth.**
        region of, down into bladder and urethra,
           left : **Berb,** tab.
           right : **Lyc.**
        ureters : **Berb, Lyc,** *med, oci, tab.*

calculus, with sensation of passage : **Berb, Lyc,** *med,* oci.
drawing : **Clem, Ter.**
    region of : berb, **Ter.**
nail, as from : **Coff,** *ign, nux-v,* **Thuj.**
needle, pricking : (See Stitching).
pressing, region of : *berb.*
shooting : (See Stitching).
sore, bruised : **Berb** (agg in bed in morning).
    region of : **Berb.**
stinging, stiching : **Berb.**
    radiating : **Berb.**
    region of, down ureter into bladder and urethra,
        left : **Berb,** tab.
        right : **Lyc.**

STIFFNESS : *berb.*

SUPPRESSION of urine : am-c, **Arn,** *arum-t, bell, colch, dig,* dulc, *hell,*
    merc-c, sec, **Stram.**
        brain troubles, in : *hell.*
        catarrhal, in grown up children : *dulc.*
        dropsy, in : hell.
        wading with bare feet in cold water, from : **Dulc.**

URAEMIC condition : *calc.*
        cold, from : *calc.*

❑❑❑

Larynx and Trachea

ANAESTHESIA larynx : kali-bi.

CATARRH, larynx : all-c, *brom*, dros, *hep*.

COLD sensation on inspiration : **Brom**, *rhus-t*, *sulph*.
    shaving amel : *brom*.
        agg : carb-an.

CONSTRICTION : dros.
    larynx : *all-c*, *dros*, **Iod**, med, *naja*.
    lying on face, amel : *med*.
    protruding tongue, amel : med.
    spasm of epiglotis, from : med.
    weakness of epiglotis, from : med.

CRAWLING, larynx : *dros*.

CROUP : acet-ac, **Acon**, **Brom**, **Calc-s**, dros, **Hep**, *iod*, **Kali-bi**, **Spong**.
    morning **Hep**.
    night : **Spong**.
    anxious : spong.
    expiration, during : acon.
    exposure to cold dry wind : **Acon**, **Hep**.
    inspiration, during : spong.
    membranous and diphtheritic : **Brom**, *chlor*, **Diph**, **Kali-bi**,
        lac-c, *merc-cy*.
        extending upwards towards nose : **Brom**.
    urticaria, in place of : ars.
    wheezing : spong.
    whooping, during : **Brom**.

DIPHTHERIA : (See Croup).

DRYNESS, larynx : **Con**, *dros*, *phos*, **Spong**.
    trachea : dros, *spong*.

DUST, as from : **Dros**.

FEATHER-LIKE sensation : dros.

FOOD easily gets into larynx : *kali-c*.

F-13

FOREIGN body : (See Dyspnoea, Respiration).

GRASPED (See Constriction), child grasps the larynx : *all-c*, **Iod**.

HEMMING : (See Scraping).

HOARSENESS : (See Voice).

INFLAMMATIONS, larynx : **Acon, All-c, Arg-n, Dros,** spong.

        singers, in : *arg-met,* **Arg-n.**

        speakers, in : **Arum-t.**

IRRITATION in air passages,

        larynx : **Arg-met, Arg-n, Bell,** *brom,* **Bry, Caust, Dros.**

        talking : **Arg-met, Dros.**

LARYNGISMUS stridulus : **Bell,** *cupr,* **Gels.**

MUCUS : *arg-met, brom,* kali-bi.

        larynx : *arg-met,* **Brom,** *canth,* **Kali-bi,** *sel, stann.*

        copious : *arg-met.*

        ejected with difficulty : *canth.*

        trachea : *arg-met,* **Kali-bi.**

OBSTRUCTED, larynx, lying on face, amel : med.

        protruding tongue, amel : med.

        spasm, from : med.

PAIN larynx : *arum-t,* **Bell,** *brom,* dros, **Phos.**

        coughing, on : **All-c, Bell,** *brom,* dros.

        grasps the larynx : **All-c.**

        talking, while : **Phos.**

PAIN, raw : alum, **Arg-met,** *caust,* **Phos.**

        larynx : **Arg-met,** *caust,* **Phos, Rumx.**

        morning : **Caust.**

        evening : *carb-v,* **Phos.**

        coughing, from : **Arg-met, Caust,** *rumx.*

        inspiration, during : **Acon, Hep, Phos,** rumx.

        swallowing, on : *arg-met.*

        talking, from : **Arg-met.**

        trachea : **Arg-met, Caust, Phos, Rumx.**

        coughing. on : **Arg-met,** *caust, rumx.*

        swallowing, on : *arg-met.*

PAIN, raw, trachea, talking : **Arg-met**.

over bifurcation : arg-met.

soreness : alum, *arg-met*, *arum-t*, *caust*, *med*, **Phos**.

larynx : **Arg-met**, *caust*, **Dros**, **Phos**, *spong*.

clergyman's sore throat : **Arum-t**, *dros*.

coughing, on : **Arg-met**, *caust*, *dros*.

swallowing, on : *arg-met*.

talking painful : *phos*

trachea : *caust*.

coughing, on : **Caust**.

tearing, larynx, coughing, on : med.

PARALYSIS of larynx : **Caust**.

PHTHISIS larynx : *dros*, *sel*.

whooping cough, after : **Dros**.

POLYP, larynx : *arg-n*, *sang*.

RATTLING, larynx : *ant-t*, **Brom** (no choking as in hep).

trachea (See Respiration) : **Ant-t**.

ROUGHNESS : dros, *phos*.

larynx : dros, *phos*.

trachea : dros, phos.

SCRAPING, clearing larynx : *arg-met*, *dros*, *sel*, *stann*.

reading aloud, from : *arg-met*.

SMOKE sensation of, larynx : *brom*.

SULPHUR vapour, as from : *brom*.

TICKLING in air passages : **Acon**, **Cham**, **Hyos**, **Nux-v**, rumx.

larynx in : **Rumx**.

throat pit, in : caust, **Rumx**.

VOICE, barking : bell, brom, dros, spong.

change or alteration in timbre of voice in singers and public speakers : *arg-met*, **Arum-t**.

changeable : **Arum-t**, rumx.

cracked : dros.

deep : **Dros**, *stann*.

VOICE, hoarseness : alum, *ambr*, **Arg-met**, **Arum-t**, **Brom**, **Calc**, **Carb-v**, **Caust**, **Dros**, *euphr*, **Hep**, **Iod**, **Kali-bi**, *nux-m*, *rumx*, *spong*, **Stann**.

morning : **Calc**, carb-v, **Caust**, *eup-per*.

evening : **Carb-v**, phos, *rumx*.

cold, after : rumx.

cough, amel : *stann*.

damp weather, in : *carb-v*.

expectorating mucus, amel : *stann*.

over-use of voice : alum, *arg-met*, **Arum-t**.

painless : **Calc**.

singing, singer professional : *arg-met*, alum, **Arum-t**.

speakers, actors, public : alum, *arg-met*, **Arum-t**.

sudden : nux-m.

talking, from : alum, **Arg-met**, **Arum-t**.

walking in open air : euphr, **Hep**, *nux-m*.

> against the wind : euphr, hep, **Nux-m**.

warm wet weather agg : *carb-v*.

hollow : *stann*.

husky : *sel*, *stann*.

> begining to sing, when : sel.

lost : **Ant-c**, **Arg-met**, arum-t, **Brom**, **Carb-v**, **Caust**, *dros*, lach, *sel*.

morning : *caust*.

evening : **Carb-v**.

exertion, on : **Carb-v**.

heated, from being : *ant-c*.

long use of voice, from : sel.

singers, professional : **Arg-met**, **Caust**, **Phos**, *sel*.

wind, after exposure to north-west : *acon*, *arum-t*, **Hep**.

toneless : **Dros**.

uncertain : (See Changeable)

uncontrollable : **Arum-t**.

❑❑❑

Mind

ABASHED : *ph-ac.*

ABSENT-MINDED (See Forgetful) : anac, *agn*, *kali-br*, kreos, *lac-c*, **Lach**, **Nat-m**, **Nux-m**.

ABUSIVE : croc, *hyos*, *nux-v*, *verat*.

ACTIVE : tub.

ACTIVITY, desires : (See Industrious).
           lack of, or of 'boyish-go' : aur.
           overactivity : **Coff**, phys.

ACUTENESS : (See Memory).

AFFECTIONATE : *croc, puls.*

AIMLESS : (See Ambition, Loss of).

AMBITION, loss of (See Indolence) : lil-t (no ambition, though desires to do something), phos (in brain or nervous troubles).

AMOROUS : (See Lewdness and Lascivious).

AMUSEMENT, averse to : bar-c, lil-t, sulph.

ANGER, irascibility (See Irritability and Quarrelsome) : **Ars**, **Aur**, *bell*, **Bry**, *calc-p*, *caps*, **Cham**, *cocc*, *coloc*, *con*, hell, **Hep**, *hyos*, **Ign**, **Lach**, **Lyc**, *mez*, *mur-ac*, *nat-m*, **Nux-v**, **Petr**, *ph-ac*, **Staph**.
           ailments after anger, vexation, etc. : acon, *apis*, *aur*, *bry*, *calc-p*, caust., **Cham**, **Cocc**, **Coloc**, hyos, **Ign**, *lach*, *lyc*, *nat-m*, nux-v, *ph-ac*, **Plat**, **Staph**.
                after anger with indignation : *aur*, **Coloc**, nat-m, **Staph**.
                   with silent grief : aur, **Ign**, **Lyc**, *nat-m*, **Staph**.
           attention, at every little : *ant-c*, *nat-m*.
           but soon sorry for it : mez.
           complaints about ones own : aloe.
           contradiction, from : **Aur**, con, **Ign**, **Lyc**.
           constipation, agg : aloe.
           disposition, to : cocc.
           fault finding, from : *ign*.
           harmless things, at : mez.

      himself about : aloe, *ign*.

      questioned, when : *coloc*.

      suppressed, from : aur, cham, *ign*, **Staph**.

      things refused, when : **Cham**.

      trembling, with : *aur*, **Staph**.

      trifles at : *caps*, cocc, *hep*, **Ign**, mez, **Plat**, *staph*.

ANGUISH : **Acon**, *arg-n*, **Ars**, *bism*, canth, *coff*, hell, iod, nit-ac.

      driving from place to place : **Ars**.

      loss of dearest friend, from : nit-ac,

      restless (he sits, then walks, then lies, never long in one place) : **Bism**.

ANSWERS, abruptly, shortly, curtly : cham, *hyos*.

      aversion to : sul-ac.

          inaptness, from : sul-ac.

      correctly : *ph-ac*.

          but unconsciousness and delirium returns at once : **Arn**, **Bapt**, **Hyos**.

      falls asleep in the midst of sentence : **Bapt**.

      hastily : bell, *lyc*.

      incoherently : *hyos*.

      irrelevantly : *hyos*, **Phos**, **Sulph**.

      peevishly : *cham*.

      refuses to : *arn*, bell, *hell*, *hyos*, **Phos**, **Sulph**.

      repeats questions first : ambr, *caust*, zinc.

      slowly : *hell*, **Ph-ac**, **Phos**.

      spoken to, when, yet knows no one : *cic*.

      stupor returns quickly after : **Arn**, bapt, **Hyos**, *ph-ac*.

ANTICIPATION, complaints from : *arg-n*, *gels*, med

ANXIETY : **Acon**, *ambr*, *anac*, *ant-c*, *ant-t*, **Arg-n**, **Ars**, *asar*, **Aur**, *borx*, **Cact**, **Camph**, **Caust**, *crot-h*, *cupr*, *gels*, *hep* (unreasonably), iod, kali-br, *lach*, *lil-t*, med, **Nat-c**, **Nit-ac**, *nux-v*, **Phos**, **Psor**, **Rhus-t**, *samb*, *sep*, *sil*.

      evening : **Nit-ac**, **Sep**.

      night : **Ars** (driving out of bed).

          midnight after : **Ars**.

      apprehension when on engagement : **Arg-n**.

bed, in : **Ars**, **Rhus-t**.

business : nux-v.

business failures of : psor.

children, in : ant-t.

    clings to those around : **Ant-t**.

conscience, of : cycl.

disease, about : lil-t, nit, ac.

    incurable : **Ars**, *cact*, *lil-t*.

downward motion, from : **Borx**, *gels*.

evils about, real or imaginary : *sep*.

fears, with : **Acon**, **Ars**, nat-c, **Psor**, *sep*.

    disease with prove fatal : **Acon**.

flushes of heat, during : *sep*.

future about : aur, **Phos**.

hungry, when : **Cina**, **Iod**, *sulph*.

ineffectual desire for stool, from : **Ambr**.

motion, downward, from : **Borx**, *gels*.

music, from : *nat-c*, **Sabin**.

riding on horse back, while : **Borx**.

salvation, about : **Lach**, **Lil-t**, *lyc*, *sulph*, **Verat**.

sleep, on going to : *lach*.

    from loss of : *cocc*, *nit-ac*.

thunderstorm, during : *nat-c*, *phos*.

unconquerable, attacks of : *cupr*.

walking, while : *anac*.

APATHY : (See Indifference).

APPROACHED, aversion to being : **Arn**, bell, cina, *thuj*.

    insane women will not be approached : *thuj*.

    children : (See Fear).

APPREHENSION : (See Fear, Anxiety).

    imagines, going to be very ill : *ars*, podo.

ARDENT : nux-v.

ARROGANCE : (See Haughty).

ATTENTION : (See Concentration).

ATTITUDE, assumes strange : plb.

AVARICE : Ars, *lyc*, *sep*.

AVERSION approached to being : cina.

business, to : con.

child averse to any body near him : *cham*.

husband, to : **Sep**.

members of family, to : **Sep**.

mental exertion, to : *bapt*.

motion, to : **Bry**.

strangers : (See Company).

study, to : con.

BAD news, ailments from : *apis*, **Calc**, **Gels**, *ign*, ph-ac.

BEAUTIFUL, everything looks, even rags : **Sulph**.

BED, desire to remain in : *arg-n*, *hyos*, psor.

feels hard : **Arn** (moves in search of soft parts).

BELIEVES, disease incurable : (See Despair).

BEMOANING : (See Lamenting).

BENUMBED : (See Stupefation).

BESEECHING : (See Entreating).

BEWILDERED : (See Confusion).

BITING : **Bell**, *hell*, **Stram**.

attendants : **Bell**, **Stram**.

fingers or nails : *arum-t* (until it bleeds).

fists, child gnaws : acon.

spoon : *bell*, *hell*.

BOLDNESS : (See Courageous).

BOOKWORM, adapted to : *cocc*.

BRAIN-FAG (See Prostration of Mind) : *coca*, **Pic-ac** (of literary and business people).

BREAK things, desire to : *apis*, *stram*, *tub*.

BROODING : (See Anxiety and Sadness) : aur, cocc, **Ign**, *naja*.

over imaginary trouble : aur, **Ign**, *naja*.

BUSINESS, averse to : *con*, *lach*, lil-t, **Sep**, *sulph*.

incapacity for : *anac*.

loss of, or embarrassment : **Ambr**, cimic, sep.

BUSY : (See Occupied, Delirium).

CAPRICIOUSNESS : Bry, **Cham**, **Cina**, keros, *rheum*, **Staph**.

CAREFULNESS : *nux-v*.
                children and girls, yet let things fall : *apis*, bov.

CARES full of (See Anxiety) : caust.
                ailments, from : *ph-ac*.

CARESSES, averse to : **Cina**.

CARRIED, desires to be : ant-t, *ars*, **Cham**, **Cina**.
                which does not amel : **Cina**.
                rapidly : **Ars** (in teething children).
                dislike to be : **Bry**.

CAUTIOUS : graph.

CENSORIOUS, critical : **Ars**, helon, verat.

CHAGRIN : (See Mortification).

CHANGEABLE : (See Mood).

CHEERFUL, gay, happy (See Mirth) : alum, caust, **Coff**, **Croc**, ferr, gels,
      Hyos, **Lach**, *phos*, *plat*, sil, verat.
                ailments from sudden : caust, **Coff**, gels.
                alternating with sadness : croc, ign, *nat-m*, *nux-m*.
                leucorrhoea worse, when : murx.

CHILDISH behavior (See Foolish) : **Bar-c**, **Cic**.

CLINGING to person or furniture : ant-t, *borx*, *gels*, sanic.
                children while lying, clings to nurse : **Borx**.
                child awakens, screams and clings to nurse or cradle : apis,
                      bell, *borx*, cina, stram.

CLOUDINESS : (See Confusion, Stupefaction).

CLUMSY : *caps*.

COMPANY, aversion to : *ambr*, **Cham** (cannot endure anybody near him),
      coca, *con*, *cycl*, **Gels**, **Ign**, kali-c, lyc, **Nux-v**.
                amel when alone : con, *lyc*.
                delights in solitude : *coca*, kali-c, lyc.
                desire to be alone : *caps*, **Gels**, **Ign**, nux-v.
                desires solitude to practise masturbation : bufo.

does not wish to have any one near her even if the person is silent : *gels*, *ign*.

dreads being alone, yet : *con*.

ill at ease in society : *coca*.

presence of strangers, to : **Ambr**.

people intolerable during stool : **Ambr**.

desire for : **Ars**, **Bism**, **Hyos**, **Kali-c**, **Lyc**, *stram*, verat.

yet refuses to talk : verat.

alone, while agg : *bism*, *stram*.

child holds on to mother's hand for company : **Bism**, kali-c, lil-t, lyc.

COMPLAINS of nothing : **Op**.

COMPREHENSION, difficult : (See Dullness).

CONCENTRATION, difficult : *agn*, bapt, **Bar-c**, gels, graph, *lac-c*, **Lach**, *nat-c*, **Sep**.

studying, reading while : *agn*, lac-c.

CONFIDENCE, want of self : **Anac**.

want of, in others : *anac*.

CONFUSION of mind (See Concentration) : aeth, agn, *anac*, bapt, *dulc*, gels, *hyos*, **Lach**, lil-t, **Nux-m**.

cannot find right word for anything : *dulc*, lyc, nux-m.

cannot recognise well-known streets : **Cann-i**, lach, *nux-m*.

premature old age, in : agn.

sleep, after : lach.

uses wrong words : (See Cannot Find Right Words).

CONSCIENCE, terror of : cycl.

duty not done or bad act committed : cycl.

CONSCIENTIOUS about trifles : **Ign**.

CONSOLATION agg : *hell*, **Ign**, *lil-t*, **Nat-m**, Sep, Sil.

amel : *puls*.

CONTEMPTUOUS (See Scorn) : **Plat**.

everything of : **Plat**.

looking down upon people usually venerated : **Plat**.

self : agn.

unwillingly : *plat*.

CONTRADICT, disposition to : anac, *aur*, ferr, **Ign**.

CONTRADICTION, is intolerant of : anac, aster, **Aur**, *cocc*, con, *ferr*, *helon*, **Ign**, **Lyc**.

      least contradiction excites wrath : *aur*, con.

COSMOPOLITAN : Tub.

CONTRARY : (See Irritable).

COWARDICE : Gels, **Lyc**.

CRAZY feeling on vertex : *lil-t*.

CRUELTY : abrot.

CURSING : Anac, *lac-c*, *lil-t*, **Nit-ac**, stram.

      on slightest provocation : *lac-c*, *lil-t*, **Nit-ac**.

CUT things : verat.

DANCING : *croc*, **Tarent**.

DARKNESS, agg (See Fear) : **Stram**.

      cannot walk in dark room : **Stram**.

DARK side, looks only : aur, caust.

DEATH, desire (See Loathing of Life) : **Aur**, *chin*, **Lac-c**, syph.

      fearless of : lac-d.

      presentiment of, or predicts death : **Acon**, *agn*, ars, lac-d, *med*, podo.

            believes that she will die : *agn*.

            predicts time of death : *acon*.

      thoughts of : **Acon**, *ars*, cann-i, **Graph**, *psor*.

      during disease, surely going to die : **Ars**.

DECEITFUL : *nux-v*.

DECIDE, unable to, anything : *graph*, *puls*.

DELIRIUM : Agar, anthraci, arn, **Bell**, **Bry**, **Cann-i**, **Hyos**, **Lach**, mur-ac, nat-s, **Op**, ph-ac, *plb*, podo, ran-b, sabad, **Stram**.

      alternating high and low : **Hyos**.

      animals, of : *bell*.

      bed, tries to get out of (See Escape) : *agar*, bry, *cimic,* hyos.

      business, constantly talks : **Bry**.

      constantly talking : op.

      faces, sees : **Bell**.

         hedious : *bell*.

fever, during : **Stram**.

frightful : **Bell**.

furious : (See Violent).

ghosts, spirits, etc, sees : **Bell**.

go home, wants to : **Bry**, *cimic,* **Hyos**.

headache, from : syph.

insects, sees : **Bell**, *stram*.

intermitent fever, during : podo, sabad.

loquacious : **Lach, Stram**.

maniacal : **Bell, Hyos, Stram**.

muttering : *arn, bell,* **Bry, Hyos,** *mur-ac, lach, phos,* ph-ac.

pursued, thought he was being : anac.

raving, raging : **Agar, Bell, Hyos, Stram**.

restless : hyos.

sings and makes verses : **Stram**.

tremens : *cann-i, hyos,* **Lach, Nux-v, Op,** *ran-b*.

unintelligible : ph-ac.

violent : **Bell, Canth, Hyos, Stram**.

wild : **Bell, Stram**.

wrongs, of imaginary, but has no wants and make no complaints : hyos.

DELUSION, imagination, halucination, illusion : aeth, anac, *bapt,* **Bell,** cimic, **Hyos,** *kali-br,* lac-c, op, **Petr,** plat, **Sabad,** thuj.

night : tub.

air, when walking seems to be walking on : lac-c.

that he is hovering in, like a spirit : asar.

airy, light and, as if not resting on bed : **Stict**.

animals are in abdomen : *thuj*.

animals, sees : **Bell**, *stram*.

black : *bell*.

babies, are two in bed : *petr*, valer.

bed feels as if not lying on : asar, lac-c.

body scattered about bed, tossed about to get pieces together : *bapt*.

cloud, heavy black, enveloped her : *cimic*.

demon, thinks himself : *anac*.

disease, has horrible : *sabad.*

      will be fateful : *sabad.*

dogs sees : **Bell**, *stram.*

    black : *bell.*

    double, of being : *petr, stram.*

        one limb, of : petr.

faces, sees hedious : **Bell.**

fancy, illusions of : **Stram.**

floating in air, as if : asar, lac-c, valer.

        legs, as if : *stict.*

friendless, that he is : lac-c.

ghosts, spirits, etc., sees : **Bell**, *stram.*

glass, that limbs are made of, and would break : **Thuj**.

growing larger in every direction, senstion of : plat.

head feels scattered about, as if : *bapt, stram.*

home, thinks, is away from : **Bry**, *op.*

inferior, all persons are physically and mentally : plat.

insane, that she is going to be : **Cimic**.

insects, sees : **Bell**, *stram.*

larger physically : plat.

lying crosswise : petr, stram.

melancholy : kali-br.

mice, sees : aeth, *cimic*, lac-c.

mind and body seperated : thuj.

person, strange, were at his side : *thuj.*

    that she is three : *bapt, petr*, nux-m.

    that another person in same bed : petr.

pregnant, thinks herself : *sabad, verat.*

shrunken, parts are : sabad.

sick, that she is : *sabad.*

small, things appear : *plat.*

    everything looks, only she is, tall, elevated : plat.

soul and body seperated : thuj.

strange, everything seems : tub.

superior physically : plat.

superior power, under control of, is : *thuj.*

well, thinks he is : **Arn**.

wolves, sees : **Bell**, *stram*.

wrong place, thinks he is in : *hyos*.

DEPRESSION : (See Sadness).

DESIRE, things immediately which are not to be had : **Bry**.

but when offered refused : *ant-t*, **Bry**, **Cham**, **Cina**, *staph*.

DESERTED : (See Forsaken).

DESPAIR : Ant-c, **Ars**, **Aur**, cact, *caust*, **Hell**, Psor.

religious (of salvation) : **Ars**, **Aur**, mill, *psor*.

recovery of : **Ars**, *cact*, lac-c, ph-ac, *psor*.

DESPONDENCY : (See Sadness).

DESTRUCTIVENESS, clothes of : **Tarent**, *verat*.

cuts them up : verat.

DICTATORIAL : con.

DISCONTENTED, displeased, dissatisfied : aloe, apis, *aur*, *staph*, **Sulph**.

complaints about one's own : aloe.

himself about : aloe, *sulph*.

reserved displeasure : *aur*, **Staph**.

DISCOURAGED : *apis*, *ars*.

DISGUST (See Loathing) : canth (drink, food, tobacco).

DISLIKE to be carried : **Bry**.

to be raised : **Bry**.

DISINCLINED to see friends : coloc.

DISPUTIVE : ferr, *lyc*.

DISPLEASED : (See Discontented).

DISSATISFIED : (See Discontented).

DISTANCE, inacurate judge of : *cann-i*.

DISTRACTIONS : (See Confusion, Concentration Difficult).

DISTURBED, functional activity of brain : *caust*.

exhausting disease, from : caust.

mental shock, from : **Caust**.

DISTURBED, averse to being : *bry*, *gels*, *hell*, nat-m.

DISTRUSTFUL : (See Suspicion).

DOMINEERING : (See Dictatorial).

DOUBTFUL, recovery of : **Ars**, *cimic*.

DREAD : (See Fear).

DREAM, as if in a : *anac*.

DULLNESS, sluggishness, difficulty of thinking and comprehending :
agn, aeth, **Bapt, Bar-c, Bry, Carb-v**, diph, **Gels, Hell, Lyc**, med,
Nat-c, Ph-ac, Pic-ac, *sel*, **Sep, Sil, Stram, Sulph, Zinc**.

> children, in : **Bar-c**, *lyc*, zinc.

>> cannot be taught, because they cannot remember :
Bar-c.

>> repeats everything said to it : zinc.

> old people : **Ambr, Bar-c**.

> reading, while : agn, **Con**, *lyc*, *nat-c*, nat-p, *nux-v*, **Op**, *ph-ac*,
sil, *sulph*.

>> read a sentence twice before he comprehends : agn,
Lyc, Ph-ac, sep.

> think long, unable to : *gels*, *ph-ac*, **Phos**, *pic-ac*, sil.

> understands questions, only after repetition : ambr, *caust*,
cocc, *phos*, *sulph*, *zinc*.

EAT, refuses to : **Hyos**, *ign*, **Ph-ac, Verat**.

ECSTACY (See Exilaration) : ant-c (love), *lach*.

EMOTIONAL : (See Excitement).

ENTREATING : Stram.

ENVY : *staph*.

ESCAPE attempts to : *agar*, **Bell**, *bry*, hell, **Hyos**, *op*, rhus-t, *stram*.

> run away, to : *bell*, *bry*, hyos, op, rhus-t.

> spring suddenly from bed : bell.

EXAGGERATION of distance (See Distance) : *cann-i*.

> time (See Time) : *cann-i*.

EXCITEMENT, excitable : **Acon**, ambr, *anac*, *asar*, aster, **Bell**, *caust*, **Cham**,
chin, **Coff, Coll**, con, cocc, *ferr*, gels, glon, ign, **Hyos, Lach**, *lyss*,
mag-m, *mosch*, **Nux-v**, *valer*.

> bad news, after, : **Gels**, ign.

emotional, ailments from : aster, *caust*, *cocc*, **Coff**, **Coll**, **Gels**, *glon*, *ign*, *lyss*, samb.

depressing : ph-ac.

excitable news : **Gels**.

pleasurable surprise, from : *caust*, **Coff**.

sudden : *caust*, *cocc*, **Coff**, **Gels**, *glon*.

EXERTION, from mental : aml-ns, **Arg-n**, **Aur**, **Calc**, **Calc-p**, *cocc*, *cupr*, *nit-ac*, **Nux-v**.

nursing the sick, from : *cocc*, *nit-ac*.

amel : *ferr*.

EXHILARATION : Cann-i, **Lach**, med, *op*.

night : med.

and depression alternate : lach.

FASTIDIOUS : *apis*, **Ars**.

FAULT finding : (See Censorious)

FEAR (See Anxiety) : **Acon** (life rendered miserable by fear), **Arg-n**, *ars*, **Aur**, **Bell**, **Borx**, *cact*, **Calc**, *caust*, cimic, coff, *gels*, *hyos*, **Ign**, *kali-br*, *kali-c*, lach, *lil-t*, **Nat-c**, nit-ac, *op*, **Psor**, *rhus-t*, **Sep**, **Stram**.

night : **Rhus-t**.

ailments from sudden : caust, coff, *gels*, *glon*.

alone, of being (See Company) : bism, **hyos**, **Kali-c**, *lac-c*, lil-t, **Lyc**, *sep*, *phos*, *stram*.

approaching him, of others : **Arn**, *bell*, *thuj*.

children cannot bear to have anyone come near them : *cina*.

lest he be touched : **Arn**.

bitten, of being : *hyos*, *lyss*.

business failures, of : psor.

calamity, of impending : *lil-t*.

cholera : *ars*, **Nit-ac**.

church or opera, when ready to go : **Arg-n**, *gels*.

crossing street, of : **Acon**.

crowd in a : **Acon**.

dark : **Cann-i**, phos, **Stram**.

death : **Acon**, **Ars**, *cact*, *cann-i*, **Gels**, **Lac-c**, med, **Plat**, *psor*, rhus-t.

alone, when : **Ars**.

apprehension of approaching death : **Acon**, *cann-i*, med.

bed, when in : *ars*.

die, of being poisoned : *rhus-t*.

die, sure she will : *ars*, *phyt*.

disease will be fateful : **Acon**.

predicts the time : **Acon**.

pregnancy, during : **Acon**.

disease being serious, of : *lil-t*.

incurable : **Ars**, *cact*, *lil-t*.

downward motion, of : **Borx**, gels, sanic, *stann*.

dream, of : **Arn**.

drink, of : (See Water).

eating, of : hyos.

evils, of : *sep*.

falling, of, in children, grasp the crib or seize the nurse : *borx*, *gels*, sanic.

fear of fright remaining : **Op**.

falling, of : *borx*, *gels*, *lac-c*.

friends, of meeting : sep.

going out, of : acon.

heart disease, of : *lit-t*.

will cease to beat unless constantly on the move : *gels*.

imaginary things, of : **Bell**, stram.

wants to run away from them : **Bell**.

insanity, of : **Calc**, **Cann-i**, *cimic*, *lac-c*, *lil-t*, lyss, syph.

jar, of, he has to walk carefully : **Bell**.

losing reasons or senses : **Calc**.

men, of (See People) : **Lyc**, **Nat-c**, sep.

mirrors in room, of : *lyss*.

move, to : **Bry**, **Gels**.

night, of, because of mental and physical exhaustion on awakening : *syph*.

observed, of her condition being : **Calc**, *cimic*.

paralysis, of : syph.

people, of : *acon*, **Lyc**.

pins, needles of : *sil*, *spig*.

poisoned, of being : *hyos*.

public places, nervous dread of : **Arg-n**, *gels*.

riding on horse back : *borx*.

sold, of being : *hyos*.

stage fright : **Arg-n**, *gels*.

struck being, by persons coming near : *arn*.

suffering, of : syph.

> awakening from exhaustion, on : *lach*, syph.

take, to, what is offered : hyos.

thunder-storm, of : *nat-c*, **Phos**, psor, *rhod*, sil.

touch, of : *arn*.

uterine troubles, with : sep.

waking, on : *stram*.

> awakens with a shrinken look as if afraid of first object seen : stram.

water, of : **Hyos, Lyss, Stram,**

work of : caps.

FEARLESS of death : lac-d.

> but is sure he is going to die : lac-d.

FIDGETY : (See Restless).

FOOLISH behaviour (See Childish) : *apis*, *bar-m*, **Hyos, Stram**, *verat*.

FOREBODINGS : (See Anxiety and Sadness).

FORGETFUL (See Memory) : *agn*, *anac*, **Bar-c, Cann-i**, *kali-br*, **Lac-c**, *lach*, nux-m, sel.

> begining sentence, when, forgets what he intends to speak : **Cann-i**.
>
> child cannot be taught for he cannot remember : **Bar-c**.
>
> his ideas : **Cann-i**.
>
> how to talk, forgets : kali-br.
>
> inability to recall thought, on account of other thought crowding his brain : anac, **Cann-i**, *lac-c*.
>
> name, his own : *med*.
>
> purchases, of, and walks away without them : agn, *anac*, caust, *lac-c*. nat-m.

sleep, during, he remembers all he had forgotten : sel.

words, of, while speaking : **Cann-i**, *med.*

FORSAKEN feeling : lac-c (feels has no friend living).

FRETFUL : (See Irritable).

FRIGHTENED easily (See Starting) : **Borx**, calad, kali-c, op, **Stram.**

cough, by : *borx.*

cry, by : *borx.*

lighting a match : asar, *borx*, calad.

noise, at a : (See Starting),

sharp shound, from : *borx.*

sneezing, at : *borx.*

wakens with a shrinking look, as if afraid of first object seen : *stram.*

wakens in a fright from sleep : tub.

FRIGHT, complaints from : **Acon**, *apis, aur, caust, coff, gels, glon, hyos, hyper,* **Ign**, *lach,* **Lyc**, **Nat-m**, **Op**, **Ph-ac**, *plat,* verat.

GENTLENESS : (See Mildness).

GESTURES, makes : *bell*, cann-i, *hyos, stram, tarent.*

gnashes teeth : **Bell**, stram, zinc.

grasping or reaching at something : *hyos.*

motions, involuntary, of the : *hyos.*

quick : *bell.*

picks at bed clothes : *hell*, **Hyos**, *op.*

sleep, during : *op.*

awake, while : *bell, hyos.*

and bores on raw, painful surfaces, screams with pain, still bores, in typhoid etc : **Arum-t.**

GLOOMY : (See Sadness).

GREEDY : (See Avarice).

GRIEF : ars, **Aur**, **Caust**, cimic, **Ign**, *lach*, **Nat-m**, *ph-ac*, samb.

ailments from : **Aur**, *calc-p*, **Caust**, **Cocc**, colch, cycl, *hyos*, **Ign**, **Lach**, **Nat-m**, *plat*, **Ph-ac**, **Staph.**

GRINNING : (See Gestures).

GRIMACES : agar, bell.

GROANING : (See Moaning).

HALLUCINATIONS : (See Delusion).

HAPPY : (See Cheerful).

HASTY : (See Hurry).

HATRED (contempt) : agn, *lac-c*, nit-ac.

> persons of, unmoved by apologies : **Nit-ac**.
>
> premature old age, in self contempt : agn.

HATEFUL, feels : *aur*.

HAUGHTY : **Plat**, *staph*.

HEADSTRONG : (See Obstinate).

HESITATING : *graph*, *puls*.

HOME desire to go : **Bry**, *op*.

> constantly thinking of : bry, *op*.

HOME-SICKNESS : **Caps** (of indolent and melancholic), *ign*, **Ph-ac**.

> red cheeks, with : *caps*.
>
> sleeplessness, with : caps.
>
> thin, tall, in : **Ph-ac**.

HOPEFUL : *tub*.

HOPELESS : (See Sadness. Despair).

HUMOR : (See Mood).

> ill : *caps*, **Cina**.
>
>> coition, after : *sel*.
>
> ill, increases, as coldness of body increases : *caps*, *cycl*.

HUMOROUS : (See Jesting, Mirth).

HURRY : acon, anac, *arg-n*, aur, *coff*, *hep*, iod, **Lil-t**, **Med**, **Merc**, **Sulph**, **Sul-ac**.

> cannot do things fast enough : **Arg-n**, *aur*, *sulph*, *sul-ac*.
>
> doing anyting when in such a hurry she gets fatigued : med.
>
> drinking , while : anac, *bell*, bry, *coff*, *hep*.
>
> eating while : anac, coff, **Hep**.
>
> speech : (See Speech).
>
> waking, in : **Arg-n**.

HYDROPHOBIA : *bell*, **Lyss**, **Stram**.

HYPOCHONDRIACAL : (See Sadness).

HYSTERIA : *bar-c*, *caul*, caust, *cimic, croc*, **Gels**, *hyos*, **Ign**, **Mag-m**, **Mosch**, **Nux-m**. **Plat**, **Puls**, **Tarent**, **Valer**.

> metrorrhagia, from : *caul, cimic, mag-m.*
>
> puberty, at : *caul.*

IDEAS, abundant, clearness of mind : **Coff**, **Lach**.

IDIOCY : *bar-c* (chronic), *hell* (acute).

ILL at ease in society : coca.

ILL-HUMOR : **Cina**, cycl.

> during wet stormy weather : **Am-c**.

ILL-NATURED : abrot.

ILL-WILLED : nit-ac.

> unmoved by apologies : **Nit-ac**.

ILLUSION : (See Delusion).

IMAGINATION : (See Delusion).

IMBECILITY : **Aloe**, **Bar-c**, **Lyc**, *nat-c*.

IMPATIENCE : *acon*, **Cham**, *coloc*, **Ign**, *med*, **Nux-v**, rheum.

IMPERIOUS : (See Haughty).

IMPERTINENCE : graph.

IMPETUOUS : (See Hurry, Impatience).

IMPRUDENCE (See Indiscretion) : graph.

IMPULSE to destroy himself : (See Suicide).

> to jump : (See Jumping).
>
> to kill : (See Kill).

IMPULSIVE : **Arg-n**.

INCONSOLABLE : *cham*, *cina*, *nat-m*.

INCONSTANCE : **Ign**.

INDECISIVE : **Puls**.

INDIFFERENCE, apathy : *agn*, *ars*, bapt, **Chin**, *con*, *diph*, *hyos*, **Lil-t**, **Mez**, *nit-ac*, *nux-m*, **Ph-ac**, **Phos**, *phyt*, pic-ac, plb, **Puls**, **Sep**, **Staph**.

> affairs of life, to : *ph-ac.*
>
> business affairs, to : *fl-ac, ph-ac, sep.*
>
> everything, to : mez, nux-m, **Ph-ac**.
>
> family, to, one's own : chin, lyc, merc, *ph-ac*, **Sep**.

fever, during : **Ph-ac**.

life, to : *phyt*.

loved ones : **Phos, Sep**.

relations, to : **Ph-ac, Phos, Sep**.

her children : **Phos, Sep**.

says 'nothing matter with him' : *arn, ph-ac*.

things, to, that used to be of most interest : *ph-ac*.

INDIGNATION, : *coloc*, ign, **Staph**.

bad effects following : *coloc*, **Staph**.

things done by others or himself about : **Staph**.

INDOLENCE, aversion to work : aloe, am-c, *caps*, *chin*, con, *cycl*, helon, *hep*, **Lach, Nux-v, Sep**.

INDUSTRIOUS : Aur.

INHUMANITY : (See Cruelty).

INJURE tries to, herself : *cimic*.

INSANITY, madness : **Bell, Hyos**, *ign*, meli, naja.

on the borderland of, but previously of sweet disposition : tub.

early stages, in : meli.

menses, from suppressed : verat.

puerperal : *cimic, hyos, stram, verat*.

suicidal : *naja*.

INSENSIBILITY : (See Unconsciousness).

INSIGHT, power reduced : **Agn**.

IRRESOLUTION : Ign, *mez*.

IRRITABILITY : (See Anger) : abrot, **Acon**, *aesc*, **Ant-c**, *ant-t*, **Apis**, *arg-met*, *arg-n*, *ars*, *asar*, aster, aur, **Bell, Bry**, camph, *caps*, caust, **Cham, Chel, Cina**, coca, *coloc*, con, *cycl*, *dulc*, *ferr*, *gels*, hell, *helon*, **Hep**, *hyos*, *lach*, *lac-c*, **Lil-t, Lyc, Mag-c**, *med*, *mur-ac*, ph-ac, **Nat-m**, *nat-s*, **Nit-ac, Nux-v**, op, **Petr**, *psor*, rheum, sanic, sec, **Sep, Sil, Sulph**, *tarent*, *tub*, *valer*.

daytime : lyc, med.

cross during, but exhilerated at night : *med*.

morning : *nat-s*.

cannot return a civil answer : **Cham**.

children, in : **Ant-c**, ant-t, ars, **Cham**, cina, *nat-m*, **Rheum**.

complaints, from : *apis*.

consolation, agg : (See seperate-section).

dentition, during : *cham*, cina, kreos, rheum.

miserably cross : **Aesc**.

noise, from : *ferr*.

even cracking of papers drive him to despair : asar, *ferr*.

perspiration, during : **Rheum**.

questioned, when : coloc.

spoken to, when : **Cham**, nat-m.

temper, loses easily and gains control slowly : aesc.

trifles, at : *med*, nat-m.

waking, on : **Lyc**.

JEALOUSY : *apis*, **Hyos**, ign, **Lach**, *nux-v*, ph-ac.

complaints, from : *apis*.

JESTING : cann-i.

JOVIAL : caps.

yet get angry at trifles : *caps*.

JOY, ailments from excessive : caust, *coff*, gels.

JUMPING : *croc*, hyos.

bed, out of : **Bell, Hyos**.

KEEN intellect : **Lyc**.

but weak physique : lyc.

KICKS : *bell*, *lyc*, sanic.

child is cross, kicks and screams : *cina*, lyc.

KILL desire to : **Hyos**.

barbar wants to kill his customer : ars, hep.

sudden impulse to : *ars*, *ars-i*, *hep*, iod, *nux-v*.

impulse to, herself : *nat-s*, thuj.

KISSES every one : *croc*, verat.

LASCIVIOUSNESS, lustful : **Hyos, Lach**, *verat*.

LAUGHING : **Cann-i**, *anac*, *bell*, *hyos*, **Ign, Mosch, Stram**.

fits of laughter, breaks into : **Bell**.

immoderately : **Cann-i, Mosch**.

inclined to laugh at everything : hyos.

reprimands, at : **Graph**.

serious matter, over : *anac*.
spasmodic : **Ign**.
   grief, from : **Ign**.
trifles, at : *cann-i*.

LEWDNESS (See Shameless) : *hyos*, verat.
   lewd talk : *hyos*, verat.
      thought : anac, lil-t, lac-c, *sel*.
      songs : *hyos*, *stram*, verat.

LIE : op, verat.

LIFE burdensome : **Aur**.
   makes intolerable his own and those around him : psor.

LIGHT desire for : **Stram**.

LISTLESS : (See Indifference).

LIVELY : (See Mirth).

LOATHING : canth (drinks, food, tobacco).
   life (See Desires, Death) : **Ant-c, Aur, Chin**, lac-c, lac-d, podo,
   Nat-m, nat-s, thuj.
      nothing worth living for or does not care to live : lac-c,
      lac-d.
   tired of life : (See Loathing Life).

LONGING for things which are rejected when offered : (See
Capriciousness).

LOOKED at, cannot bear to be : **Ant-c**, ant-t, cham, cina.

LOQUACITY (See Speech) : agar, *cann-i*, **Hyos, Lach**, *podo*, **Stram**, *verat*.
   chill, during : *podo*.
   changing quickly from one subject to another : agar, cimic,
   Lach.
   continually talks : cic, cimic, **Lach**, *stram*.
   heat, during : podo.
   jumps from one idea to another : agar, **Lach**.
   rhymes and verses, in : *ant-c*.

LOSE minds, feels as if : kali-br.

LOVE ailments from disappointed : ant-c, *aur*, *calc-p*, **Hyos, Ign**, *lach*,
Ph-ac.
   ecstatic : *ant-c*.
   with jealousy, rage, incoherent speech : hyos.
      silent grief : **Ign, Nat-m, Ph-ac**.

LOW-SPIRITED : (See Sadness).

MAGNETISED, desires to be : **Calc, Phos, Sil**.

    which amel : **Phos**, sil.

MALICIOUS : *anac*, cham, *lyc*, *nit-ac*, **Nux-v**.

MANIA, madness (See Delirium, Insinity, Rage) : **Bell**, *cimic,* **Hyos, Stram**,
   tarent, **Verat**.

    acute disease, after : **Hyos**.

    injure herself, to : cimic.

    lascivious : **Hyos**.

    menses suppressed, from : verat.

    neuralgia, after : cimic.

    puerperal : cimic, verat.

    suspicious : **Hyos**.

MELANCHOLY : (See Sadness, Despair, Grief).

MEMORY, active : (See Ideas).

    loss of : **Anac**, bry, **Kali-bi**, lac-c, *lyc*, **Nux-m**, nat-m, *plb*, sulph,
     syph.

     had to be told the word before he could speak it : *anac*,
     Kali-br.

     sudden : **Anac**.

    weakness (See Mistakes and Forgetfulness) : *agn, anac, aur,*
     Bar-c, *carb-v*, **Con**, *kali-br, lac-c,* **Lach, Lyc, Med, Nux-
     m**, plb, **Ph-ac**, *staph, syph, zinc*.

     arithmatical calculations : syph.

     book : syph.

     difficulty in stating symptoms, questions to be repeated:
     med.

     friend, has to ask the name of intimate : *med*.

     letters, initial, for : *med*.

     loses thread of conversation : *med*.

     names, for : *med*.

       even one's own : med.

     persons : syph.

     places : syph.

     say, for what he is about to : *med*.

     words, for : *anac*, lac-c, med, **Plb**.

     sexual abuse, from : *anac, aur, nat-m,* **Ph-ac**, *staph*.

MEN dread of (See Company) : *aur*.

MENTAL traumatism, mental efferts from head injury : **Nat-s**.

MENTAL efforts inability to sustain : (See Prostration of Mind).

> symptoms alternating with physical : *cimic*, *plat*.

> suffering, menses during : *act*.

>> suppressed, bad effect : **Ign**.

MESMERISED, bad effects : hyper.

MILDNESS : alum, *ign*, op, ph-ac, **Puls**, *sep*, **Sil**.

MIRTH, hilarity, liveliness : *aur*, **Bell**, **Cann-i**, caps, **Coff**, *croc*, *ferr*, **Hyos**, *ign*, **Lach**, *nux-m*.

> lacking in children : *aur*.

> lacking in boyish-go : **Aur**.

> lively and entertaining when well, but violent when sick : **Bell**.

MISCHIEVIOUS : **Cann-i**.

MISDEEDS of others, ailments from : *coloc*, **Staph**.

MISERLY : (See Avarice).

MISTAKES, spelling, in : *lyc*, *med*.

> words misplacing or too many : *lac-c*.

> writing, in : *lac-c*, **Lach**, **Lyc**.

>> omitting letters : *lac-c*.

> wrong words, using : lac-c, **Lyc**.

MOANING, groaning, lamenting : ant-t, **Cann-i**, *cham*, kali-br, *mur-ac*, podo.

> sleep, during : *bell*, kali-br.

MOOD, humor,

> alternating : *croc*, **Ign**, *nux-m*, **Plat**, *puls*, sanic.

> changeable, variable : acon, **Croc**, *coff*, **Ign**, lach, **Nux-m**, plat, **Puls**, sanic, *tub*, *valer*.

MOONLIGHT : *ant-c*.

MORAL, loose : cocc.

MOROSE : **Aur**, **Bry**, **Con**, *cycl*, **Nux-v**, **Puls**, **Sil**, tub.

MORTIFICATION, ailments after : *aur*, *bry*, **Coloc**, **Ign**, **Lyc**, lyss, mur-ac, **Nat-n**, nux-v, **Ph-ac**, **Staph**.

MOTIONS : (See Gestures).

MUSIC, aversion to : (See Sensitive).

MUTTERING : (See Delirium).

NACKED, wants to be : **Hyos**.
      lies nacked in bed and chatters : *hyos*.

NERVOUS : (See Restless).

NEWS, bad, complaints from : apis, *gels*.

NYMPHOMANIA : **Hyos, Lach**, lil-t, *murx*, **Plat**, *tarent*.
      puerperal : *plat*.
      virgins, in : kali-p, plat.

OBSTINATE : **Anac, Cham**, *nit-ac*, sanic, *sil*.
      children, yet cry, when kindly spoken to : iod, sil.
      unmoved by apologies : **Nit-ac**.

OCCUPATION, amel : *helon, kali-br, lil-t* (must keep busy to repress sexual desire).
      constantly changing : sanic.

OFFENDED, easily (See Sensitive) : *cocc, coloc, ign*, **Nux-v**, *petr*.
      harmless words offend : ign, med, *nux-v, petr, staph*.
      questioned, when : *coloc*.

OVERSENSITIVE : (See Sensitive).

PEEVISH : (See Irritability).

PERCEPTION, prophetic, almost : *lach*.
      quickness of : **Ign, Phos**.
      slow : *plb*.

PHLEGMATIC : (See Indifference).

PICKING : (See Gestures).

PRAYING : aur, *stram*.

PRECOCIOUS : *tub*.

PRIDE : (See Haughty, Mortification).

PROPHESYING : *acon*.

PROSTRATION of mind : agar, *alum*, anac, **Aur**, *bar-c*, bapt, *calc*, camph, coca, **Con**, *cocc*, **Cupr**, *fl-ac*, helon, ign, **Lach**, *lyc*, med, **Nat-c**, **Nit-ac**, *nux-m*, **Nux-v**, **Ph-ac**, **Pic-ac**, **Sil**, stann, *staph*, zinc.
      over-exertion of body and mind, from : *cupr*.
      grief, long continued, from : **Ign, Ph-ac**.
      loss of sleep, from : **Cocc**, *cupr*, **Nux-v**, *nit-ac*.

menses, after : **Alum**.
over-exertion of mind : *cocc*, **Cupr**, **Nux-v**.
meal, after, for 2 or 3 hours : **Nux-v**.
nursing the sick, from : *cocc*, *nit-ac*.
reading, from : *sil*.
writing, after : *sil*.

QUARRELSOME : Aur, *con*, ferr, **Ign**, *lyc*, **Nux-v**, **Petr**.

QUICK, to act (See Thought, Rapid) : **Bell**, **Coff**, *ign*, lach.
   motioned : **Bell**, **Sulph**.
   tempered : (See Irritability).

QUIET, disposition : *gels*.
   cannot remain quiet : **Cina**.
   carried, only by being : **Cham**.
   wants to be : bell, **Bry**, **Gels**.
      desires repose and tranquility : **Nux-v**.

RAGE : apis, **Bell**, **Canth**, **Hyos**, **Lac-c**.
   complaints, from : apis.

READING, averse to : con.

REFUSES things asked for (See Capriciousness) : **Bry**, **Cham**, **Cina**, kreos.
   to take medicine : hyos.

RELIGIOUS affections (See Anxiety, Despair, Fear) : **Hyos**. **Lach**, **Lil-t**,
   meli, *psor*, *stram*, **Verat**.

REPROACHES, ailments, after : coloc, *ign*, **Op**, *staph*.
   himself : *ign*.
   others : staph.

RESERVE : aur, chin, ph-ac, *plat*, tub.

RESTLESSNESS, nervousness : **Acon**, ambr, aml-ns, *ant-t*, *apis*, **Arg-n**,
   arn, **Ars**, asar, aster, *aur*, **Bell**, bism, borx, *bov*, bry, calad, **Camph**,
   Caps, *caust*, *cham*,chin, *coff*, *colch*, **Coloc**, croc, *dulc*, eup-per,
   gels, glon, *graph*, helon, **Hyos**, *ign*, kali-br, *lac-c*, *lach*, lac-d, *lil-
   t*, **Lyc**, mag-c, *med*, mur-ac, *nat-c*, *nit-ac*, nat-m, nux-m, *nux-v*,
   phos, *psor*, phyt, **Puls**, pyrog, rheum, **Rhus-t**, ruta, **Sec**, **Sep**, **Sil**,
   Sulph, **Tarent**, valer, verat, **Zinc**.
      evening : acon.
      night : acon, **Caust**, **Psor**.

unable to get an easy position or lie still a moment :
Caust, euphr, **Rhus-t**.

anxious : **Ars**, **Tarent**.

bed, driven out of : **Ars**, caust, **Rhus-t**.

> tossing about in : **Acon**, **Ars**, *caust*, mag-p, psor, *puls*,
> **Rhus-t**, rheum, **Tarent**.

> wants to go from one bed to another : **Ars**, *rhus-t*.

business embarassment, from : hyos, kali-br.

children, in : ant-t, *cham*, *jal*, rheum.

> wants to be carried : *ant-t*.

convulsion, before : arg-n.

convulsive attacks, between : cupr.

grief, from : kali-br.

mentally, but physically too weak to move : **Ars**.

move, constantly : kali-br, phos.

> must, constantly : caust, helon.

>> but motion does not amel : *caust*.

> wants to : iod.

music, from : nat-c, **Sabin**, tarent.

property, loss of, from : kali-br.

reputation, loss of, from : kali-br.

sitting, while : *caust*, *phos*.

> at work, while : **Graph**, *zinc*.

standing, while : phos.

thunderstorm, during : nat-c, *phos*, *psor*, *rheum*.

> before : nat-c, *phos*, *psor*, rheum, sil.

walk, does not like to, yet : lil-t.

weak, too, to move physically : **Ars**.

working, while : **Graph**, zinc.

worry, from : kali-br.

young people, of : verat.

REVENGEFUL : (See Malicious).

ROMANTIC girls : *cocc*.

RUNS about : (See Escape).

SADNESS, mental depression, melancholy : abrot, **Acon**, aesc, *agn*, *alum*,
ambr, *am-c*, *anac*, **Ant-c**, apis, *arg-n*, Ars, asar, **Aur**, calad, **Calc-ar**, *caps*, **Caust**, **Chin**, coca, cocc, *con*, *croc*, *cycl*, dios, **Graph**,

Hell, *helon,* **Ign,** *hep,* **Kali-br, Lach, Lac-c,** lac-d, **Lil-t, Lyc,** nux-m, **Mez, Murx, Nat-c, Nat-m, Nat-s, Nit-ac,** *nux-v, ph-ac, phos,* podo, **Psor, Puls, Sep, Stann,** *staph,* tab, tarent, tub.

  morning : **Lach,** *nat-s,*

  evening : **Nit-ac.**

  ailments, from : ph-ac.

  children : caust.

    low spirited : *aur.*

  climaxis, during : psor.

  constipation, with : anac.

  excitement, after : *con.*

  future, about : (See Anxiety).

  fever, in intermittent : ant-c.

  girls at puberty : *hell.*

  haemorrhoids, with : anac.

  menses fail to return after appearing after puberty : *hell.*

  menses, before : am-c, *nit-ac,* **Stann.**

    during : am-c, aur, nat-c.

  music, from : *acon, nat-c, nat-s, sabin.*

  nervous exhaustion, from : *coca.*

  premature old age, in : *agn.*

  sexual desire, from suppression of : **Con.**

  typhoid, after : hell.

  uterine affections, with : *aur.*

SANGUINE : (See Cheerful).

SATIETY of life : *nat-s,* plat.

SCOLDS : con, mosch, verat.

SCORN : Cham, Nux-v.

SCREAM : (See Shrieking).

SENSES, acute, quick : **Bell,** *chin,* **Coff.**

  dullness : *agn.*

SENSITIVE, oversensitive (See Offended) : aml-ns, *acon, ars, asar, aur,* **Bell,** *canth,* **Cham, Chin,** *cocc, caust,* **Coff,** *ferr,* gels, glon, hep, **Ign,** *lac-c,* **Lyc, Lyss,** *mag-m,* med, *nat-c,* **Nux-v, Phos, Op,** *sabin, sep,* **Sil,** *staph,* **Ther, Valer.**

  bad manners, to : *colch,* **Nux-v.**

climacteric years, during : ther.

coffea, after : **Cham**.

external expression, to all : *cocc, colch, nux-v, phos*.

light : **Bell**, *colch*, nux-m, **Phos**.

mental impressions, to : staph.

music, to : *acon*, **Nat-c** (intolerable), **Nux-v**, **Sabin** (intolerable,
  goes through bone and marrow),
    amel : tarent.

narcotics, after : **Cham**.

noise, to : **Asar**, *aur*, **Bell**, **Borx**, calad, **Coff**, colch, **Con**, *ferr*,
  ign, *mag-m*, nux-m, **Nux-v**, *phos*, *spig* **Ther**, verat-v.

  cracking of paper or linen unbearable : **Asar**, *ferr*, tarax.

  scratching of linen : **Asar**.

  slightest noise startles from sleep : *asar*, calad, **Nux-v**,
    Ther.

  water splashing : **Lyss**, stram.

odor, to : **Colch**, nux-m, **Nux-v**, phos.

pain, to : **Cham**, chin, **Coff**, hep, ign.

  driven to despair : **Cham**.

pregnancy, during : ther.

senses, to (smell, taste, touch, hearing, etc.) : anac, *aur*, **Bell**,
  Cham, **Coff**, *colch*, nux-m, **Op**, phos, *valer*.

slightest thing, affects, : *ant-c*, *borx*, *ferr*, hep, **Puls**.

touch, to : *apis*, **Bell**, colch, chin, **Lach**, **Hep**.

SENTIMENTAL : Ant-c.

  moonlight, in : **Ant-c**.

SERIOUS : anac.

  laughable things over : *anac*.

SEXUAL excess, mental symptoms from : **Calc**, con, **Lyc**, **Nux-v**, **Phos**,
  Staph.

SHAMELESS : bell, **Hyos**.

  exposes the person : **Hyos**, phos.

SHINING objects, agg : **Bell**, **Lyss**, *stram*.

  surface of water : **Lyss**.

SHRIEKING : acon, ant-c, **Apis**, *borx*, **Cic**, *cina*, *hell*, *hyos*, **Lyc**, nux-v,
  rheum, sanic, stram, *zinc*.

  brain cry : **Apis**, *hell*.

children in : *apis*, **Borx**, *hell*, *jal*, **Lac-c**, nux-v, psor, rheum, zinc.

night : *jal*, **Lac-c**, nux-v, **Psor**.

lying on couch, when : **Borx**.

washing in cold water, when : **Ant-c**.

convulsions, before : **Apis**, hell, *op*.

during : *apis*, *hell*, *op*.

imaginary appearanes, about : kali-c.

pain, with : **Acon**, **Bell**, *cact*, **Cham**, **Coff**, *colch*.

hard stool, during : **Lac-d**.

sleep, during : *apis*, *cina*, *hell*, kali-br, **Lyc**, **Zinc**.

spoken to, when kindly : iod, sil.

sudden : *apis*, *hell*.

urinating, before : **Borx**, **Lyc**, *sars*.

while : **Borx**, **Lyc**, *sars*.

waking, on : apis, hell, tub.

SHY : (See Timid).

SIGHING (See Respiration) : **Calc-p**, cimic.

SILENT : (See Talk).

SINGING : *croc*, tarent.

alternating with anger or rage : croc.

obscene songs : *hyos*.

SLOWNESS : *carb-v*, **Hell**, *puls*.

action, in : hep.

tought, of : *carb-v*.

SLUGGISHNESS : (See Dulness).

SMALLER, things appear : **Plat**.

SOLITUDE : (See Company).

SOMNAMBULISM : kali-br, *sil*.

SORROWFUL : (See Sadness).

SPEAK wish to, does not : *gels*.

SPEECH hasty : anac, bry, *bell*, cocc, **Hep**, **Hyos**, **Lach**, **Merc**.

incoherent : **Bry**, **Cann-i**, **Hyos**, **Lach**, **Stram**.

SPITS : **Bell**.

SPITEFUL : (See Malicious).

SPOKEN to, averse to being : ant-t, **Cham**, *gels*, *iod*, *nat-s*, sil.
of his loss, when : gels.

STARTING, startled : *acon*, bell, *borx*, cina, calad, hell, *kali-c*, *med*, psor, *sil*, zinc.
easily : **Borx, Kali-c**, *sil*.
fright, from : **Borx**.
noise, from : **Borx**, calad, *med*, **Nux-v, Sil**.
sleep, during : *bell*, calad, *cina*, **Lyc**.
from : asar, *calad*, *nux-v*, tarent.
sneezing, at : **Borx**.
sound sharp, from : *borx*.
touched, when : **Kali-c** (especially on the feet).

STRIKING : Bell, lil-t.
attendants : *bell*, *cina*, **Stram**.

STUDIOUS : *nux-v*.

STUDY : (See Work, Mental).

STUPEFACTION (stunned) : **Apis, Bapt**, diph, **Hell, Hyos**, nat-c, **Ph-ac, Rhus-t**.
grief, whith : **Ph-ac**.

STUPIDITY : (See Dullness).

STUPOR : (See Unconsciousness).

SUGGESTIONS, will not receive : helon.

SUICIDAL, disposition : *ant-c*, **Aur, Aur-m**, *chin*, naja, **Nat-s**, *nux-v*, *psor*.
constantly dwelling on : **Aur**, naja.
drowning, by : ant-c, aur.
lacks courage, but : **Chin, Nux-v**.
liver troubles, in connection with : aur (in men).
shooting by : nat-s.
thoughts : **Aur** (thinks she is not fit for this world).
womb troubles, in connection with : aur (in females).

SULKY : Ant-c, *plat*, tub.

SURPRISES, pleasant affections, after : **Coff**.

SUSPICIOUS : *anac*, *hyos*.
plot, of some : *hyos*.
talking about her, that people are : *bar-c*.

F-15

SWEARING : (See Cursing).

SYMPATHETIC : *caust*.

TACITURN : (See Reserved).

TALK, desires to : ant-c.

      constantly : (See Loquacity).

      irresistible in rhymes and verses : ant-c.

   indisposed to : *ant-c*, **Aur**, *bell*, *bry*, *cham*, coloc, cocc, *hell*, iod, **Ph-ac**, **Phos**, sil, **Verat** (if irritated gets mad).

TALKATIVE : (See Loquacity).

TEARS, things : **Bell**, *stram*, *tarent*, *verat*.

      clothes : tarent, **Verat**.

TEASING : graph.

TENACIOUS : nux-v.

THEORIZING, : **Cann-i**.

THINKING, aversion to : *bapt*, caps.

      complaints, of, agg : bar-c, *calc-p*, *gels*, *helon*, *med*, **Ox-ac**.

           amel : *camph*, *hell*.

      difficulty or want of power to : (See Dullness).

THOUGHTS of death : (See Death).

      disease, incurable : **Ars**, *cact*, lil-t.

      obscene things : anac, lil-t, lac-c.

        alternates with uterine irritation : lil-t.

      past troubles, about : nit-ac.

      persistent : **Cann-i**, **Nat-m**, nit-ac, phys.

        sexual subjects, of : **Staph**.

      rapid : *coff*, *ign*, *lach*,

      sad : nat-c.

      sexual pleasures, constantly thinking of : **Staph**.

      slowness : (See Dullness of Mind).

      thinks, mind and body seperated : anac, thuj.

      thinks, she is not fit for this world : aur.

        she is going insane : cimic.

      thinks, nothing the matter with him : **Arn**.

        useless to take medicine : *ars*.

        surely going to die : **Acon**, **Ars**.

two trains of thoughts : anac, lyss.

vanishing of : hell, **Nux-m**.

reading, talking, writing, while : camph, cann-i, lach, *nux-m*.

THROWS things away : bry, cham, *cina, kreos,* **Staph**.

TIME a few seconds seems ages : *cann-i*.

passes too quickly : **Cocc**, sulph, *ther*.

too slowly : alum, *arg-n*, **Cann-i**, *med, nux-m*.

TIMIDITY : Calc, *coca, graph*, lil-t, *puls*.

TORPOR : gels, **Nux-m, Op**, *plb*.

TOUCHED aversion to being : **Ant-c**, *ant-t, arn, bry*, **Cham**, *cina*, **Kali-c**, sanic, *thuj*.

averse to caresses : **Cina**.

will not allow to feel the pulse : *ant-c*, **Ant-t**, sanic.

UGLINESS : Cham, Cina, *lac-c, lyc, staph*.

UNCONSCIOUSNESS : Acon, *apis*, apoc, *arn*, bapt, cic, *diph*, **Hell**, **Hyoc, Lach**, *mosch, mur-ac, nat-m*, **Nux-m, Op, Ph-ac**, phos, tab, rhus-t.

answers correctly when spoken to, but unconsciousness and delirium returns at once : *arn, bapt, hyos*.

aroused easily when spoken to : *bapt, diph, sulph*.

falls asleep midst of sentence or when spoken to : *arn, bapt*.

conscious when aroused, answers slowly and correctly and relapses into stupor : **Ph-ac**.

concussion, from : **Arn**.

lies like a log : ph-ac.

UNDERTAKES, lacks will-power to undertake anything : phos, *pic-ac*.

manythings, perseveres in nothing : *acon, lach. lac-c*.

nothing, lest he fails : *arg-n*.

things opposed to his intensions : sep.

VEXATION : (See Irritability and Anger).

easily vexed : *ars, con*.

VINDICTIVE : (See Milicious).

VIOLENT vehment (See Anger, Rage, Wildness) : abrot, **Bell**, *bry*.

VISIONS : (See Delusions).

WANTS nothing, durng ailments : **Op**.

        something, he knows not what : **Bry**, **Cham**, **Cina**, kreos.

        to do something, yet no ambition : lil-t.

WEAKNESS : (See Prostration of Mind).

WEARY of life : **Ars**, **Aur**, *nit-ac*, **Phos**.

WEARISOME or easily wear out under mental strain : aloe, calc, **Coca**, *helon*.

WEEPING, tearful mood, etc. : ambr, *ant-c*, alum, **Apis**, *aur*, **Calc**, cann-i, **Caust**, *cimic, cina, coff*, croc, cycl, **Graph**, **Ign**, **Kali-br**, **Lac-c**, lach, *lil-t, med, mosch*, **Nat-m**, *ph-ac, phos*, **Plat**, **Puls**, sabin, **Sep**, stann, thuj.

        aggravates : *arn, bell, stann, verat*.

        all day, cannot calm herself : **Lyc**.

        alternating with laughter : *coff, ign*, **Nux-m**, *puls*.

        carried when, child cries piteously if taken hold of or carried : cina.

            is quiet, only when caried : **Cham**, cina.

        causeless : **Apis**, *nat-m*, **Puls**, **Sulph**.

        children, in, cries all day sleeps all night : **Lyc**.

            cries all night : **Jal**, **Psor**.

        consolation, agg : *calc-p, ign*, **Nat-m**, **Sep**, **Sil**.

        joy : *coff*.

        least thing makes the child cry : *caust*.

        music, from : **Graph**.

        pains, with the : *coff*.

        pitiful, when awake : **Cina**.

        sits for days : *ambr*.

        speaking, while : *med*.

        spoken to when kindly : iod, *med*, sil.

        sleep, during : **Kali-br**.

        telling of her sickness, when : *med*, **Puls**, **Sep**.

        thanked, when : **Lyc**.

        uncontrollable, fits of : *kali-br*.

WHINING : ant-t. (child whines if any one touches it), cham (because he cannot have what he wants).

WHISTLING : stram.

WILD feeling on vertex : lil-t.

WILL contradiction, of : **Anac**.

two, feels as if he had two wills : **Anac**.

WORK, aversion to mental : **Aloe**, **Bapt**, *aur*,con, *gels lach*, *lyc*, *nat-c*, *pic-ac*.

complaints from : lyc, colch, pic-ac.

desire for mental : aur.

fatigues, mental labor, from : aloe, pic-ac.

impossible : **Nat-c**, nat-s, *pic-ac*.

inability to fix mind on : **Bapt**, **Nat-c**, nat-s, nux-m.

YIELDING : (See Mildness).

Mouth

ABSCESS, gums : *hep*, merc, *sil*.

    frequently recurring : **Caust**, *sulph*.

APHTHAE : ars, **Bapt, Borx,** hydr, **Merc, Merc-c, Sulph, Sul-ac.**

    bleeding easily : **Borx**.

    children : **Borx**.

        prevents children in nursing : **Arum-t, Borx, Merc.**

    gum : **Nat-m**, *sul-ac*.

    tongue : **Borx**, hydr.

        bleeding : **Borx**.

BITING, cheek when talking or chewing : **Ign**.

BLEEDING : *arum-t*, borx, canth, **Chin,** cupr, dros, ham, *ip*, indg, kreos, *sul-ac*.

    black blood : anthraci, *crot-h, carb-v*.

    continuous, does not coagulate : anthraci, crot-h, *chin*.

    cough, when : cupr, dros.

    easily : **Hep**, lach, **Phos.**

    oozing of blood : *anthraci*.

        decomposing rapidly : anthraci, crot-h.

    thick tar-like : anthraci, crot-h.

    whooping cough, in : dros, ip, indg.

    gum : **Bov, Carb-v, Crot-h,** *ham*, kreos, lach, *sul-ac*.

        black blood when teeth extracted : *ars*.

            oozes out : bov, kreos, ham.

        blood coagulates quickly : kreos.

        easily : **Carb-v, Crot-h,** *ham*.

        extraction of teeth, after : **Arn**, *bov, ham, kreos,* **Lach, Phos,** tril-p.

    tongue : **Arum-t, Borx.**

        easily : *borx*.

        eating while : *borx*.

        touched, when : borx.

BREATH : (See Odour, Cold).

CANCER tongue : *mur-ac.*

CANKER sores : ant-c, arg-n, *ars, sulph.*

CARIES palate : **Aur.**

CATCHES on the teeth tongue : (See Protruded Tongue).

CHEWING motion : (See Face).

CLEAN, tongue : *cina* (in worms), dig (in heart disease), **Ip**, mag-p, **Pyrog.**

COATED white (See Discolouration, Membrane) : *lac-c, sul-ac.*

COLDNESS, sensation of : *camph.*

        tongue : **Camph.**

COLD breath : **Camph, Carb-v,** jatr-c, **Verat.**

        tongue : **Camph, Carb-v.**

CRACKED, tongue fissured : **Arum-t,** *bapt,* borx, *bry, crot-h,* **Hyos,** kali-i, *lach, lyc, merc, mur-ac,* **Nit-ac, Phos,** *pyrog,* **Rhus-t.**

        centre : **Bapt.**

DISCHARGE, putrid : anthraci, carb-ac, diph, psor, *pyrog.*

DISCOLOURATION, paleness : ferr.

           redness : *nit-ac, sulph.*

      gums, blue : *plb.*

         bluish-red : **Kreos, Lach.**

         blue line on margin : **Plb.**

         lead coloured line : **Plb.**

         pale : **Plb.**

      palate, red : *bapt.*

      tongue, coated black : *ars, lach.*

           blue : **Arum-t, Dig,** thuj.

           brown, : ars, **Bapt.**

           dirty : **Nat-s.**

               clears during menses but returns when flow ceases : sep.

               base : **Nat-s.**

           green : **Nat-s.**

           greenish-brown : nat-s.

               gray : **Nat-s.**

         pale : *ferr.*

         raw : *arum-t.*

red : ant-t, *crot-h*, bell, *diph*, **Merc**, **Rhus-t**, *ter*.

    fiery-red : **Apis**, *crot-h*, **Pyrog**.

    glistening (See Smooth) : **Kali-bi**, ter.

    papillae : ars, ant-t, bell.

    red and white alternate : **Ferr**.

    spots : ter.

    streaks : ant-t.

    brown, down centre : *arn*, **Bapt**.

    strips down centre : ant-t, **Caust**, **Verat-v**.

    edges : ant-t, bell, **Chel**, *merc-i-f*, **Sulph**.

    tip : *merc-i-f*, **Rhus-t**.

    triangular : **Rhus-t**.

white : **Ant-c**, *ant-t*, ars, *bapt*, *bry*, diph, **Merc**, *mur-ac*, *puls*, **Tarax**.

    middle, in the : bell.

    milk white without coating : glon.

    milky : **Ant-c**.

    red papillae with : *bapt*.

    red and white alternate : **Ferr**.

    thick, pasty : ant-t.

    sides, red in middle : caust.

yellow : *bapt*, **Chel**, *kali-bi*, *merc-i-f*, *verat-v*.

    centre : bry.

    yellow-brown, in : *bapt*.

    base : kali-bi, **Merc-i-f**, **Nat-p**.

    golden yellow : **Nat-p**.

DRYNESS : aesc, *ant-t*, *apis*, **Ars**, **Bell**, **Borx**, **Bry**, **Hyos**, **Lach**, **Mur-ac**, nat-m, **Nux-m**, *puls*, **Rhus-t**, *tarent*, **Verat**, **Verat-v**.

    morning : *nux-m*, **Puls**.

    walking, on : **Lach**, *nux-m*.

    menses, during : **Nux-m**, tarent.

    sensation of : **Nux-m**, nat-m.

    with moist mouth : acon, sulph.

    sleeping, when : *nux-m*, *tarent*.

    thirst, with : **Bry**, **Nux-m**, **Puls**.

    without : **Bry**, **Nux-m**, **Puls**.

    tongue : *ant-t*, ars, *bapt*, **Bry**, **Hyos**, **Lach**, **Mur-ac**, **Nux-m**,

Puls, pyrog, Rhus-t, tarent, Ter, *verat*, verat-v.

night : Nux-m.

menses, during : *nux-m*, tarent.

sensation of, without actual dryness : Nux-m.

sleeping, when : *nux-m*, *tarent*.

thirst, without : Puls.

centre : ant-t.

FISTULA, gum : Fl-ac.

FLABBY tongue : Camph, *hydr*, hyos, Merc, *pyrog*, sanic.

FROTH, foam, from : aeth, Cupr, Hyos, *mag-m*.

GLOSSY tongue : (See Smooth).

HAIR on tongue : kali-bi, *nat-m*, Sil.

HEAT : Bell, Borx, Cham.

INDENTED, tongue : ars, Chel, *hydr*, mag-m, Merc, med, *podo*, Rhus-t, stram.

INFLAMMATION, gum : Kreos.

LARGE tongue : Merc, Pyrog.

LEATHER-like tongue : Mur-ac.

MAPPED tongue : ars, *lach*, merc, *nat-m*, nit-ac, Tarax.

MUCUS, slime (See Saliva) : Chel, *kali-c*.

flies from mouth when coughing : bad, *chel*, kali-c.

ropy (See also Saliva) : Kali-bi.

stringy : Kali-bi, *hydr*.

viscid : Kali-bi, *hydr*, lach, merc.

MUCOUS membrane, bleeding : *arum-t*.

excoriation : Arum-t.

pale : *eup-per*, *ferr*.

raw, : *arum-t*.

red and white alternate : Ferr.

ulceration of : *bapt*.

NUMBNESS of tongue : nat-m.

ODOR (breath),

offensive : *ambr*, *aur*, *bapt*, borx, Carb-ac, *diph*, lach, Merc-c, *mur-ac*, sang, *sul-ac*, ter.

puberty, at : aur.

onion-like : sin-n.

putrid : ambr, *bapt*, *mur-ac*, psor, pyrog.

OPEN : Lach, Lyc, *mur-ac.*

PAIN tongue : merc.

    root : *phyt.*

        putting out the tongue : cocc, phyt.

        swallowing, on : *phyt.*

    gum : *kreos.*

    burning : aesc, **Ars, Arum-t, Bell,** canth, **Iris, Mez,** *sulph.*

        tongue : **Ars, Arum-t, Iris,** sanic.

            protrudes it to cool it : sanic.

            tip : ter.

    burnt, as if : *verat-v.*

        tongue : *sang,* **Verat-v.**

    rawness : aesc.

    sore : alum, **Arum-t,** borx.

        children refuse food and drink : **Arum-t, Merc.**

        eating salty or sour food, agg : *borx.*

        old people, of, from plate of teeth : alum, borx.

        touch, agg : borx.

        tongue : **Nit-ac,** rhus-t.

PAPILLAE, tongue, elevated : ter.

PARALYSIS, tongue : **Caust,** *cupr,* dulc (after damp cold), *mur-ac.*

PROTRUDED, Tongue : **Crot-h,** *lach.*

    difficulty, with : gels, **Lach.**

        catches on the teeth : **Lach.**

    rapidly darting in and out like a snake : *cupr,* lach.

PERCHED, tongue : *bry.*

RANULA : Ambr, Thuj.

RETRACTED, gum : **Carb-v, Sulph.**

RINGWORM, tongue : *nat-m,* sanic.

SALIVA, acid : (See Sour).

    acid : arum-t, sulph.

    copious : **Merc,** *lob.*

    coppery : cupr, merc.

cotton-like : *nux-m*, **Puls**.

fetid : carb-ac, **Merc**.

frothy : lyss.

metallic taste : cupr, *merc*.

offensive : diph, psor.

ropy (vicid) : **Kali-bi**, *lyss*, merc.

saltish : **Cycl**.

soapy (See Frothy) : merc.

sweet : *cupr*.

tenacious or tough : (See Viscid).

viscid : bov, *hydr*, **Kali-bi**, **Lyss**, **Merc**.

SALIVATION : acet-ac, **Arum-t**, **Borx**, *cupr*, **Ip**, *kreos*, lac-ac, lob, merc, rhus-t.

 night : **Merc**.

 day and night : acet-ac, *arum-t*, *ip*, lac-c.

 dentition, during : **Borx**.

 profuse : *acet-ac*, *arum-t*, *ip*, lac-ac, lob, **Merc**, psor.

 wets pillow in sleep : *merc*, lac-ac.

SCORBUTIC gum : **Carb-v**, **Kreos**, **Mur-ac**, *staph*.

SENSITIVE, tongue : **Tarax**.

 spots : ran-s, *tarax*.

SHRIVELLED, tongue : mur-ac.

SMOOTH, shining, glazed, glistening, varnished tongue :
 apis, *ars*, crot-h, *glon*, **Kali-bi**, **Lach**, **Pyrog**, *ter*.

SOFTENING gum : **Kreos**.

SPEECH, difficult : bov, *crot-h*, *kali-br*, **Nat-m**, pyrog, **Stram**, ter.

 hasty : (See Mind, Speech).

 heaviness of tongue : nat-m.

 imperfect : cupr.

 inability to speak : naja.

 indistinct : caust, gels.

 slow : bov, kali-br, stram.

 stammering : *bov*, *cupr*, *kali-br*, *spig*, **Stram**.

  abdominal ailments in : spig.

  exerts himself a long time before he can utter a word :
   Stram.

 repeats first syllable 3 or 4 times : spig.

 thick : **Gels**, **Nux-v**, *verat-v*.

SPITTING of saliva, constant : hydr, lyss.

SPONGY gum : *carb-v*, **Kreos**, lach.

STIFFNESS, jaw and tongue : dulc (after damp cold).

SWELLING : Merc, Nit-ac.

   gums : lach, **Merc-c, Plb**.

   palate : diph.

   tongue : *diph*, **Crot-h**.

TASTE, acute : *bell*, **Coff**.

  bad : **Bry, Nat-s, Nux-v, Puls**.

     morning : **Nat-s, Nux-v, Puls**.

  bitter : *bry*, *nat-m*, **Puls**.

  bloody : ham.

  coppery : (See Metallic).

  ingesta : ant-c.

  loss of : cocc, nat-m, *puls*.

  metallic : **Cocc**, *cupr*, **Merc, Rhus-t**.

  pus-like as from an abscess : **Pyrog**.

  putrid : **Psor**, *pyrog*.

  saltish : *cycl*.

  sour : **Lyc, Mag-c, Nux-v**.

  sulphur-like : *ham*.

  sweetish : **Cupr, Dulc, Merc, Puls**, *pyrog*, rhus-t.

  eggs, rotten : arn.

THICK, tongue : *merc-i-f*.

THREAD sensation : (See Hair on Tongue).

TINGLING of tongue : nat-m.

TREMBLING tongue : **Camph, Gels, Lach**.

  protruding it, when : **Gels, Lach**.

ULCERS : Ars, *bapt*, *hydr*, **Lach**, *merc*, **Mur-ac**, *sul-ac*.

  bases, black : mur-ac.

    lardaceous : **Merc, Nit-ac**.

  deep : *mur-ac*.

  dirty looking : merc.

  edges undefined : merc.

  painful : *sul-ac*.

        perforating : mur-ac.

        shape irregular : merc.

        syphilitic : **Hep, Kali-bi, Merc**.

        unhealthy looking : merc.

     gum : **Kreos, Merc**.

VARNISHED : (See Smooth).

VEINS, distended, tongue : *dig*.

VARICOSE, veins, tongue : *dig, thuj*.

VESICLES : ars, sulph.

        burning : **Kali-i**, sulph.

UNWIELDY tongue : hyos.

❏❏❏

Nose

BLOOD, congestion of, to the : am-c, sulph.
>> on stooping : am-c.

BLOW constant inclination to : am-c, *borx*, lac-c, mag-m, stict.

BORING in with fingers (See Picking Nose) : **Arum-t, Cina**, hell.

CARIES (See Ozaena) : **Asaf, Aur**.

CATARRH : **Ars, Bell, Brom, Carb-v**, Eup-per, *euphr*, **Kali-bi, Lyc, Merc, Merc-c**, *nat-c*, **Nux-v, Psor, Puls, Rhus-t, Sel, Sep**, *stict, ther, thuj*.
> blows blood from nose : *phos*.
> dry : lyc ,**Stict**.
> exanthamata after : *thuj*.
>> extends to frontal sinuses : *kali-bi,* **Lyc**.
>>> posterior nares : *nat-c*.
>>> throat : *nat-c*.
>>> downwards to larynx, bronchi, etc : **Hep**.
> root of the nose : lyc.
> nares : merc-d.
> post-nasal : *cor-r*, **Hep, Kali-bi**.

COLDNESS : **Camph, Carb-v, Verat**.
> icy cold : *verat*.
> tip of : *verat*.
>> icy coldness : **Verat**.

CONGESTION : (See Blood).

CORYZA : aesc, **All-c**, *am-c, am-m, arg-met*, **Ars, Eup-per, Euphr**, *kali-bi*, kali-i, *lac-c, lyc*, **Merc**, *nat-c, nat-m*, **Nux-v, Phos**, *sabad*, sel, **Sil, Sulph**.
> morning : euphr.
> evening : *all-c*.
> acrid : (See Discharge, Acrid).
> air, cold, agg : aesc.
>> amel : Nux-v.
> open, agg : Nux-v.
>> amel : *all-c*.

annual (hay fever) : **All-c**, **Nat-m**, **Psor**.

    August in : **All-c**.

    spring in : *all-c*.

    same day of the month, appearing : **Psor**.

chronic : am-c.

cough, with : **Bell**, **Euphr**, **Ip**.

diarrhoea, followed by : *sang*, sel.

discharge, with (fluent) : **All-c**, **Arg-met**, *arum-t*, **Euphr**, **Merc**, **Merc-c**, **Sabad**.

    day time : **Nux-v**.

    morning ; *euphr*, **Nux-v**.

    alternating sides : **Lac-c**.

    ceases after a meal : nat-c.

discharge, without (dry) : *am-c*, *lyc*, **Nux-v**, **Samb**.

    night : **Nux-v**.

        fluent during the day : **Nux-v**.

peaches, from the odor of : **All-c**.

sensitive to cold air : *aesc*.

sitting in cold places or on cold stones : nux-v.

spring : *all-c*.

warm room : **All-c**, *nux-v*.

    south wind, agg : euphr.

water, from putting hands in : lac-d, *phos*.

wind, caused by cold dry : **Acon**, *spong*.

    north-east wind after : **All-c**.

CRACKS in nostrils : **Ant-c**.

CRUSTS : (See Discharges).

DIPHTHERIA : *am-c*, diph, *kali-bi*.

    extending downwards to larynx and trachea : kali-bi, lac-c.

    nose stopped up, when : **Am-c**.

DIRTY : (See Sooty).

DISCHARGE, daytime : nat-c.

    acrid : **All-c**, *am-c*, **Am-m**, **Arum-t**, *lac-c*, **Merc**, *merc-c*, *sulph*.

        bland from eyes, with : **All-c**.

        water dropping from tip of nose : **All-c**, **Ars**, **Ars-i**.

    bland : **Euphr**, **Puls**.

with acrid tears : **Euphr**.

bloody : **Am-c, Alum**, *hydr*, *kali-bi*, med, *sep*, teucr, *thuj*.

burning : *aesc*.

clear masses, in : kali-bi.

copious : **All-c**, arum-t, euphr, hydr, *nat-c*, *spig*.

crusts, scabs, plugs, clinkers : ant-c, *borx*, aur, **Kali-bi** (plugs, clinkers), *lyc*, nat-c, *nit-ac*, stict, teucr, thuj.

excoriating : (See Acrid).

gray : med, **Puls**.

green : **Kali-bi**, *nat-c*, **Puls**, *ther*, *thuj*.

every morning : *nit-ac*.

posterior nares, from : merc-i-r.

hard : **Alum, Kali-i, Sep**, teucr.

ichorus : all-c, ars, arum-t.

excoriating upper lips : all-c, ars, arum-t.

musty : nat-c.

offensive : diph, **Merc, Nat-c, Puls**, spig, *ther*, *thuj*.

fetid : *merc-c*, nat-c.

plugs : (See Crusts).

purulent : **Merc**, *puls*, *thuj*.

putrid : anthraci, *carb-ac*, **Psor, Pyrog**.

stringy : **Bov,** *cor-r,* **Hydr, Kali-bi**.

tenacious (viscid) : **Bov**, *canth*, **Kali-bi**.

thick : cor-r, **Hydr**, *kali-s*, **Lac-c**, med, *nat-c*, **Nat-s, Puls**, *ther*, *thuj*.

thin : aesc.

tough : **Bov, Kali-bi**.

posterior nares, from : merc-i-r.

watery : aesc, **All-c**, am-m.

white : **Lac-c**.

yellow : **Calc, Hep, Hydr, Kali-bi, Kali-p, Kali-s**, *nat-s*, **Puls**. *ther*, *thuj*.

yellow-green : **Kali-bi, Kali-s, Merc**, *nat-c*, *nat-s*, **Puls**.

posterior nares : *ant-c*, hydr, med, *spig*.

DISCOLOURATION,

red : agar, *borx*, merc, **Sulph**.

young women of : borx.

shining : borx.

    tip : borx.

yellow : chel.

    saddle across the nose : **Sep**.

DRY nostrils : hell.

DRYNESS : bry, **Spong**.

EPISTAXIS : acet-ac, **Am-c**, **Arn**, **Bov**, *bry*, **Cact**, canth, **Carb-v**, **Chin**, **Croc**, **Crot-h**, *erig*, ferr, **Ham**, **Ip**, indg, *kali-bi*, *kreos*, **Meli**, **Mill**, **Merc**, nat-s, **Phos**, *tril-p*.

    daily attack for weeks : carb-v.

    left : am-c.

    morning : *am-c*, arn, *kali-c*.

      washing face and hands : (See Washing Face).

    night : merc.

    blood bright : **Bell**, **Ip**, **Phos**, trilp.

      black : anthraci, crot-h.

        dark : **Croc**, **Carb-v**, *crot-h*, *ham*.

          and thin : **Crot-h**, **Ham**.

      cloted : *croc*, **Ip**.

      copious : *ham*, tril-p.

      decomposing rapidly : anthraci, crot-h.

      non-coagulable : crot-h, *ham*.

      passive : *ham*, *kreos*.

      stringy : **Croc**, *merc*.

      tenacious : *croc*.

      thick, tar-like : anthraci, crot-h.

    blow, from : *acet-ac*, **Arn**, diph.

    blowing the nose, when : am-c.

    children, in : *ham*,

      who developed too rapidly : *calc*, *croc*, *phos*.

    cough, with : cupr, **Dros**, merc.

      whooping cough : **Arn**, **Dros**, **Ip**.

    eating, after : *am-c*.

    exertion, from : carb-v.

    flushing of face, preceded by : **Meli**.

    headache, amel : ham, **Meli**.

    idiopathic : *ham*.

long-lasting : *ham*.

menses, during : *nat-s*.
>   instead of : *bry*, puls.
>   suppressed : **Bry**.

oozing of blood : anthraci, crot-h.

passive : *ham*.

profuse : *ham*.

perpura haemorrhagica, with : crot-h, *ham*, *lach*, **Phos**.

redness of face, preceded by : **Meli**.

sleep, during : **Merc**.

stooping, when : am-c.

traumatic : **Arn**, *ham*.

throbbing of carotids, preceded by : **Meli**.

vicarious : acet-ac, **Bry**, **Ham**, **Phos**.

washing face, when : **Am-c**, **Arn**, mag-c, *kali-c*.

ERUPTIONS : (See Face).

FAN-like motion : *ant-t*, *brom*, **Lyc**.

>   pneumonia, in : *ant-t*, *kreos*, **Lyc**.

FROST-BITTEN : *agar*.

HAY Fever : (See Coryza).

HEAT : agar.

INFLAMMATION : borx.

ITCHING : *agar*, **Arum-t**, **Cina**.

NECROSIS : (See Caries).

NUMBNESS : nat-m.

OBSTRUCTION : *am-c*, **Arum-t**, *aur*, *borx*, **Kali-bi**, **Lyc**, **Nat-c**, **Nux-v**,
   Samb, **Stict**.

>   right : borx.
>>   then left : *borx*.
>   left : am-c, lac-c, *mag-m*.
>   night : **Am-c**, **Lyc**, *nat-c*, **Nux-v**.
>>   must breathe though mouth : **Am-c**, **Lyc**, **Nux-v**, *samb*.
>   alternate sides : **Lac-c**.
>   children : am-c, *samb*.
>>   nursing infant : **Lyc**.
>   cold air, every time goes into : **Hep**.

diphtheria, in : *am-c.*

sleep, during : *am-c,* **Lyc.**

stopped feels, inspite of watery discharge : **Am-c, Arum-t,**
Samb, sin-n.

ODOR cheese, of old : *merc.*

herring (imaginary) : agn.

musk (imaginary) agn.

offensive : diph.

putrid : anthraci.

bad effects of inhaling or poisoning by : **Anthraci, Pyrog.**

OZAENA : *am-c,* **Aur, Kali-bi, Merc,** *nit-ac.*

syphilitic : **Aur, Hep, Nit-ac.**

PAIN in : **Aur, Graph, Hep, Kali-bi.**

bones : **Aur, Hep, Kali-bi.**

root : **Kali-bi.**

burning : *aesc, agar.*

pressing : *kali-bi.*

bones : **Kali-bi.**

root : **Kali-bi,** stict (amel by discharge).

rawness : *aesc,* **Arum-t.**

nostrils : *merc.*

sore, bruised inside (nostrils) : ant-c.

PICKING nose : **Arum-t, Cina,** hell.

boring with the finger into side of nose : **Arum-t.**

brain affections, in : **Cina.**

constant desire : *arum-t, cina, hell.*

until it bleeds : **Arum-t, Cina.**

PINCHED nose : *camph.*

POINTED nose : **Camph,** *verat.*

POLYPUS : *all-c, psor,* **Sang, Teucr.**

RUBS nose (See Itching), pillow on : **Cina,** teucr.

child starts out of sleep and : lyc.

shoulder of nurse, on : **Cina,** teucr.

SMELL, acute : *ars,* **Bell, Coff,** *colch,* **Ign,** *nux-m.*

sensitive to odor of, cooking food : **Colch.**

food : **Ars, Colch,** Sep.

egg : **Colch**.
fish : *colch*.
meat : *ars*, *colch*, sep.
strong odor : **Bell**, **Coff**, **Colch**.

SNEEZING : *all-c*, *arg-met*, arum-t, **Cina**, **Merc**, *phos*, **Sabad**, squil, **Stict**.
morning : *all-c*.
rising, after : all-c.
night : *arum-t*.
paroxysmal : *sabad*, tab.
violent : all-c.
water, from putting hands in : lac-d, phos.

SNUFFLES (See Obstruction) : am-c, **Hep**, **Lyc**, **Nux-v**, **Samb**, stict.
new born in : **Lyc**, **Nux-v**, **Samb**.

SOOTY nostrils : *ant-t*, **hell**.

STOPPAGE of : (See Obstruction).

SWELLING : agar, **Hep**, **Merc**.
bones : *merc*.

TENSION, root : meny.

TINGLING : nat-m.

ULCERS : *kali-bi*.
inside : **Aur**, **Kali-bi**.
nostrils : merc.
septum : *aur*, **Kali-bi**, *sep*.

WARTS : **Caust**, *nit-ac*, **Thuj**.

□□□

Perspiration

PERSPIRATION, in general : *acet-ac*, **Ant-t**, *ars*, bapt, **Calc**, *carb-v*, **Chin**, *cocc*, con, crot-h, **Hep**, kali-c, lach, lob, *mag-c*, *merc*, *ph-ac*, **Phos**, *podo*, **Psor**, rheum, **Samb**, sang, spong, stann, staph, *sulph*, sul-ac, tab, tarax, thuj, **Verat**, *verat-v*.

    daytime : *hep*.

    morning : **Hep**, *ph-ac*, *stann*.

        after 4 a. m. : stann.

    afternoon : hep.

    evening : **Hep**.

    night : *acet-ac*, **Con**, ferr-p, **Hep**, **Kali-ar**, **Kali-c**, **Kali-s**, **Merc**, myos-s, **Puls**, **Samb**, sang, **Sep**, **Sil**, **Sulph**, **Tarax**, **Thuj**.

        convalescence from fever, during : **Tarax**.

ACUTE disease, after : **Psor**.

    which amel : calad, *nat-m*, *psor*.

AFFECTED parts, on : **Ant-t**, *cocc*.

BLOODY : **Crot-h**, **Lach**, *lyc*.

CHILL, immediately after : lyc.

CLAMMY : **Ars**, pyrog, **Verat**, *verat-v*.

CLIMACTERIC, at : sep.

CLOSING the eyes, on : chin, **Con**.

COLD : **Am-c**, **Ant-t**, **Ars**, bov, *calc-p*, **Camph**, carb-ac, **Carb-v**, castm, croc, *lach*, med, pyrog, sul-ac, **Tab**, **Verat**, **Verat-v**.

    bathed in : **Camph**, *carb-ac*, **Carb-v**, med, **Verat**.

    whole body, over the : **Tab**.

COVERED parts : **Acon**, **Bell**, thuj.

COVERING agg : chin.

EXERTION during slight (See Walking) : **Calc**, **Calc-p**, *hep*, **Psor**, **Sep**.

    mental : **Calc**, **Hep**, *psor*, **Sep**.

HEAD, general sweat except the : *bell*, **Thuj**.

HOT : **Acon**, aml-ns, bism, **Cham**, con, lach, **Op**.

ODOR : carrion-like : (See Putrid).

    fetid : **Hep**, thuj.

honey, like : thuj.

musty : *stann*.

offensive : *bapt*, **Hep**, **Merc**, **Psor** (even after bathing), *pyrog*,
    Sil, **Thuj**.

    night : **Merc**, thuj.

putrid : *bapt*, **Psor**, *pyrog*.

sour : ars, **Bry**, calc, *cham*, **Hep**, kreos, lyc, mag-c, **Rheum**, *thuj*,
    sul-ac.

    night : **Hep**, *thuj*.

sulphur : phos.

sweetish : *calad* (attract flies).

PROFUSE : aloe, aml-ns, **Calc**, **Chin**, **Chin-s**, crot-h, con, **Hep**, **Lob**, **Merc**,
    Samb, *stram*, thuj, **Tub**.

    night : acet-ac, **Hep**, *lob*, thuj, *tub*.

    covered parts, on : **Chin**, *thuj*.

    day and night without relief : **Hep**.

    every complaint, with : **Merc**.

    walking, on : **Samb**.

SCANTY : apoc.

SIDES, one sided : **Puls**

SINGLE, parts : **Calc**.

    upper part of the body : **Calc**, **Sil**.

    nape of neck : **Calc**.

SLEEP, during : **Chin**, **Con**, *op*, *podo*, **Thuj**.

    amel : **Samb**.

even when closing the eyes : chin, **Con**.

on going to, amel : **Samb**.

walking, amel after : **Thuj**.

STAINING the linen : **Lach.**,

    bloody : **Lach**, lyc.

    yellow : **Lach**.

STOOL, after : aloe.

SUPPRESSED, complaints, from : *acon*, bar-c, **Calc**, **Dulc**, *graph*, **Psor**,
    sanic, **Sil**.

UNCOVERED parts, only on : **Thuj**.

WALKING, while (See Exertion) : **Calc**, *hep*, **Psor**, **Sep**, **Samb** (but dry heat
    while asleep).

❑❑❑

Prostate Gland

EMISSION, prostatic fluid : *agn,* **Sel, Staph.**

dribbling : **Sel.**

sitting, while : *sel.*

sleep, during : *sel.*

stool, at : **Sel.**

ENLARGEMENT : Bar-c, *benz-ac,* **Con, Dig,** *iod,* **Puls,** *staph.*

senile : **Bar-c, Dig, Sel.**

INDURATION : *bar-c, con, iod.*

INFLAMMATION : merc-d, **Chin.**

maltreated stricture, after : merc-d.

suppressed gonorrhoea, from : *med, merc,* **Nit-ac, Thuj.**

Rectum and Anus

BALL in rectum, sensation of : (See Lump).

CANCER : *alum, nit-ac,* spig.

CAULIFLOWER excrescence : *thuj.*

CHOLERA : **Camph** (first stage), **Cupr**, colch, ip (when nausea and vomiting predominate), **Verat**.

> infantum : **Aeth**, ant-t, *bism*, kali-br, kreos, nux-m, phyt.
>> before effusion, with reflex irritation of brain : *kali-br.*
>
> morbus : ant-t, bism, *camph, cupr,* **Podo**, **Verat**.
>
> cholera. like symptoms at commencement of menses : **Am-c**, bov, verat.

CONDYLOMATA : Cinnb, Nit-ac, Thuj.

> flat : **Thuj**.
>
> moist : *thuj.*
>
> sensitive, extremely : **Staph**.

Constipation (See Inactivity) : **Aesc**, aloe, **Alum**, *am-m*, *anac*, ant-c, **Apis**, arn, aster, **Bry**, **Calc** (better when constipated), cann-s, *carb-ac*, **Caust**, *chel*, **Coll**, *ferr*, epig, **Graph**, *hydr*, *ign*, *iris*, *iod*, *kali-c*, **Lach**, **Lac-d**, *lil-t*, **Lyc**, **Mag-m**, med, meli, **Nat-m**, **Nux-v**, **Op**, **Phos**, **Plb**, *psor*, *ptel*, *pyrog*, *rat*, **Ruta**, sang, *sel*, **Sep**, **Sil**, **Sulph**, tab, **Thuj**, **Verat**.

> Addison's disease, in : nat-m.
>
> alternating with diarrhoea : (See Diarrhoea).
>
> atony, intestinal, from : *ferr*, *hep*, ign, *plb*.
>
> carriage riding, from : *ign*.
>
> children (nursing), of : *alum, caust, hydr, lyc*, **Op**, **Nux-v**, *verat.*
>> artificial food, from : *alum.*
>>
>> bottle-fed babies, of : *alum.*
>>
>> dentition, during : **Mag-m**.
>>
>> nocturnal eneuresis, with : **Caust**.
>
> coffee, after : *mosch.*
>> habitual drinkers, in : ign.

confinement, after last : lyc.

> unless there is large accumulation : **Alum**, meli.

ineffectual desire : *caust*, **Nux-v**.

desire wanting until large accumulation : *alum*, meli, sanic.

difficult stool (See Inactivity) : aesc, **Alum, Bry, Caust**, *ferr*,
Graph, *kali-c*, **Lac-d**, meli, **Nat-m, Op**, *phos*, *psor*, **Ruta,
Sanic, Sep, Sil, Thuj**.

> natural stool : **Psor, Sil**.

> soft stool : **Alum, Hep, Nux-m**.

> > require great straining : **Alum**, *anac*, **Plat,
> > Sil, Sep**, *verat*.

stool recedes : **Op, Sil**, *sanic*, *thuj*.

drugs, after abuse of : **Nux-v**.

dryness of rectum, from : **Aesc**, *alum*, nat-m, plb.

enema, after abuse of : *lac-d*.

emigrants, of : plat.

excessive urging, felt more in upper abdomen : *ign*, verat.

fevers, during : *pyrog*.

hard stool, from (See Stool) : **Plb**.

haemorrhoidal : nat-m.

home, when away from : *lyc*.

impaction of faeces, from : *arn*, op, *plb*, *ruta*, *sel*, *sil*.

> requiring mechanical aid : aloe, calc, *sanic*, *sel*, sep, sil.

impeded by haemorrhoids : **Caust**.

ineffectual urging and straining : *alum*, **Ambr, Anac**, aster,
Caust, *ferr*, *iod*, *lac-c*, **Lil-t, Lyc, Nux-v, Plat**, *rat*, *sanic*,
Sil.

injury, after : **Arn, Ruta**.

insufficient stools : *sep*.

lactation, during : **Sep**.

lead poisoning, from : **Op**, plat.

lean far back to pass a stool, must: *med*.

menses, during : **Sep, Sil**.

obstinate : am-m, aster, cann-s, **Coll**, lac-d, **Nat-m**, plat (after
nux-v), plb (after plat fails), psor (after sulph fails), pyrog,
syph.

> accompanied by flatus : am-m.

old people : *alum*, **Lyc**, *op*.

sudden : ant-c.

painful : med, meli, **Sulph**.

so as to bring tears : med.

child is afraid to pass stool due to pain : **Sulph**.

paralysis, from (See Atony) : ign, **Plb**.

periodic, several weeks without evacuation : *lac-d*.

portal stasis, from : **Aesc**.

pregnancy, during : *alum*, **Plat**, **Plb**, **Sep**.

puberty, since : lyc.

rectum loaded : **Arn**.

sedentary habits : **Nux-v**.

sea, on going to : *bry*, plat.

serious illness, after, enteric, etc : *sel*.

standing, passes stool easier, when : **Caust**.

stool remains long in rectum : (See Impaction of Faeces).

straining, great, must grasp seat of closet : **Alum**.

travelling, while : *plat*.

at sea : *bry*.

unable to pass in presence of nurse : **Ambr**.

CONSTRICTION, contraction : *cact*, *cann-s*, caps, **Caust**, **Ign**, **Lach**, **Lyc**, med, meli, nat-m, **Nit-ac**.

CRACKED anus : (See Fissure).

DIARRHOEA : *acet-ac*, **Aloe**, alum, am-m, **Ant-c**, **Ant-t**, **Apis**, **Arg-n**, **Ars**, aster, bism, **Bry**, *calc-p*, carb-ac, chel, *crot-h*, **Crot-t**, **Ferr**, gels, **graph**, **Hep**, **Ip**, **Iris**, jal, *kreos*, *mag-c*, *med*, **Merc**, *merc-d*, merc-sul, mur-ac, nat-m, **Nat-s**, **Nit-ac**, *nux-m*, *petr*, **Ph-ac**, **Phos**, **Podo**, *psor*, ptel, pyrog, rhus-t, rumx, *sang*, *sanic*, **Sec**, sel, *sep*, **Sil**, **Sulph**, tab, ter, **Thuj**, *valer*, **Verat**.

daytime only : **Petr**.

morning : aloe, ant-c, **Bry**, **Nat-s**, **Phos**, **Podo**, **Rumx**, **Sulph**, *thuj*, *tub*.

until forenoon : *aloe*, **Nat-s**, *podo*, **Sulph**.

followed by natural stool in the evening : *aloe*, *podo*.

bed, driving out of : *aloe*, psor, *rumx*, **Sulph**.

moving about, after : **Bry**, **Nat-s**.

old people, in : *phos*.

rising, after : **Nat-s**.

afternoon : **Calc**.

night : *chel*, *ferr*, **Lach**, **Merc**, **Podo**, **Psor**, **Puls**, **Sulph**.

    only : **Puls**.

    midnight, after : **Sulph**.

acid, after : bry, *ph-ac*.

acute disease, after : *psor*.

aged persons : **Ant-c**, **Nit-ac**, phos.

alternate days, on : (See Periodical).

alternating with constipation : *abrot*, **Ant-c**, **Chel**, **Nux-v**, *sulph*.

    aged people, in : **Ant-c**.

anger, after : *cham*, **Coloc**, *staph*.

anticipation, after : *arg-n*, *gels*.

autumn, in : **Colch**, *nux-m*.

bad news, from : *gels*.

bathing, after : *podo*.

breakfast, after : **Thuj**.

cabbage, after : petr.

castor oil, after : bry.

cathertics, after : **Nux-v**.

chagrin, after : *cham*.

change of diet : nux-v.

    weather : bry, *dulc*, *psor*.

child bed, in : cham.

children, in : **Aeth**, bapt (especially when very offensive), *benz-ac*, **Calc**, **Calc-p**, carb-v, *mag-c*, **Merc-d**, **Podo**, **Psor**, *puls*, **Rheum**, *valer*.

choleraic : ph-ac.

cholera epidemic, during : crot-h, *phos*.

coffee, after : *thuj*.

cold drink, after : *bry*, *nux-m*, *puls*.

    in summer : **Nux-m**.

cold, after taking ; *cham*, **Dulc**.

    from damp : **Dulc**.

consumptives, of : *ferr*.

damp basements or cellers : **Nat-s**.

damp foggy weather : dulc.

dentition, during : *bell*, **Calc-p**, **Cham**, hell, *mag-c*, nux-m, Podo, *psor*, rheum.

downward motion, from : cham, **Borx**, sanic.

drinking water, from : *aloe* (immediately), **Arg-n**, **Ars**, *crot-t*, **Ferr**, *staph*.

impure water, from : camph, zing.

drinks as soon as : *arg-n*, *ars*, crot-t, thromb.

dropsy, in : acet-ac.

drunkards, in old : *apis*.

dysentry like : **Coloc**.

eating, while : *crot-t*, **Ferr**, puls.

as soon as they eat : *crot-t*, **Puls**.

after : **Aloe** (immediately), *arg-n*, **Ars**, **Crot-t**, Podo, **Puls**, sanic, *staph*.

must hurry from table : sanic.

effluvia, from noxious : *crot-h*, *pyrog*.

eruption, suppressed, from : apis, bry, *graph*, *psor*, **Sulph**.

eruptive disease, in : apis.

excitement, from : **Arg-n**, *gels*, *ph-ac*, *thuj*.

fever, typhoid, typhus, etc. : *bapt*, crot-h.

yellow : *crot-h*.

food, cold, agg : **Ars**, **Dulc**, *puls*.

fat : *puls*, thuj.

fright, after : acon, ph-ac, verat.

fruit, after : **Bry**, **Puls**, *crot-t*.

game, high, after : *crot-h*, *pyrog*.

hot weather : aloe, *ant-c*, **Bry**, **Crot-t**, merc-c, **Podo**.

hungry, when : aloe.

hurry, to stool : (See Morning, Driving Out of Bed).

hydrocephalus, during acute : *apis*, hell.

ice-cream, after : **Ars**, bry, dulc, *puls*.

involuntary : **Apis**, **Phos**.

anus wide open as if : **Apis**, **Phos**.

jarring of cars, from : med.

lactation, during : sep.

long-standing, of : *podo*.

measles, during : am-m.

menses, before : am-c, **Bov**, *verat*.

        during : am-c, *am-m*, **Bov**, **Verat**.

milk, after : aeth, **Calc**, *mag-c*, **Mag-m**, **Nat-c**, *nux-m*, *nicc*, *sep*, *sulph*.

motion agg : aloe, apis, **Bry**, *crot-t*, **Verat**.

nursing, after : *crot-t*.

onions, after : puls, thuj.

opium, after : **Puls**.

oysters, after : *brom*, *lyc*.

painless : bism, **Chin**, **Ferr**, *ph-ac*, **Phos**, **Podo**, *pyrog*, **Rumx**, sec, **Sulph**.

pears, after : chin, *verat*.

periodical, on alternate days : **Chin**.

        every three weeks : mag-c.

phthisis, in : acet-ac.

pregnancy, during : hell, *nux-m*, petr, *sep*.

ptomain poisoning, from : (See Septic Condition).

quinine, after abuse of : **Puls**.

septic condition : *crot-h*, *pyrog*.

smoking : borx.

sour krout, from : bry, petr.

sphincter-ani, weakness of : **Aloe**.

stormy weather, during : petr.

sudden : (See Urging).

sugar, after : **Arg-n**, crot-t, gamb.

summer : (See Hot Weather).

tobacco, after : cham, tab.

typhus, in : acet-ac.

urinating agg : **Alum**.

vaccination, after : ant-t, sil, *thuj*.

walking agg : *aloe*, **Bry**.

washing, while : *podo*.

weakness, without : **Ph-ac**.

wet weather, after spell of : **Nat-s**.

DRYNESS : Aesc, Bry, *nat-m*, **Op**.

DYSENTRY : Aloe, *arn*, *bapt*, *caps*, *carb-ac*, **Colch**, **Coll**, ferr-p, **Ip**, **Merc**, **Merc-c**, **Nux-v**, **Rhus-t**, **Sulph**.

autumnal : *colch*, **Ip**, **Merc**.

blood, more, the better indicated : ferr-p (first stage), **Merc**.

cold, from taking : *dulc*.

cold nights after hot days : colch, ip, merc.

day, worse during : **Petr**.

food or drink, from least : *staph*.

long interval between stools : **Arn**.

old people, of : *bapt*.

ERUPTION about anus : **Nat-m**, petr.

herpetic : *nat-m*, *tab*.

eczema about anus : graph.

EXCORIATION : **Lac-d**, *sanic*, **Sulph**.

stools, from the : **Lac-d**, nit-ac, sulph.

extending to genitals : sanic.

FISSURE : *ars, fl-ac*, **Graph**, **Nit-ac**, nat-m, **Rat**, syph, **Thuj**.

painful to touch : thuj.

FISTULA : **Berb**, **Calc-p**, **Nit-ac**, **Sil**.

alternating with chest symptoms : *berb*, *calc-p*, *sil*.

FLATUS : **Aloe**, **Am-m**, ant-c, **Arg-n**, **Chin**, **Dios**, **Nat-s**, olnd, pyrog, *thuj*.

amel : aloe, **Carb-v**, **Lyc**.

burning : **Aloe**.

diarrhoea, during : **Aloe**, *arg-n*.

loud : **Aloe**, **Arg-n**.

offensive : **Aloe**.

stool, before : **Aloe**.

during : **Aloe**, *arg-n*, calc-p, *chin*, nat-s.

small with much flatus : agar, *aloe*.

sensation as if stool would pass with : **Aloe**,
mur-ac, *nat-m*, olnd.

urging for stool but flatus is passed : *aloe*.

FULLNESS : **Aesc**, **Ham**, meli.

stool, after : **Aesc**.

rectum full of liquid, feels, will fall out if not go to stool :
Aloe.

HAEMORRHAGE from anus : aesc, *aloe*, am-m, anthraci, **Cact**, canth,
chin, **Crot-h**, **Coll**, erig, iod, **Ham**, **Lach**, *mill*, **Nat-m**, **Phos**.

black : anthraci, crot-h, *ham*.

blood decomposing rapidly : anthraci, crot-h, lach.

    thick, tar-like : anthraci, crot-h.

    clots, large, looking like liver : **Alum, Alum-n**.

    charred straw-like or in flakes : **Lach**.

menses, during : *am-m*.

oozing of blood : anthraci, crot-h.

profuse : ant-c (mixed with solid faeces), **Ham**.

stool, during : **Am-c, Ham**, iod, **Nat-m**.

    after : **Am-c**, nat-m.

    from hard : **Nat-m**.

typhoid, in : **Alum, Alumen, Ham**, *lach*.

vicarious : phos.

HAEMORRHOIDS : **Aesc, Aloe**, am-m, anac, *ant-c*, **Ars**, *bar-c*, **Caust, Coll, Ham**, *ign*, **Lach**, lob, **Lyc, Mur-ac, Nit-ac, Nux-v**, *rat*, **Sep, Sulph**, *thuj*.

    bleeding : (See Haemorrhage from Anus).

        as soon as rheumatism is better : *abrot*.

    blind : **Aesc**, ars.

    bluish : **Aesc**, *aloe, ham*, **Lach, Mur-ac**.

    children, in : *mur-ac*.

    chronic : **Aesc, Coll, Nux-v, Sulph**.

    climaxis, at : **Lach**.

    cold water, amel : *aloe*.

    congestion, from : *coll*.

    drunkards, in : lach, **Nux-v**.

    external : **Aloe, Aesc, Ham, Lach, Mur-ac, Rat, Sulph**.

    grape, like bunch of : *aloe*, **Mur-ac**.

    heat, amel : **Ars**, *mur-ac*.

    internal : **Ars, Cham, Ign, Nux-v, Podo, Puls, Sulph**.

    itching : (See Itching).

    leucorrhoea, after suppressed : *am-m*.

    'little hammers' sensation : **Lach**.

    menses, during : *lach*.

        after agg : *cocc*.

    mucous piles : *ant-c*.

ointment, after abuse of : *sulph*.

painful : *coll*, thuj.

painful when sitting : thuj.

pregnancy, during : *coll*, sep.

purplish : **Aesc**.

raw : caust.

sitting, preventing : *ars*.

sleep, preventing : *ars*.

smarting : am-m, caust.

sore : am-m, caust.

stool, preventing : *aesc*, *caust*, *lach*, *thuj*.

    protruding during : ign (ham, to be replaced).

strangulated : **Lach**.

suppressed leucorrhoea, after : am-m.

swollen : caust, *mur-ac*, *thuj*.

touch, agg : **Mur-ac**, nit-ac, thuj.

urination, protrude during : **Bar-c**, *mur-ac*.

walking amel : **Ign**.

    agg : **Aesc**, **Caust**, **Carb-an**, **Mur-ac**, **Sulph**.

HEAT : Aesc, Aloe.

    stool during : *aloe*.

HEAVINESS : Aesc, **Aloe** (before stool), ham.

HURRY to stool, must : *aloe*, *psor*, rumx, **Sulph**.

    loss of control of sphincter, from : **Aloe**.

INACTIVITY of rectum (no desire) : **Alum**, **Anac**, **Bry**, *coll*, **meli**, med, **Op**, *psor*, pyrog, **Ruta**, **Sanic**, **Sil**, **Sulph**, *tab*, *thuj*, verat.

    requires mechanical removal : aloe, calc, sanic, sep, sel, sil.

    soft stool even requires great straining : **Alum**, **Anac**, *plat*, **Sil**, *verat*.

INFLAMMATION : aloe, *hep*, *merc*.

INSECURITY of rectum : **Aloe**.

INVOLUNTARY stool or mucus : **Aloe**, *apis*, **Arn**, *carb-ac*, *chel*, *dig*, *hell*, **Hyos**, *mur-ac*, **Nat-m**, **Olnd**, **Op**, **Ph-ac**, **Phos**, *plat*, *psor*, *pyrog*, **Rhus-t**, *sanic*, **Sec**.

    night, 1 to 4 a.m. : psor.

flatus, on passing ; **Aloe**, iod, mur-ac, **Olnd**, **Podo**, **Ph-ac**, *nat-m*, sanic.

fright, after : *gels*, **Op**.

paralysis, from : *op*.

solid stool or lumps of : **Aloe**, *carb-ac*.

urination, while : *mur-ac*.

and stool : **Mur-ac**.

IRREGULAR stool : nat-m.

IRRITATION : canth, erig, lil-t, **Nux-v**.

ITCHING : **Aesc**, **Aloe**, *berb*, caust, bov, ferr, **Sulph**, ter.

night : *ferr*.

burning : aloe.

coccyx, tip of : **Bov** (must scratch till raw and sore).

LACERATION, anus, from hard stool : **Lac-d**.

LUMP, sensation of : *cann-i*, *chim*, lil-t, med, **Sep**.

posterior surface of sphincter : med.

stool, not amel by : **Sep**.

MOISTURE : **Ant-c**, **Caust**, **Hep**, med, sep.

acrid : *act-c*.

herring-brine, smelling like : *calc*, **Caust**, *hep*, *med*.

oozing : *ant-c*.

staining yellow : *ant-c*.

MUCUS : (See Moisture).

OPEN anus : apis, *phos*, *sec*.

sensation of : *apis*, *phos*.

PAIN : **Aesc**, *aloe*, *alum*, **Am-c**, am-m, anac, *ars*, bry, carb-ac, **Caust**, **Coll**, ferr, **Graph**, ham, ign (dreads to go to closet) med, *merc*, *rat*, *sep*, sil, *spig*, **Sulph**, syph, **Thuj**.

atrocious : (See Pain, Atrocious).

menses, during : *aloe*, ars.

stool, before : àloe.

during : aloe, **Graph**, med, *merc*, **Rat**, *sep*.

after : **Aesc**, **Aloe**, **Graph**, ign, **Mur-ac**, *nit-ac*, **Rat**, *sep*, sil, **Sulph**.

intense pain for hours : **Aesc**, **Aloe**, *graph*, ign,

Mur-ac, Nit-ac, Rat, Sulph.

amel : aloe.

tears, so as to cause : med.

atrocious : alum, *spig*.

bearing-down : aloe.

burning : **Aesc**, *am-m*, **Ars**, canth, caps, erig, **Graph**, ham, merc-sul, *rat*, **Sulph**.

heat, amel : **Ars**.

stool, during : **Alum, Ars**.

after : **Aesc, Aloe, Ars**, *am-m*, gamb, graph, **Rat, Sulph, Iris**, caps.

intense burning for hours, after, with haemorrhoids: *aesc, am-m*, **Rat, Sulph**.

anus, during diarrhoea : **Iris**.

cramping : ferr, *plb*.

spasm of anus, from : *plb*.

stool, after : *ferr*.

cutting : aesc, **Alum**, *merc-c*, *nat-m*, *rat*.

stool, during : **Merc**.

after : *merc*, **Nit-ac**.

for hours, after : **Nit-ac, Rat**, *sulph*.

labor-like, from passage of enema in constipation : **Lac-d**, *syph*, tub.

lancinating : (See Cutting).

rawness : *aesc*, ham.

sharp : med.

shooting : (See Stitching).

smarting (See Burning) : *am-m*, nat-m (after stool).

sore : **Aesc, Aloe**, am-m, **Ars**, *bry*, **Caust, Coll, Graph**, ham, *merc-d*, merc-sul, **Mur-ac, Rat**.

menses, during : *mur-ac*.

stool, during : *graph*.

hard, during : **Lac-d**.

after : **Aesc**, *am-m*, **Graph**, ign, nat-m, **Sulph**.

for hours, after : **Aesc**, *am-m*, **Sulph**.

splinter-like : *aesc*, coll, **Nit-ac, Rat**, thuj.

sticking : **Aesc**, *coll*.

stinging : **Aesc**, *am-m*, **Apis**.

    stool, after : **Aesc**, *am-m*.

        for hours, after, with haermorrhoids : **Aesc**, *am-m*, **Sulph**.

stitching : **Aesc, Ars, Ign, Kali-c, Lach**, *med*, *nat-m*, **Nit-ac**.

    sitting, when : **Ars**.

    walking, when : **Ars**.

    extending upwards : aesc, **Ign**, *lach*, **Nit-ac**, sulph.

tearing : nat-m, **Nit-ac**.

    stool, during : **Nat-m, Nit-ac**.

        after : aesc, *nat-m*, **Nit-ac**.

tenesmus : **Aloe**, alum, **Aesc**, *carb-ac*, **Canth**, *caust*, *coll*, *lac-d*, med, **Merc, Merc-c, Nit-ac**, phos, *sil*.

    diarrhoea, during : *alum, nit-ac*.

    difficult, from sensation of prolapse of rectum : alum, med.

    dysentery, during : **Merc, Merc-c**.

    great straining, but passes little : *nit-ac*.

    finish, cannot, sensation : **Merc, Merc-c**.

    incessant : **Merc-c**.

    stool, before : *kali-c*.

        during : **Aloe, Merc, Merc-c**.

        after : **Merc, Merc-c**, *rheum, nit-ac*, rat.

        stool does not amel : **Merc-c**.

            amel : **Nux-v**.

    urinating, when : alum, med.

PARALYSIS (See Inactivity) : aloe, *anac*, **Mur-ac, Op, Plb, Sil**, *tab*.

    sensation of : **Aloe**.

PLUG sensation : anac.

PROLAPSE : *ferr*, **Ign**, lil-t, *lyc*, med, **Mur-ac, Nux-v, Podo, Ruta**, sep, syph, tab.

    children : *ferr*, **Podo**.

    diarrhoea, during : **Dulc, Merc, Podo**.

    lifting, while : ign, nit-ac, podo, ruta.

    parturition, after : *podo, ruta*.

    stool, before : *podo*.

after : **Podo**.

during : **Ign**, lyc, **Podo**, *ruta*.

loose, when : ign.

stooping : ign, nit-ac, podo, ruta.

sensation of, cannot strain from : alum, med.

urging, unsuccessful from : *ruta*.

urinating, while : aloe, **Mur-ac**.

PULSATION : Lach, meli.

RECEDES, stool : (See Constipation).

REDNESS of anus : **Sulph**.

SENSITIVE : *aloe*, **Mur-ac**.

SPASM : *tab*.

STRAINING : (See Tenesmus).

SWELLING of anus : *aesc*.

sensation as if sitting on a ball : cann-i.

TENESMUS : (See Pain).

TICKLING : (See Itching).

UNCERTAIN : Cham, pyrog.

UNSATISFACTORY stool : nat-m, nux-v.

URGING : Aesc, *aloe*, *anac*, *ars*, *bell*, cham, chel, crot-t, *dulc*, ham, **Ign**, lach, **Lil-t, Nux-v, Plb, Rheum, Sil**, *tab*.

anxious : nux-v.

constant : **Crot-t**, *lil-t*, **Merc, Merc-c**, *nux-v*.

sudden evacuation, followed by : **Crot-t, Gamb, Grat, Podo**, thuj.

effort, great desire passes away without : **Anac**.

flatus, passing when : **Aloe**, sanic.

frequent : *ambr*, **Lil-t, Merc, Nux-v**.

morning, after rising : *nux-v*.

in epigastrium : *ign*, *verat*.

ineffectual : ambr, arn, **Nux-v**.

labor pain, with every : nux-v.

mental exertion, after : *nux-v*.

must cross legs to, prevent faeces escaping : sanic.

must desist, it hurts so : lach.

pressure in rectum, from : lil-t.

stool, before : *aloe*.

for, but with effort desire passes away : **Anac**.

amel : **Nux-v**.

sudden : aloe, **Camph**, **Crot-t**, *nat-s*, *psor*, rumx, **Sulph**, tab.

WARTS : (See Condylomata).

WATER, drops of cold, were falling from anus, sensation as if : cann-s.

WEAKNESS, feeling : anac, podo.

WORMS sensation of : (See Crawling).

complaints : *cic*, **Cina**, *sabad*, *sil*, **Spig**, *stann*, **Sulph**, *ter*.

ascarides : cina, **Sabad**, sil, *spig*, ter, **Teucr**.

lumbricoids : **Cina**, *sabad*, *sil*,**Spig**, stan, ter.

tapeworm : ter.

❑❑❑

Respiration

ACCELERATED : *coca.*

ANXIOUS : Acon, Ars, *hep.*

ARRESTED : *cic.*

> as if dead : **Cic.**
> convulsions, during : *cic.*
> coughing : **Ant-t, Cupr, Dros, Ip.**

ASPHYXIA : **Ant-t.**

> coma and drowssiness, with : **Ant-t.**
> gas, from : bov.
> mechanical, drowning, foreign body in trachea or larynx,
> > etc. : ant-t (before sil in foreign body).
> mucus in bronchi : ant-t.
> newborn infant : **Ant-t.**
> paralysis of lungs : **Ant-t.**

ASTHMATIC : **Ars,** aral (after first sleep), *brom, cann-s, carb-v, erio*(from accumulation of mucous), *hep, iod,* **Ip, Kali-c,** *med, nat-s, psor, sang,* **Samb.**

> night : **Ars.**
> > midnight, after : **Ars.**
> > > must spring out of bed : **Ars.**
> > > 2 to 4 a. m. : **Kali-c.**
> air, open agg : *psor.*
> bend forward, must : **Ars,** *kali-c.*
> cardiac : pyrog.
> > septic condition from : pyrog.
> children : **Ip, Nat-s, Puls.**
> cold, damp weather : **Dulc,** *nat-s.*
> expectoration, amel : zinc.
> humid : (See Rattling).
> lying, agg : **Ars.**
> > amel : *psor.*
> measles, after : *carb-v.*
> old people : carb-v.

paroxysmal : tab.

rocking, amel : kali-c.

'rose cold' after : sang.

sailors as soon as they go ashore : **Brom.**

sit up, must : **Ars,** *kali-c.*

sitting up, agg : *psor,* laur.

spasmodic : **Ars, Ip, Lob.**

standing, can only breathe when : cann-s.

stretching of arms away from body, amel : **Psor.**

agg : ars.

suppressed eruption, after : **Ars,** *hep,* **Psor.**

wet weather, in : *dulc, nat-s.*

whooping cough, after : *carb-v.*

DEEP : Arg-n, Aur, Bry, Hep, Ign, Nat-s, Op.

desire to breathe : **Bry, Ign, Nat-s.**

damp cloudy weather, during : *nat-s.*

DIFFICULT, dyspnoea, breathlessness : acet-ac, act, am-c, **Ant-t. Ars,** *brom,* cann-s, cimic, *coca,* **Crot, Cupr,** *dig,* **Hep, Ip,** *kali-bi,* **Lach, Lob,** lyc, med, *merc,* mosch, **Nat-s,** *nux-v,* psor, **Puls,** *samb, seneg, spig,* **Spong, Sulph.**

night : am-c, **Ars,** *nux-v,* **Samb, Sulph.**

suffocative attack, wants doors and windows open : **Sulph.**

midnight : **Ars.**

after : **Ars.**

2 a. m. : **Ars.**

air, in open : **Psor.**

ascending : *am-c, ars,* **Calc, Ip,** *iod, lob.*

atheletes, in : *coca.*

bending head backward, must rise up and : hep.

cold exposure, from : lob.

constriction of middle of chest, from : lob.

cough, with : **Ant-t, Cupr, Dros.**

croup, as in last stage of : samb.

exertion : am-c, **Ars, Calc, Ip, Lob.**

expiration : *med,* **Samb.**

child inspires but cannot expire : chlor, meph, **Samb.**

fanned, wants to be : **Carb-v.** (rapidly), *lach* (slowly and at a distance), *med.*

foreign body, from, in larynx and trachea : ant-t (before sil).

heart trouble, from : cimic.

haemorrhage, during : ip.

hysterical : asaf, lac-d.

infant, new born : **Ant-t.**

inspiration, during : *brom.*

labour pain, from : lob.

least thing near mouth or nose interferes with breathing : *lach.*

lying, while : aral, **Ars,** *lac-c.* (as if breath would leave her), *lach,* merc-sul.

    amel : kali-bi, **Psor.**

    get up must and walk : am-c, **Grind, Lach,** *lac-c.*

    head high, with, amel : cact, spig, spong.

    impossible or unable to lie down : **Ars,** merc-sul.

    on face, amel : med.

        side, right, amel : *spig*

menses, during : alum, carb-an, *cocc, iod.*

metrorrhagia, during : **Ip.**

motion agg : ars.

mucus in the trachea, from : **Ant-t, Ip.**

old people, in : coca.

palpitation, with : am-c.

protruding tongue amel : med.

sinking sensation in abdomen, from : acet-ac.

sitting : *laur, psor.*

    amel : merc-sul.

sleep, during : **Lach,** samb.

    after : **Lach.**

    falling asleep, when : am-c, dig, **Grin,** lac-c, **Lach, Op.**

smoke, as from : *brom.*

sponge, breathing though, as if : *brom, spong.*

stairs, going down : *ip*, lob.

standing, can only breath when : cann-s.

suffocative : apis (feels as if every breath would be his last especially in dropsy and fever), cact, *ip, lob,* **Laur** (about heart).

sulphur vapour, as if air-passages filled with : brom.

suppressed eruption, after : *hep,* **Psor.**

          tobacco smokers, in : *coca.*

          violent : **Ip.**

          waking with : *samb, spong* (with loud cough, alarm).

          waking with a start : **Grin.**

          warm room, agg : am-c, **Puls.**

          wet weather : **Nat-s.**

          whisky drinkers, in : *coca.*

GASPING : ant-t, *brom,* laur, *spong.*

          newborn, in : *ant-t.*

HISSING : acet-ac.

IRREGULAR : Dig.

          inspiration : samb.

LOSES, breath : (See Arrested, Coughing).

OPPRESSED : (See Difficult Breathing),

OPPRESSION : (See Chest).

RATTLING : **Ant-t,** *brom,* dulc, **Hep, Ip, Kali-s,** lyc, *nat-s, op.*

          cough, during : (See Rattling Cough).

          death-rattle, relieves : **Ant-t,** *tarent.*

          inspiring, when : **Ant-t, Ip.**

          sounds loose but no expectoration : **Ant-t, Brom.**

ROUGH, crowing : (See Croup).

          sawing : *ant-t,* **Brom, Iod, Spong.**

SAWING : (See Rough).

SHORT (See Difficult) : *hep,* lyc.

SIGHING : arn, cimic, **Dig, Ign,** lach.

          expiration : samb.

          involuntary : **Ign,** lach.

SNORING : Op.

          loud : **Op.**

STERTOROUS : Am-c, *arn,* **Op.**

          sleep, during : **Op, Puls.**

SUFFOCATIVE : (See Difficult).

WANT of breath : (See Difficult).

WHEEZING : Ars, aral, hep, *iod,* **Ip,** spong.

❑❑❑

Sensation As If

ABDOMEN, in, something alive moving in abdomen, stomach, uterus, etc. : **Croc,** sabin, sulph, **Thuj.**

        something tight would break if much efforts for stool were used : apis.

        wall drawn by a strin to the spine : **Plb.**

BACK, small of, were falling to pieces : tril-p.

BAND, drawn tightly around the body : **Anac, Cact, Carb-ac,** mag-p, *sulph.*

BLUNT instrument pressing : anac.

BODY feels caged, each wire being twisted tighter and tighter : **Cact.**

        lifted high up into air, great anxiety lest she falls from this height : hyper.

BRAIN, torn to pieces : verat.

BREATH would leave her, when lying down, : *lac-c.*

CALVARIUM, opening and shutting : **Cann-i,** *cimic.*

CLOUD, heavy black had settled all over her : **Cimic.**

COLD air blowing on her, even when covered, as if sheets were damp : *lac-d.*

        severe, in throat : med.

EYES, in, they would be pressed inward or outward when reading : *asar.*

        cold bathing of eyes, amel : *asar.*

        room filled with smoke : **Croc.**

        weeping : **Croc.**

        cold wind blowing across eyes : **Croc.**

        closing lids tightly, amel : **Croc.**

        too large for orbit : cimic, *com, spig.*

HEAD elongated : *hyper.*

        feels large and skull too small for brain : *glon.*

        wood, made of : petr.

HEART, blood, all gone to heart : lil-t.

        feels full to bursting : lil-t.

feels as if clasped and unclasped by iron band : **Cact.**

bound, no room to beat : **Cact.**

grasped and squeezed by iron band : **Cact, Iod, Lil-t,** sulph.

would stand still : aur, lob.

> as though ceased to beat and then suddenly gave one hard thump : aur, sep.

would stop beating, if she moved : cocaine, **Dig.**

> if not moved : gels.

HIPS were falling to pieces : tril-p.

pelvic bones were broken : aesc, tril-p.

sacro-iliac synchondrosis were falling apart : tril-p.

HOT iron, thrust through back : alum.

needles falling on body : **Agar.**

ICE touched or ice-cold needles piercing skin : **Agar.**

SHEETS were damp : lac-d.

SPARKS, fire, of, falling on body : **Ars, Sec.**

STICKS, sand, gravel, lodged in rectum : **Aesc, Coll.**

STOMACH, burst, would : **Carb-v, Colch.**

> pressing, digging, of , when waking in the morning (after a debauch) : *asar.*

STOOL would pass when passing flatus : **Aloe,** mur-ac, *nat-m,* **Olnd.**

SWELLING in perineum, as if sitting on a ball : **Cann-i.**

with ropy mucus in urine : **Chin.**

TENDONS, to short : *cimx.*

VAGINA, in, warm water flowing down : borx.

WATER, drops of cold, were falling on or from single part : cann-s.

Sensation of

BAND, in forehead : **Carb-ac,** cact, **Gels, Sulph.**
  or hoop, of, around a part : (See Hoop).

BALL of, in forehead : *staph.*
  of, rolling in bladder : *lach.*

BURNED, lime being, in stomach : **Caust.**

BLUNT or dull instrument pressing : anac.

BURNING, of, to examining hand : **Bell.**

COBWEB, on face : *bar-c,* borx, *brom,* **Graph,** *ran-s.*

COLD and heat, of, at same time on scalp : verat.

COLDNESS, of, between scapulae : *am-m,* lachn.

CONGESTION in chest, as if blod from extremities filling in : lob.

CORD, of, tied round the chest : **Cact.**

HEAT and cold, of, at same time on scalp : verat.

HOLLOWNESS, of, in head and other parts : *cocc,* ign.

HOOP or band, of, around a part : **Anac, Cact, Carb-ac,** mag-p, **Sulph.**

LUMP of ice, on vertex : verat.

MICE creeping under : sec.

PLUG, of, in inner part : anac.
  of, in ear : **Asar.**

PRESSING and digging, of, in stomach when waking in morning : asar
  (after a debauch).

PROLAPSE, of, rectum, on : alum, med.

SINKING, of, in abdomen : *acet-ac.*

SPLINTERS of : **Arg-n, Hep, Nit-ac.**

SWASHING, in intestine as from water : **Crot-t.**

SHARP stones, of, on movement : *cocc.*

WRETCHEDNESS, of : *tab.*

TREMBLING, of all over : **Sul-ac.**

❑❑❑

Skin

AFFECTIONS, prone to : **Psor, Sulph.**

    suppressed chancre, from : syph.

    cold weather agg : *alum*, **Petr.**

        amel : *kali-bi.*

ANASARCA : (See Swelling).

ANAEURISM, capillary : *fl-ac.*

ANTHRAX : (See Eruption, Pustule-Malignant).

BED-SORE : (See Sore).

BITING : *merc.*

BLEEDING : petr.

BURNING : Acon, agar, *anthraci* (when ars or best selected remedy fails), **Ars, Bell,** caps (not amel by heat), cham, *dulc,* **Lach, Rhus-t,** sabin, **Sulph.**

    intolerable complants, with : **Anthraci.**

    scratching, after : agar, *am-c,* **Caust,** *dulc,* **Lach, Merc, Rhus-t, Sulph.**

    sensation of, to the examining hand : **Bell.**

    sparks, as from : agar, *calc-p,* **Sec.**

    spots, in : agar, *fl-ac,* **Ph-ac, Sulph.**

CHILBLAIN (See Part Affected) : abrot, **Agar.**

    burn intolerably : **Agar.**

    complaints from : **Agar.**

    itch intolerably : abrot, **Agar.**

CICATRICES, blue : sul-ac.

    break open : *caust,* fl-ac, **Graph.**

    green : led.

    painful : sul-ac.

    red become : *fl-ac, sul-ac.*

        around edges : *fl-ac.*

    sore, become : caust, *fl-ac,* **Graph.**

COARSE : psor.

COLDNESS : arn, **Ars**, **Camph**, *chin*, *ferr*, *hell*, *led*, med, *phos*, pyrog,
           Sec, spig, sul-ac, tab, **Verat**.
           convulsions, during : *hell*.
           except head which may be hot : **Arn**, *hell*.
           icy : **Camph**, **Carb-v**, *tab*.
           injured parts : **Led**.
           suffering parts : *led*.
           touch, cold to, but not cold subjectively : *led*, **Sec**, spig.
           yet throws off cover : **Camph**, med, *sec*.

CONDYLOMATA : (See Excrescences).

CRACKS : **Graph**, **Petr**, **Sars**.
           and burns : *sars*.
           painful : sars.
           winter, in : *graph*, petr.

DELICATE : *bell*, *brom,* dulc.

DIRTY : (See Filthy).

DISCOLOURATION,
           ashy : pyrog, sec.
           black and blue places become green, after injury : *led*.
           blue : *ant-t*, *ars*, *carb-an*, **Carb-v**, **Dig**, **Lach**.
                capillary circulation, deficient from : **Carb-v**.
                newborn, of : *ant-t*.
                spots : **Sul-ac**.
           brown, liver spots : *plb*, sanic, *thuj*,
                white spots : *thuj*.
           dirty : psor, sanic, **Sulph**.
           earth-coloured : **Acet-ac**, **Ars**, spig.
           green, injury after : led.
           jaundiced : phos.
           mottled : hydr.
           pale : *acet-ac*, *ars*, *carb-ac*, *carb-v*, **Lyc**, **Ph-ac**, *plb*, pyrog,
              spig, **Verat**.
                newborn, of : *ant-t*.
           red : **Agar**, *am-c*, **Apis**, **Bell**, **Stram**.
                spots : **Sul-ac**.
                    white, became : ferr, valer.

fiery red : tub.

scarlet : **Bell**.

white : **Ars**, kali-c (milky).

yellow, jaundice : *ant-t*, aur-m-n, *berb*, *caust*, **Chel**, chin, dig, dol, **Crot-h** (malignant), **Plb**, podo, *spig*, tarax.

gray : *chel*.

DRY : acet-ac, *acon*, alum, *am-c*, **Ars**, **Bell**, **Bry**, **Colch**, **Nux-v**, **Petr**, *psor*, pyrog, *sabad*, sars, **Sil**.

burning : **Acon**, **Bell**, pyrog.

inability to perspire : *alum*, **Ars**, **Bell**, **Colch**, **Graph**, **Nux-m**, **Plb**, *psor*.

exercising, when : arg-met, *calc*, *nat-m*, **Plb**.

and perspiring alternately : apis.

ECCHYMOSIS : **Arn**, *carb-v*, *crot-h*, **Led**, **Sec**, **Sul-ac**, *ter*.

ERUPTIONS : *am-c*, alum, *apis*, arn, **Ars**, bell, bov, *bry*, canth, **Caust**, *con*, cupr, *dulc*, *graph*, *hell*, lach, **Merc**, **Mez**, **Nat-m**, **Petr**, **Psor**, **Rhus-t**, **Sil**, **Sulph**, *thuj*, tub.

covered portion only, on : *thuj*.

blisters : *anthraci*, **Ant-c**, **Rhus-t**.

black or blue : **Anthraci**, **Lach**, **Pyrog**.

often fatal in 24 hours : **Anthraci**, **Lach**, **Pyrog**.

blood : *sec*.

blotches : sul-ac.

boils : **Arn** (extremely sore, one after another), *crot-h*, dulc, *graph*, **Lach**, *sec*, **Sulphaci**, tarent.

blood-boils : anthraci, arn, *bell*, crot-h, *sil*.

crops, coming in : *sulph*.

greenish pus : sec.

maturing slowly and healing slowly : hep, sec, sil, sulph.

one heals, another comes : *sulph*, *tub*.

small : **Arn** (painful, one after another).

burning : **Apis**, **Ars**, *canth*, dulc, **Graph**, **Rhus-t**, thuj

scratching after : (See Burning).

ERUPTIONS, carbuncle : *anthraci*, *arn*, **Ars**, **Bell**, *crot-h*, lach, **Sil**, *tarent*.

burning : **Anthraci**, *ars*, **Tarent**.

purple with small vesicles around : **Lach**.

chicken-pox : **Ant-c**, *ant-t*.

coppery : **Carb-an**, syph.

    turning blue on getting cold : syph.

crusty : **Calc**, **Calc-s**, *cic*, **Dulc**, **Graph**, **Mez**, *sars*, *staph*.

    bleeds on scratching : *dulc*.

    body, over whole : **Dulc**.

    lemon-coloured : *cic*.

    moist : **Graph**, **Staph**.

    red border, with : *dulc*.

    scratching, after : *dulc*.

    yellow : *cic*, dulc, staph.

damp weather, from : *dulc*.

desquamating : *arum-t*, **Mez**.

    scarlatina, second or third time : arum-t.

discharging, moist : **Dulc**, **Graph**, **Mez**, **Merc**, nat-m, psor, staph.

    copious : mez.

    corrosive : *graph*, staph.

    glutinous : **Graph**.

    ichorous : anthraci.

    offensive : anthraci.

    scratching, after : **Graph**, mez.

    serous : mez.

    yellow : staph.

dry : alum, *dulc*, *graph*, **Mez**, nat-m, psor, *sars*.

eczema : **Calc**, **Cic**, **Crot-t**, **Dulc**, **Graph**, **Mez**, nat-m, **Psor**, **Rhus-t**, *staph*.

    edges of hair, on : nat-m.

    inflamed : nat-m.

    itching, without : cic.

    raw : nat-m.

    red : nat-m.

    salt agg : nat-m.

    solaris : mur-ac.

    sea voyage or sea-shore : nat-m.

    tubercular : *tub*.

    vaccination, after : *mez*.

    wet weather, damp rainy, during : **Dulc**.

    winter, worse in : **Petr**.

herpetic : **Dulc**, **Graph**, *hep*, *ran-b*, *sars*, **Sep**.

    blue : ran-b.

    cercinate : **Nat-m**, **Sep**, **Tell**.

        upper part of body : **Sep**.

        in intersecting rings all over : **Tell**.

    cold water agg : *dulc*.

    corrosive : **Graph**.

    crusty : **Calc**, **Graph**, sars.

    itching : sars.

    moist : **Calc**, **Dulc**, **Graph**.

    zoster : **Ran-b**, **Rhus-t**.

ill-developed from defective vitality : *am-c*, apis.

itch : aloe, alum, dulc, **Graph**, **Mez**, *petr*, *psor*, *sars*, *sep*, sul-ac.

    night : **Merc**.

    suppressed, ailments from : *psor* (after sulph fails).

        by sulphur or mercury : sep.

    vaccination, after : *mez*.

    warmth, agg : *alum*, **Merc**, *sulph*.

        in bed, agg : *alum*, merc, *mez*, **Psor**, **Sulph**.

    winter, at approach of : aloe, *petr*, **Psor** .

leprosy : **Sec**, **Sulph**.

measles : **Acon**, **Apis**, camph.

    black : lach.

    bad effects of : camph.

    badly managed : **Puls**.

    eruptions do not appear : *camph*.

    imperfectly developed : apis, **Zinc**.

    suppressed, bad effects of : *apis*, bry, **Zinc**.

moist : (See Discharging).

non-developed : **Zinc**.

painful : *hep*, petr.

petechiae : **Phos**, **Rhus-t**, sul-ac.

pimples : *con*, *dulc*, *hep*.

psoriasis : **Ars-i**, **Phyt**, **Sep**.

pustules : *ant-t*, **Ars**, *dulc*, *hep*, lach.

    black or blue : **Anthraci**, **Lach**.

        often fatal in 24 to 48 hours : **Anthraci, Lach, Pyrog.**

        malignant : **Anthraci, Lach,** *tarent.*

        renewing constantly : sep.

rash : **Am-c, Bell,** con, *dulc, graph,* sars.

        air, exposure to open : sars.

        menses, before : *con, dulc.*

            during (disappear with flow) : *con, dulc.*

            profuse, during : **Bell,** graph.

        miliary : *am-c.*

        scarlet (red) : **Am-c, Bell.**

        slow evolution of rash in eruptive fevers : **Bry.**

red : syph.

        turning blue on getting cold : syph.

ringworm : **Rhus-t, Sep, Tub.**

scabies : **Carb-v,** *graph, hep, merc,* **Psor, Sep, Sulph.**

        suppressed : *carb-v, caust,* **Sulph.**

            mercury and sulphur, with : **Caust, Psor, Sep.**

scaly : **Ars,** *psor.*

        bran-like : tub.

        dry : **Ars,** *psor.*

            disappear in summer, return in winter : **Psor.**

scarlatina : **Am-c, Apis, Bell,** *carb-ac, crot-h,* **Rhus-t.**

        eruptions do not appear : *camph.*

        imperfectly developed : apis, **Zinc.**

        malignant : **Am-c,** *carb-ac, crot-h,* lach.

        suppression, bad effects of : *apis,* **Zinc.**

small-pox : am-c, **Ant-t,** *carb-ac,* **Merc,** vario.

        malignant : am-c, carb-ac, lach.

smooth : **Bell.**

spring : *nat-s,* psor, *sars.*

suppressed : apis, **Bry,** *caust, cupr,* op, **Psor, Sulph, Zinc.**

        bad effects of : apis, **Caust, Cupr,** *hell,* **Psor** (after failure of sulph), **Zinc.**

        by sulphur and zinc ointment : **Caust, Psor.**

suppurating : **Hep, Graph, Merc, Nit-ac,** *psor.*

tettery : alum, *bov,* nat-m (at bends of joints), sep.

tubercles : *dulc.*

urticaria : **Apis, Ars,** bov (after rhus-t fails), **Dulc, Nat-m,** rumx.

  alternating with croup-like attack : *ars*.

  cold air amel *: dulc*.

  cold, from taking : **Dulc**.

  exercise, violent, after : apis, calc, hep, *nat-m*, sanic, *urt-u*.

  scratching, after : **Dulc**.

  suppression, bad effects of : *apis*, **Zinc**.

  warmth, agg : *dulc*.

varicella : vario.

varioloid : vario.

vesicular : **Ars**, carb-ac, **Canth, Dulc**, rhus-t, rumx, staph.

  black : *anthraci*, **Ars**.

  sore : canth.

  suppurating : canth.

washing, agg : *dulc*.

winter, worse in : aloe, alum, **Petr, Psor**.

ERYSIPELAS : **Anthraci, Apis** (more oedema), **Bell**, *canth* (more blistering), **Graph, Lach, Rhus-t**.

  right to left : *apis, graph, lyc*.

  left to right : *lach, rhus-t*.

  chronic : **Graph**.

  gangrenous : **Anthraci**.

    burning, terrible : **Anthraci**.

  inflammation, with : **Rhus-t**.

  iodium, after application of : graph.

  old debilitated persons, of, where reaction weak : *am-c*.

  swelling : **Rhus-t**.

  vesicular : canth (sore and suppurating), **Rhus-t**.

    yellow : *rhus-t*.

ERYTHEMA from exposure to sun : *canth*.

EXCORIATION : **Calc, Calc-s, Nit-ac, Sulph**.

EXCRESCENCES : *ant-c*, **Caust, Graph, Nit-ac, Staph**, sulph, **Thuj**.

  condylomata : *aur*, **Med, Merc, Nat-s, Nit-ac, Thuj**.

    bleeding : **Nit-ac, Thuj**.

    moist : **Nit-ac, Thuj**.

sticking pain : **Nit-ac.**
syphilitic : **Nit-ac.**
fungus, cauliflower : **Ant-c.**
horny : **Ant-c.**

FILTHY : *caps*, lyc, **Psor**, *sanic*, **Sulph**, thuj

FLABBY : abrot, agar, bar-c, **Calc**, *caps*, *ferr*, iod, op, puls, sars.
hangs loose in folds : abrot.

FORMICATION : acon, sec.

FRECKLES : *ant-c*, lach, **Lyc**, *mur-ac*.

GANGRENE : *agar*, **Anthraci**, **Ars**, *rhus-t*, **Sec**, *tarent*.
cold : **Ars**, **Plb**, **Sec**.
dry : **Sec**.
heat, agg : *sec*.
moist : **Chin**.
senile : **Sec**.

GREASY : (See Face).

HARD, like callosities : *ant-c*.
perchment, like : **Ars**, psor, sabad, *sars*.
thickening. with : **Ant-c**.

HEAT without fever : acet-ac, bell, sulph.

HOT needles, sensation of : *agar*.

HYPERAESTHESIA : (See Sensitiveness, Sore).

ICE or ice-cold needles, sensation of : *agar*.

INDURATIONS, nodules, etc : **Ant-c**, **Calc**, sars.

INTERTRIGO : Caust, *lyc*.
during, dentition : **Caust**, *lyc*.

ITCHING : Agar, *alum*, **Bov**, *calad*, *crot-t*, *dulc*, **Graph**, *kreos*, merc, **Mez**,
Rhus-t, rumx, sabin, **Sep**, **Sulph**.
evening : **Kreos** (so violent as to make one wild), *merc*.
bathing agg : tub.
biting : merc.
burning : **Ars**, **Rhus-t**, *sep*, **Sulph**.
scratching, from : sep, **Sulph**.
cold, from : *hep*, olnd, nat-s, *rumx*.

despair, driven to, from : **Psor**.

eruption, without : dol, **Mez**.

heat of bed, agg : merc, **Sulph**.

intense or intolerable : *alum*, **Calad**, **Crot-t**, merc, *mez*, tub.

    but so tender unable to scratch : **Crot-t**.

        gentle rubbing amel : crot-t.

        genitals, of : *crot-t*, **Rhus-t**.

        insect or mosquito bites : *calad*.

        insect bite, as from : merc.

        eruption, without any visible : dol.

scratch until it bleeds : *alum*, **Ars**, *med*, *psor*,

    until it is raw : **Graph**, merc, **Petr**.

scratching agg : **Ars**, **Caps**, **Rhus-t**, **Sulph**.

        amel : merc, *sulph*.

        not amel. by : sep.

        changing place, on : *staph*.

touch, agg : mez

undressing agg : **Hep**, *olnd*, *nat-s*, **Rumx**, *tub*.

voluptuous : **Sulph**.

warm, becoming : **Merc**, mez, **Psor**, **Sulph**.

    in bed, on becoming : *alum*, *merc*, merc-i-f. *mez*, **Psor**,
    Sulph.

    amel : rumx.

JAUNDICE : (See Discolouration, Yellow).

MEDICATED soaps and washes, after : *sulph*.

MOISTURE : **Bell**, *cham*, *petr*.

MOLES : **Puls**.

NAEVI : **Fl-ac**, thuj.

ODOUR : (See Perspiration).

PERCHMENT, like : (See Hard).

PETECHIAE : (See Eruption).

PURPURA haemorrhagica : *crot-h*, **Lach**, **Led**, **Phos**, **Sec**, **Sul-ac**, **Ter**.

RAWNESS : (See Excoriation).

RHAGADES : (See Cracks).

ROUGH : Calc, Petr, Sep, Sulph.
 hands, of : **Petr.**

SCALY : (See Eruption).

SENSITIVENESS : Apis, Bell, Chin, *coff*, **Hep, Lach,** *nux-m*, **Petr**, plb, rumx, **Sulph**, tarent.
 atmospheric changes, to : **Hep, Kali-c, Psor, Sulph.**
 clothing, to, of the affected part : **Bell, Chin, Hep, Lach**, petr.
 slightest touch, to, but can bear hard pressure : **Chin.**
 touch, to, skin affection, even fainting : **Hep, Nux-m.**
 cold to : **Dulc.**

SHINING : Apis, Bell, bov.

SMOOTH : Bell.

SORE becomes (decubitus) : **Ars**, bapt, carb-ac, fl-ac, **Graph, Lach**, mur-ac, nux-m, pyrog.
 in folds of skin : lyc, sulph, tub.
 rapid : carb-ac, pyrog.

SPHACELUS : ars.

SPLINTER, pain, as from : **Hep, Nit-ac.**

STINGING : *rhus-t*, **Apis, Urt-u.**

STINGS of insects : *anthraci* (even suspicious), merc.
 if swelling changes colour and red streaks map out : *anthraci*, *lach, pyrog.*

SUN-BURN : (See Erythema).

SUPPURATES, slight injury : *calen*, **Borx, Graph, Hep,** *merc*, *petr*, **Sil.**

SWELLING : ant-c, **Apis,** *dulc*, **Sulph.**
 dropsical : *dulc.*
 ague, after : *dulc.*
 rheumatism, after : *dulc.*
 scarlet fever, after : *dulc.*

TENDENCY to skin disease : **Psor, Sulph.**

TENDER : Crot-t.

ULCERS : *anthraci*, *arn*, **Ars,** *aur*, calad, carb-ac, **Carb-v**, chel, *fl-ac*, *graph*, **Hep, Lach, Merc-c,** *mez*, **Nit-ac,** *sars*, **Sil.**
 black or dark : **Anthraci, Ars, Lach.**

bleeding : **Ars, Hep, Lach**, *mez*, **Nit-ac**.

    touched, when : **Hep, Lach**, *mez*, *nit-ac*.

bluish : ars, **Lach**, lyss.

burning : **Anthraci, Ars**, *carb-ac*, **Carb-v**, *hep*, *mez*.

    after ars fails : anthraci.

cancerous : **Ars, Bufo, Hep, Lyc, Sil, Sulph**.

cold, amel : *fl-ac*.

crusty : **Calc, Mez**.

    thick : mez.

    yellowish-white : mez.

    with thick yellow pus beneath : **Mez**.

discharges, brown : nit-ac,

    copious : *calen, fl-ac*.

    corrosive : **Merc**, *nit-ac*.

    gluey, sticking the linen : *graph*, mez.

    ichorous : **Merc-c**.

    malignant : *tarent*.

    offensive : **Nit-ac**, pyrog, psor, **Ars, Bapt**.

    putrid : **Chel**.

    thin : nit-ac.

    yellow : *nit-ac*.

        green : nit-ac.

elevated, indurated margins, with : **Ars, Sil**.

exuberant granulations, with : arg-n, nit-ac, sabin, thuj.

fistulous : **Caust**, *fl- ac*, *hep*, *sil*.

gangrenous : am-c, *anthraci*, **Ars, Lach**.

glistening : (See Shining).

indolent : fl-ac.

inflamed : *calen*.

irritable : calen.

itching : **Mez**.

jagged margin, with : **Merc**.

    zig-zag : *nit-ac*.

lardaceous : ars, **Merc**.

malignant : *anthraci, lach,*

mercurial : **Hep**, hydr, **Nit-ac, Sars**.

obstinate : *fl-ac*.

old : *fl-ac*.

old persons, of : pyrog.

painful : **Arn**, **Calen**, *fl-ac*, *lach*.

    beaten, as if : **Arn**, **Calen**.

    like streaks of lightening : *fl-ac*.

painless : **Op**.

pimples, surrounded by : *hep*, **Lach**.

potash chlorate, after : hydr.

pricking pain, with : ham.

purple : **Lach**.

raw flesh-like base : nit-ac.

red areola : **Mez**.

    edges : fl-ac.

scratching, after : *graph*, *hep*, **Lach**.

shining glazed : *lac-c*, mez.

sloughing : *anthraci*, **Calen**.

spreading : *ars* (in breadth), *chel*.

stinging : ham, **Nit-ac**.

    splinters, as from : *hep*, **Nit-ac**.

syphilitic : **Kali-i, Merc, Merc-c**, merc-i-r, **Nit-ac, Phyt**, *sars*.

touch, agg : nit-ac.

unhealthy : **Borx, Graph, Hep**, *lyc*.

varicose : *fl-ac*, ham.

vesicles, surrounded by : *fl-ac*, **Mez**.

warmth agg : *fl-ac*.

women, in, who have borne many children : fl-ac.

UNHEALTHY : **Borx, Calc, Graph, Hep**, *lyc*, merc, **Sil**, *thuj*.

VARICOSE veins : (See Generalities).

WARTS (See Excrescences) : anac, *ant-c*, **Caust, Calc, Nit-ac**, *nat-m*, sabin, staph, **Sulph, Thuj**.

    bleeding : **Caust, Thuj**.

        from washing : *nit-ac*.

    cauliflower-like : *staph*.

    dry : *staph*.

    horny : **Ant-c**.

    jagged : **Caust, Nit-ac**.

    large : *caust*, **Nit-ac, Thuj**.

mercury, after abuse of : *aur*, *nit-ac*, sabin, *staph*, thuj.

moist : *caust*, **Nit-ac**.

oozing : *nit-ac*.

palms of hands, on : *anac*, *nat-m*.

pedunculated : **Caust**, **Nit-ac**, *staph*, *thuj*.

small, all over the body : **Caust**.

seedy : **Thuj**.

sensitive : *caust*, **Staph**, *thuj*.

sticking pain : **Nit-ac**, *staph*, **Thuj**.

sycotic : **Nit-ac**, **Thuj**.

syphilitic : **Nit-ac**.

WAXY : Acet-ac, Apis, Ars, kali-c, phos.

WENS : ant-c.

WRINKLED, shrivelled : *abrot*, *ars*, *op*, spig.

hangs in folds in children : *abrot*, *iod*, nat-m, *sanic*, sars.

Sleep

ANXIOUS : (See Mind, Dreams).

COMATOSE : **Ant-t, Bapt, Bell,** *hell,* **Nux-m, Op,** *ph-ac, sulph.*

CONVULSIONS, after : *op.*

DEEP : am-c, **Ant-t, Bapt, Bell,** *hell,* **Kreos,** mur-ac, **Nux-m,** *ph-ac,* **Puls,** *sep.*

  morning, when time to get up : **Puls.**

DISTURBED : puls.

  first sleep : puls.

DREAMS, amorous : *dios* (of women), **Staph.**

  darger : psor.

  drinkng, of : med.

  exertion, of great : rhus-t.

  frightful : **Kali-br,** kali-p, **Nat-m,** psor.

    night-terror of children : **Kali-br,** kali-p.

  happy : *sulph.*

    wakes up signing : sulph.

  horrible : (See Frightful).

  robbers : **Nat-m,** psor.

    cannot believe to contrary on waking until house is searched : **Nat-m,** psor.

  rowing : rhus-t.

  swiming : rhus-t.

  thieves : (See Robbers).

  thirsty, of : **Nat-m.**

  women, of, all night : dios, **Staph.**

  working hard at his daily occupation : bry, rhus-t.

DROWSINESS (See Sleepiness) : *aeth,* **Ant-t,** bapt, gels, *helon,* **Nux-m, Op,** *sulph.*

  afternoon : **Sulph.**

    wakeful all night : **Sulph.**

  vomiting, after : *aeth,* **Ant-t.**

FALLING, asleep,

  evening : nux-v.

   reading, while : *nux-v.*

   sitting, while : **Nux-v.**

  answering, when : **Arn, Bapt.**

  coition, during : *lyc.*

  embrace, during : *lyc.*

  heat, during : *ant-t,* **Calad.**

   wakes when it stops : calad.

  sitting : mur-ac.

  vomiting, after : *aeth,* **Ant-t.**

HEAT, during intermittent : **Ant-t, Op.**

HEAVY : op.

POSITION, abdomen : acet-ac.

  back, on : ars.

   impossible : acet-ac.

  limbs crossed : rhod.

PROFOUND : (See Deep).

RESTLESS : Ars, Bell, Cina, Lyc, rhod, **Rhus-t.**

SLEEPINESS : *aeth,* **Ant-t, Bell,** caps, **Chin,** *cham,* coca, *gels, helon,*
  Nux-m, Op, Ph-ac, Phos, Sel, *stram,* **Sulph.**

  morning : **Nux-v, Sulph.**

   from which it is hard to arouse : **Nux-v.**

  afternoon : **Sulph.**

   after sunset : **Nux-v,** sulph.

    sleepless whole night : **Sulph.**

  but cannot sleep : **Bell,** *cham,* **Op,** *stram.*

  convulsion, after : aeth.

  dinner, after : nat-m, **Nux-v.**

  intoxication, as from : **Nux-m.**

  irresistible : *ant-t,* **Nux-m,** nux-v, **Op.**

   morning, at daybreak from which it is hard to arouse :
    Nux-v.

  purring in ears, from : pyrog.

  stool, after : aeth.

  throbbing in ears, from : pyrog.

  vomiting, after : *aeth, ant-t,* **Ip.**

SLEEPLESSNESS : aeth, ambr, am-c, arum-t, *bapt,* **Bell,** *caust,* canth, **Cham,** cimic, *cocc,* **Coff,** helon, **Hyos,** *ign, jal, kali-br, med,* **Op,** psor, **Puls,** rhod, **Staph,** *stict,* stram, **Sulph,** *syph.*

evening : **Puls.**

ailments from, or night watching : *caust,* **Cocc,** *ign.*

babies, in : (See Sick Babies).

business embarrassment, must sit up : **Ambr,** cimic, **Hyos,** kali-br, **Sep.**

cannot get herself together, because she : bapt.

excitement, physical, from, through mental exaltation : *ambr,* **Coff, Hyos.**

frightful dreams of robbers or danger, etc., from : **Nat-m.**

grief, from : *ign, kali-br.*

headache, from : syph.

imaginary cause, from : hyos.

impossible to close eyes : **Coff.**

itching, from : **Psor.**

anus, of : aloe, ind.

joy, excessive : **Coff.**

menses, during : senec.

mental strain, after : **Nux-v.**

exertion, after : *coff.*

night watching : **Cocc.**

noise, from slight : *nux-v.*

clock stricking and cocks crowing at great distance keep her awake : **Op.**

nursing the sick : **Cocc.**

obstruction of nose, from : *am-c.*

pain, from : ars, med.

prolapse uterus, from : senec.

property, from loss of : *kali-br.*

prostration, with : *aeth.*

pregnancy, during : cimic.

reputation, from loss of : kali-br.

retiring, after, but sleepy before : **Ambr.**

sexual excitement, from : *canth.*

sick babies, in : *cham,* jal, *psor.*

day and night : jal, psor.

plays all day but cries all night : jal, *psor.*

cries all day but sleeps at night : lyc.

sleepiness, with : **Bell,** *caust,* **Cham, Op,** *stram.*

in afternoon, after sunset : **Sulph.**

sleepy all day but sleeples all night, body aches all over : **Staph.**

thoughts, activity of mind, from : **Coff.**

uterine irritation, from : senec.

weariness, from : **Ars,** *helon.*

wide-awake condition : **Coff.**

worry, from : ambr, hyos, kali-br.

UNCONQUERABLE : (See Sleepiness, Irresistible).

UNREFRESHING : bry, *chin,* con, hep, **Mag-c,** *op, puls, sulph.*

more tired in the mornng than when retiring : bry, con, hep, *mag-c,* op, **Sulph.**

WAKING, 3 a.m. : **Nux-v, Sulph.**

cold limbs, from : **Carb-v.**

early : chin.

fright, as from : **Lyc,** *spong,* zinc.

sudden : sulph.

YAWNING : am-c, aml-ns, asar, *kali-c.*

constant : asar.

frequent : aml-ns, *kali-c.*

menses, during : *am-c.*

profound : aml-ns, kali-c.

□□□

Stomach

ACIDITY : (See Sour Eructation and Vomiting).

ALIVE sensation as if something, in : **Croc**.

ANXIETY : **Ars**, ip, sulph.

APPETITE, abnormal things for (See Desires) : **Alum, Cic, Psor**.

        capricious (hunger, but knows not for what) : **Bry, Chin, Cina**.

        diminished : **Alum**, *psor*.

        easy satiety : *cycl*, **Lyc**, petros.

        increased : aloe, **Calc**, casc, **Cina**, *lac-c*, **Lob, Lyc, Psor**, sel, stront.

        night, middle of : **Cina, Psor**, sel.

            must eat something : **Cina, Psor**, phos, *sulph, tub*.

        eating increases the : **Lyc**.

        eating, after : *calc*, casc, lac-c, **Lyc**, stront-c.

            does not amel : (See Emptiness).

        diarrhoea, during : *aloe*.

        headache, with : ign, lyc, **Psor**.

        stool, after : aloe.

        insatiable : **Iod, Lyc**, *zinc*.

        loss of : (See Wanting).

        ravenous, canine, excessive : *abrot*, *chin*, **Cina, Ferr, Iod**, lac-ac, **Lyc**, med, **Nat-m, Psor**, sanic, *sec*, **staph, Sulph, Zinc**.

        11 or 12 a.m. : **Sulph, Zinc**.

        night : **Chin, Psor**, sel, *staph*, **Tub**.

        cannot eat fast enough : zinc.

        diarrhoea, during : aloe.

        eating increases the hunger : **Lyc**.

            after, soon : **Cina, Iod, Lyc**, *med, psor*.

            every few hours : **Iod**.

        emaciation, with : *abrot*, **Iod, Nat-m**, sanic, *tub*.

        fever, in, for days before attack : staph.

        stomach, full when : staph.

waking while at night : **Cina**, *lyc*, **Psor**.

wanting : chel, chin, **Cocc**, **Ferr**, **Kali-bi**, *psor*, tarax, **Sulph**.

AVERSION, to acids : *bell*, *ferr*, *sulph*.

bread : **Chin**, **Nat-m**.

drinks : *canth*, **Ferr**.

fats and rich food : *colch*.

fish : colch.

food : **Ars**, *canth*, **Cocc**, **Colch**, **Ferr**, rheum.

though desires various kinds : *rheum*.

liquids : bell, **Lyss**, **Stram**.

meat : **Calc**, **Mur-ac**, nit-ac.

milk : *aeth*, *cina*, **Lac-d**, **Nat-c**.

mother's : *cina*.

tobacco : *canth*, **Ign**.

water : *bell*, *lyss*, **Stram**.

BELCHING : (See Eructation).

BURNING of : colch.

CANCER : *bism*, con.

CLOTHING disturbs : **Lach**, **Nux-v**.

COLDNESS : *calc*, *colch*, *sul-ac*.

cold drink, after : *sul-ac*.

CONGESTION : **Verat-v**.

DESIRES, acids, sour : alum, *ant-c*, chin, **Hep**, *med*, *sec*, **Verat**.

accustomed stimulants, for : coca.

alcoholic drinks : **Asar**, *coca*, *med*, **Sel**, *syph*.

unconquerable craving for : **Asar**, *calc-ar*, *carb-v*, *med*, **Sul-ac**.

which before he hated : asar, med, *sel*.

ale : *med*.

beer : **Nux-v**.

brandy : carb-v, **Nux-v**, **Op**.

whisky : asar, carb-ac, carb-v, *sel*.

wine : sel.

apples : aloe, ant-t.

chalk : *alum*, calc, cic, *psor*.

charcoal : *alum*, *cic*, psor.

bread and butter : **Ferr**.

cloves : *alum*.

coal : *alum*, *calc*, *cic*.

coffee, ground : *alum*.

cold, drinks : **Ars**, **Phos** , *podo*, **Verat**.

    food : **Phos**, *verat*.

earth : (See Lime).

eats indigestible things, chalk, coal, etc. with apparent relish:
    alum, *cic*, *psor*.

eats seldom but much : *ars*.

eggs : *calc*.

fat : **Nit-ac**, *nux-v*.

fruit : **Ph-ac**, **Verat**.

    green : *med*.

hot drink (See Warm Drink) : **Ars**, *casc*, *chel*.

ice : *med*.

ice cream : **Phos**.

indigestible things : *alum*, calc, cic, *psor*.

    with relish , children takes : *alum*, *cic*, *psor*.

juicy things : **Ph-ac**, *phos*.

lemonade : **Bell**, sec.

lime, slate pencil,earth, chalk, clay, etc. : alum, *calc*, *cic*, psor.

meat : *mag-c*.

    smoked : *calc-p*.

    in children of tubercular parentage : *mag-c*.

onion : *all-c*.

orange : med.

pickles : *ant-c*.

refreshing things : **Ph-ac**, *phos*, **Verat**.

salt thing : **Arg-n**, *calc-p*, calc-s, *caust*, *med*, **Nat-m**.

sour : (See Acid).

stimulants, accustomed : *coca*.

starch : *alum*.

sweets : **Arg-met**, *cina*, **Chin**, **Lyc**, *mag-m*, *med*, **Sulph**.

    sugar : **Arg-n**.

tea : *ant-c*.

    ground : *alum*.

tobacco : asar, carb-ac, carb-v, coca, *scaph*, **Tab**.

varieties : *cina*.

warm drinks : **Ars**, casc, *chel*.

can retain only : chel.

DIGESTION weak : carb-v, *dios*.

DISORDERED : Ant-c, Arg-n, Carb-v, Ip.

over-eating, from : **Ant-c.**

DISTENSION : ant-c, **Arg-n**, asaf, **Calc, Carb-v, Cic, Chin**, dios, iod, **Kali-c, Lyc, Nux-m.**

burst, it would feels as if : **Arg-n, Asaf, Carb-v, Kali-c.**

debauch, effects of a : **Carb-v.**

drinking, after : carb-v.

eating, after : ant-c, **Carb-v, Chin**, dios, **Lyc**, *nux-m*, **Nux-v.**

eructation amel : **Carb-v.**

do not amel : **Chin.**

everything she eats or drinks converted into gas : iod, **Kali-c, Nux-m.**

fruits, after : **Chin**, puls.

lying agg : *carb-v.*

rich food, after : *carb-v.*

supper, after : carb-v.

EMPTINESS, weak feeling, faintness, goneness, hungry feeling : *anac*, chel, cocc, *crot-h*, **Dig, Hydr, Ign**, *iod*, *Lac-c*, *lob*, **Murx, Phos, Puls**, sep, **Stann, Sulph, Tab**, tril-p.

10 or 11 a.m. : nat-c.

eating, amel : *nat-c.*

11 a. m. : **Sulph.**

digestion, during , amel : anac.

agg : *bry*, **Nux-v.**

eating, while, amel : *anac*, chel, **Iod**, murx, *phos*, sep.

not relieved by : casc, **Calc, Cina**, *hydr*, **Ign, Lyc, Sep**, stront-c.

tea, after excessive use of : *lob*, **Puls.**

tobacco, after excessive use of : *lob.*

ERUCTATIONS (belching) : acet-ac, alum, **Ambr**, *ant-c*, **Arg-n, Arn**, *asaf*, bism, *calc*, **Carb-v**, *cham*, **Chin**, *ferr*, **Iod, Kali-bi, Kali-c, Lyc**, *mag-m*, **Nux-v, Phos, Psor, Puls, Sulph.**

evening : *alum*, **Puls.**

aggravate : **Cham, Chin.**

ameliorate : **Carb-v, Kali-c, Lyc**.

bursting with wind : **Arg-n**.

coughing, after : **Ambr**.

difficult : **Arg-n**.

drinking, after : *kali-c*.

eating, after : **Arg-n**, kali-bi, *kali-c*, *nux-v*.

    over-eating, from : ant-c.

frequent : calad.

fruit, after : **Chin**, puls.

long lasting : *alum*.

meal, after every : *arg-n*.

potatoes, after : *alum*.

air rising out in volume : **Arg-n**.

bitter : **Nux-v**.

eggs, rotten, spoiled, like : **Arn**, ant-t, graph, mag-m, *psor*.

empty : **Ant-c**, *calad*, **Iod**, *kali-c*.

food (regurgitation) : aeth, alum, **Ferr, Phos**.

    after eating, an hour or so : aeth.

    mouthful, by the : alum, *ferr*, **Phos**.

        nausea, without : *ferr*.

food tasting like : **Ant-c**.

foul : **Arn**.

loud : **Arg-n**.

onion-like : *mag-m*.

putrid : *arn*.

sour : *acet-ac*, **Calc**, carb-v, *ferr-p*, lyc, **Mag-c**, *nat-p*, **Nux-v**,
    Rob, Sulph, Sul-ac.

    pregnancy, of : **Acet-ac**.

waterbrush, pyrosis : acet-ac, carb-v, *bism*, **Lyc, Nux-v**.

FAINTNESS : (See Emptines, Sinking).

FERMENTATION : *chin*.

FLATULANCE : (See Eructation).

FOOD, cold, agrees : **Nux-v**.

    hot, agrees : **Puls**.

FULLNESS, sensation of : **Carb-v, Chin, Lyc**.

    eating, while : *nux-m*.

        after : **Carb-v, Chin**, kali-bi, **Lyc**, *nux-m*, **Nux-v**.

a few mouthful, after : **Lyc**.
eructation amel : *carb-v*.
    do not amel : *chin*.

GAGGING (See Nausea) : bry, *kali-c*, *podo*, sec.
    morning : cina.
        clearing the throat, when, until vomits the breakfast just
            taken : euphr, bry.
    convulsive after laparotomy : **Bism, Nux-v, Staph**.
    coughing, from : bry, dros, ip, kali-bi, kali-c.
    mucus, viscid, in the throat, from : kali-bi.
    swallowing water, when : lyss.

GOUT, metastasis : **Ant-c**.

HAEMORRHAGE : (See Vomiting).

HANGING down, sensation of, relaxed : agar, **Ign, Ip**, *staph, tab*.

HEARTBURN : **Lyc, Mag-c**, *sul-ac*.
    pregnancy, during : *mag-c*.

HEAVINESS, weight, oppression (See Fullness) : ant-c, **Chin**, *kali-bi*.
    eating, from : *ant-c*.

HICCOUGH : **Cic, Ign, Mag-p, Nux-v**, *ran-b*.

INACTIVITY : *op*.

INDIGESTION : *ars*, **Carb-v**, *coll, mag-m*, **Nux-v**, *tab*.
    children, in, during dentition : aeth.
    cheese, strong, after : ars.
    cold fruit, after : ars.
    coffee, after : **Nux-v**.
    drugs, after abuse of : Nux-v.
    drunken debauch, from : **Carb-v, Nux-v**.
    ice cream : *ars*, **Puls**.
    ice water : **Ars**.
    mental exertion, after : **Nux-v**.
    milk, after : **Aeth**, *mag-c*, **Mag-m**.
        difficult dentition, during : **Mag-m**.
    onions, after : **Lyc**.
    over-eating, after : *ant-c*, **Nux-v**.
    potatoes, after : **Alum**.

IRRITATION : Bism.

LOATHING of food : **Ant-c, Ars, Cocc, Colch**.

MORNING sickness : (See Nausea and Vomiting).

MOVEMENTS, sensation as if : (See Sensation).

NAUSEA : *act*, aloe, **Ant-c**, apoc, **Ars**, *asar*, *bry*, chel, *cimic,* **Cocc, Colch**,
croc, *cycl*, **Ip**, *iris*, lac-d, **Lob, Nat-m**, nux-m, **Nux-v**, *phos*, puls,
Sep, *stann*, **Sulph, Tab**, *ther*, **Verat**, *verat-v*.

    morning : graph, **Nux-v, Puls, Sep**, stann.

        menses, during : graph.

        pregnancy, during : graph

    air, open, amel : **Tab**.

    closing eyes, on : *ther*.

    constant : asar, *ip*, **Nux-v**.

    deathly : **Ip, Tab**.

    eating, after : asar, **Nux-v**, puls.

    fish, smell of : **Colch**.

    food, on looking at : **Colch**, *sep*, stann.

        smell of : *ars*, **Colch**, *sep*, stann.

            thought of : *ars*, **Cocc, Colch**, *sep*.

    gastric disturbance, from : **Ip, Puls**.

    headache, during : *nat-m*, *tab*.

    looking at a boat in motion : **ars, Cocc,** *nux-m*.

    menses, before : *nat-m*.

        during : nat-m.

        after : nat-m.

    motion, on : *bry*, **Cocc**, *ip*, ther.

    noise, from : **Ther**.

    paroxysm, in : asar, *ip*.

    pregnancy, during : **Asar**, cimic, *ip*, **Kreos**, *nux-m*, **Nux-v, Sep**.

    riding in a boat, carriage, rail, or on the cars, while : *arn*,
        Cocc, *nux-m*, **Petr**, sanic, *ther*.

    sea-sickness : aml-ns, **Cocc, Tab**, ther.

        amel, on deck in fresh cold air : **Tab**.

    sitting, while : bry.

        up, in bed : *bry*.

    smoking, from : **Nux-v**.

    stooping, on : *ip*.

    tobacco, from : *ip*.

    tongue, clean : asar, **Ip**, *sulph*.

uncovering abdomen, amel : *tab*.

vomiting does not amel : *dig*.

  feels, vomiting would amel : **Nux-v**.

warm water, from placing hands, in : **Phos**.

PAIN : **Ars**, asar, **Bism**, **Bry**, **Coloc**, caul, *ip*, *mag-c*, *mag-m*, *mag-p*, **Nux-v**, *petr*, **Phos**, *staph*, **Sulph**.

morning : asar.

empty, when : (See Emptiness).

ice cream agg : **Ars**.

      amel : *phos*.

laparotomy, after : **Bism**, **Nux-v**, **Staph**.

milk, after : **Mag-m**.

violent : abics-n (after eating), **Bism**, *nux-v*.

warm drink, amel : **Nux-v**, *ph-ac*.

  food agg : **Phos**, **Puls**.

burning : *carb-v*, *bism*, canth, *colch*, iris, erig, *nux-v*, **Sulph**.

  eructation, with : *bism*, *nux-v*.

cramping, griping, constricting, spasmodic : **Bism**, *caul*, **Coloc**, **Ip**, *mag-c*, **Mag-p**.

  band, as if a, was drawn tightly around body : mag-p.

  hand, as from a, each finger sharply pressing into intestine : *ip*.

diggng : (See Gnawing).

drawing : *petr*.

gastralgia : petr.

  eating constantly amel : **Anac**, chel, *petr*, sep.

  hysterical women, in : **Ign**.

  pregnancy, of : petr.

  when stomach empty : petr.

gnawing : asar.

  morning, on waking after a debauch : asar.

griping : (See Cramping).

neuralgic : *mag-p*.

pressing : asar, *bism*, ip, kali-bi, nux-m, *nux-v*, *petr*.

  morning, on waking after a debauch : asar.

  eating, after : *kali-bi*, nux-m, **Nux-v**.

    an hour or two : **Nux-v**.

immediately : kali-bi, nux-m,
stone, as from : (See Stone).
load, as from : *bism*.
alternating with burning : bism.
stone, as if : (See Stone).
sore, bruised, tenderness : **Arn, Ars, Bry, Colch**, *ip*.
spasmodic : (See Pain, Cramping).

PRESSURE as from a load : *bism*.

PYROSIS : (See Eructation, Waterbrush).

REGURGITATION : (See Eructation, Food).

RELAXATION : (See Hanging Down).

RETCHING : *bry, dros*, erig, kali-c.
cough, with : bry, **Dros**, *kali-c*.

SATIETY : (See Appetite).

SENSITIVENESS : kali-c.

SHOCK : **Cic**.

SINKING : (See Emptiness) : *crot-h*, **Dig**, lac-c.

STONE, sensation : **Bry**, cham, **Nux-v, Puls**.
eating, after : **Bry, Nux-v**.
an hour or two after : **Nux-v**.
immediately after : kali-bi, nux-m.
eructation amel : **Bry**.

SWELLING : (See Distension).

TENSION : Nux-v.
must loosen clothing : **Nux-v**.

THIRST : **Acet-ac, Acon**, ant-c, *apoc*, **Ars**, *bism, borx*, **Bry, Cham**, chin,
Eup-per, Hell, ign, med, **Merc**, *nat-m*, petros, podo, **Rhus-t**, sanic,
Verat, lac-ac.
acid drink, for : verat.
burning : **Acet-ac**, *acon, ars, canth*.
without desire to drink : *ars*.
chill, before : **Eup-per**.
during : **Apis, Eup-per, Ign** (external heat amel).
cold water, for, cannot tolerate : **Acon, Ars**.
drinks often but little : **Ars**.
great thirst for : **Acon, Ars**, podo, **Verat**.

swallows cold water, unconscious, while : *hell*.

constant : (See Unquenchable).

diabetes, in : *acet-ac*.

diarrhoea, in : acet-ac.

dropsy, in : *acet-ac*.

extreme : **Acet-ac, Acon, Ars,** *bism,* **Eup-per, Hell,** helon, **Merc, Verat**.

moist mouth, with : **Merc**.

heat, during : **Acon, Ars, Eup-per**.

large quantities, for : acet-ac, *acon,* **Ars, Bry,** *eup-per,* podo, **Verat**.

long interval, at : **Bry**.

often, for : **Bry**.

moist mouth, with : **Merc**.

small quantities, for : **Ars,** phos, sanic.

often : **Ars,** phos, sanic.

pain, during : cham.

perspiration, after : *lyc*.

stool, after : **Caps**.

unquenchable : *acet-ac,* **Eup-per,** *med, verat*.

vanishing, on attempting to drink : petros.

vomiting, before : **Eup-per**.

THIRSTLESS : aeth, **Apis, Gels,** ign, **Nux-m, Puls,** *samb*.

anasarca, in : **Apis**.

ascites, in : **Apis**.

heat, during : **Acet-ac, Apis,** *ign*.

TIGHTNESS : (See Tension).

ULCERS : gymno, **Hydr,** kali-bi.

VOMITING : acet-ac, **Aeth,** *am-m,* **Ant-t,** *apoc,* apom, **Ars,** *bism,* **Bry,** *cact, camph,* carb-ac, **Cham,** *cocc,* coloc, **Colch,** crot-h, **Cupr,** *dros, eup-per,* **Ferr,** *graph,* **Iris,** *kali-bi,* kali-c, **Kreos,** *lac-d,* **Lob,** *nat-m, nux-m,* **Nux-v, Phos,** *sep,* **Sulph, Tab,** *valer,* **Verat, Verat-v**.

morning : graph, nux-v, sep, stann.

menses, during : graph.

pregnancy, during : *sep*.

afternoon : puls.

night, midnight, after : **Ferr**.

anger, after : **Cham, Coloc,** staph, *valer*.

appetite, with : **Lob**.

bright light, from : stram

cancer of : carb-ac,

chill, during : **Eup-per**.

cholera morbus, of : **Ant-t**, bism, kreos, **Verat**.

    with diarrhoea and cold sweat : ant-t, **Verat**.

chronic : **Lob**.

colourless : (See White).

convulsions, after : *cupr*.

convulsive : **Bism**, *cupr*.

coughing, on : **Bry, Dros, Kali-c**.

dentition, painful, during : **Aeth**, *kreos*.

diarrhoea, during : **Ars, Gamb**, verat.

drinking, after : **Ars**, *bism*, *eup-per*, **Phos, Verat**.

    immediately after : **Ars, Bism**, sanic.

    soon as water becomes warm in stomach : **Phos**.

    soon as water reaches stomach : **Bism**.

drunkards, of : *carb-ac*.

eating, after : *hyos*, **Nux-v, Puls**.

faints, until : ant-t.

headache, during : **Ip, Puls, Sang**, tab.

incessant : kreos, lac-d.

lying on back, while : crot-h.

      right side : crot-h.

        amel : ant-t.

      left side : ant-t.

malignant affections of stomach : **Kreos**.

menses, before : nat-m.

    during : *am-m*, *graph*, nat-m.

    after : nat-m.

milk, after : **Aeth, Sil, Valer**.

    mother's : **Sil**, *valer*.

      angry, after : *valer*.

motion, on : **Bry**, *colch*, **Tab**, *verat*.

odor of cooking food : ars, **Colch**, stan.

nausea, without previous : apom.

persistent : *pyrog*.

pregnancy, during : acet-ac, *carb-ac*, *ip*, **Kreos, Lac-ac**, lac-d,
    lob, **Nux-m, Nux-v**, *psor*, *phos*, **Sep, Tab** (after lac-ac, fails).

raising head from pillow, as soon as : *stram*.

riding rail, boat, carriage, etc. : *arn*, **Cocc**, nux-m, **Petr**, sanic, **Tab**.

sea-sickness, during : *carb-ac*, **Cocc**.

smoking, from : *ip*.

stool, simultaneously with : ars.

stooping, on : **Ip**.

sudden : aeth, *camph*.

suppressed eruption, from : *cupr*.

uncovering abdomen, amel : *tab*.

violent : aeth, **Ars**, **Tab**, **Verat**.

water, from sight of : *phos*.

yellow fever, of ; crot-h.

VOMITING, of acid : (See Sour).

bile : chel, *crot-h*, **Eup-per** (between chill and heat).

chill, before : *eup-per*.

during : **Eup-per**.

headache, with : arg-n.

lying on back, while : crot-h.

right side, while : crot-h.

menses, after : *crot-h*.

bitter : *eup-per*, iris, lac-d.

chill, at close of : *eup-per*.

black : *crot-h*.

blood : acet-ac, **Arn**, **Cact**, carb-v, **Crot-h**, erig, **Ham**, kali-bi, *mill*, **Phos**.

vicarious : *phos*.

brown : pyrog.

cheesy matter : aeth.

coffee ground, like : **Cadm**, crot-h, iris, pyrog.

curdled milk : (See Milk).

faecal : **Op**, *plb*, pyrog.

food : aeth, **Ars**, **Bry**, *cupr*, **Ferr**, *kali-c*, *lac-d*, **Phos**, sep.

cough, from : *kali-c*.

eating, while, leaves table suddenly and with one effort vomits everything, can sit down and eat again: **Ferr**.

immediately after : *ferr*, phos.

interval or days, after food has filled the stomach : **Bism**.

an hour or so, after : aeth.

and water : **Ars**.

retained longer but water vomited at once : **Bism**.

solid food only : cupr.

    after regaining consciousness from paroxysm of
whooping cough : *cupr*, canth.

    undigested : *ferr*, lac-d.

fluids, all, as soon as taken : **Bism**.

frothy : aeth.

glairy : ip, *iris*.

green : aeth, carb-ac, *crot-h*.

dark : crot-h.

olive, dark : *carb-ac*, pyrog.

milk : **Aeth**.

curdled : **Aeth**, **Sil**, **Valer**.

    large : **Aeth**, **Valer**.

milky : aeth.

mucus : *cupr*, **Dros**, *ip*, **Kali-bi**.

cough, from : cupr, *dros*.

offensive smelling : **Ars**, pyrog.

sour : acet-ac, **Calc**, *ferr*, *hep*, **Iris**, *lac-d*, **Lyc**, **Mag-c**, *nat-p*.

chill and heat, between : **Lyc**.

stercoraceous : (See Faecal).

stringy : **Hydr**, **Iris**, *kali-bi*.

sweetish : iris, **Kreos**.

tenacious : *kali-bi*.

water : apoc, **Ars**, **Bism**, *cupr*, *kreos*, lac-d.

soon as reaches stomach : **Bism**.

coughing, on : dros.

white : ip.

yellow : aeth.

followed by large curds : **Aeth**.

WATER drops of cold, were falling from stomach, sensation as if : cann-s.

    if : cann-s.

WATERBRUSH : (See Eructation).

WEAK : ant-c, carb-v.

WEIGHT : (See Heaviness).

◻◻◻

Stool

ACRID, : corrosive, excoriating : bry, *cham*, **Lac-d**, **Iris**, **Merc**, *nit-ac*, sanic, *sulph*.

ADHERING to anus : *alum*, plat.

ASH COLOURED : (See Gray).

BALLS, like (See Sheep's Dung) : **Alum**, chel, lach, **Mag-m**, *med*, **Op**, **Plb**, sep, thuj, Werat.

       black : **Alum**, **Op**, plb, *pyrog*, thuj, *verat*.

       small : *bry*.

BERRIES, laurel, like : alum.

BILIOUS : bry, **Crot-h**, **Merc**, **Podo**, **Puls**, *sulph*.

BLACK : ars, carb-ac, *crot-h*, **Lept**, **Op**, **Plb**, ph-ac, **Pyrog**, stram.

BLOODY : acet-ac, aloe, *am-m*, ars, **Canth**, colch, *crot-h*, **Ham**, *ip*, **Merc**, **Merc-c**, *nit-ac*, *mur-ac*, **Phos**, ph-ac, **Ter**.

       dark : *alumn*, *crot-h*, *ham*, mur-ac, **Ter**.

       fluid : *crot-h*, mur-ac.

       menses, during : am-m.

       passive : *ham*, ter.

       typhoid, septic, zymotic diseases, during : **Alum**, **Alumn**, *crot-h*, *ham*, kreos, lach, **Mur-ac**, *nit-ac*, *ph-ac*, **Ter**.

BROWN : *chel*, *graph*, *psor*, pyrog, **Rumx**, **Sec**, tub.

       dark : psor, *rheum*.

CHALKY : (See White).

CHANGEABLE : am-m, *podo*, **Puls**, sanic, sil.

CHOPPED : arg-n, *cham*.

       eggs : *cham*, merc-d.

       spinach : **Arg-n**, *cham*.

CLAY coloured : *berb*, chel, *calc*, *hep*, *podo*.

CLAY like : *alum*, med.

COFFEE grounds : *crot-h*.

COLOURLESS : (See White).

COLOUR, varying in, no two stools alike : *am-m*, **Puls**.

COPIOUS : acet-ac, *bism*, *calc*, **Crot-h**, merc-d, **Phos**, **Podo**, *rumx*, **Sec**, *ter*, **Verat**.

CRUMBLING : Am-m, *am-c*, **Mag-m**, **Nat-m**, *sanic*.

DARK : *ars*, *bry*, mur-ac, tub.

DIFFICULT : (See Constipation).

DRY : aesc, **Bry**, **Lac-d**, **Nat-m**, **Phos**, sanic, *sulph*.

        as if burnt : **Bry**, *sulph*.

FATTY, greasy : *caust*, *phos*.

FERMENTED : *ip*.

FLAKY : *arg-n*, **Verat**.

FORCIBLE, sudden gushing : aster, **Crot-t**, *gamb*, **Grat**, **Jatr**, *nat-s*, petr, *phos*, **Podo**, **Sec**, *thuj*, tub, **Verat**.

        coming out like a shot : **Crot-t**, *gamb*, grat, jatr, *podo*.

        hydrant, as from *: phos*, *thuj*.

FREQUENT : Ars, **Cham**, **Merc**, **Nux-v**, **Podo**, *ter*, **Verat**.

FROG spawn : (See Green).

FORTHY : ip, **Mag-c**, sanic.

        molasses, like : ip.

GRAY : *chel*, *dig*, sanic.

GREASY : (See Fatty).

GREEN : Arg-n, *borx*, **Cham**, calc-p, **Ip**, **Mag-c**, **Merc**, **Merc-c**, *merc-d*, **Podo**, rheum, *sanic*, tab, *ter*, **Verat**.

        grass : **Ip**, **Merc-d**, *sabin*.

        scum on frog pond, like : hell, **Mag-c**, *sanic*.

        spinach, chopped in flakes, like : **Arg-n**.

        turning green on diaper : **Arg-n**.

            on standing : sanic.

GURGLING : (See Forcible).

GUSHING : (See Forcible).

HARD : Alum, **Am-m**, aster, **Bry**, **Calc**, *chel*, **Coll**, *ferr*, **Graph**, **Lac-d**, **Mag-m**, **Nat-m**, **Op**, **Phos**, **Plb**, *rat*, **Sel**, **Sep**, **Sil**, *sanic*, staph, **Sulph**, thuj, **Verat**.

        requires mechanical removal : *aloe*, **Calc**, **Sel**, **Sep**, **Sil**, **Sanic**.

HOT : Cham, **Merc-c**.

INTERVAL long, between stools : **Arn**.

JELLY like : (See Mucous Stools).

KNOTTY : Alum, Graph, Mag-m, *sep*, **Sulph**.
mucus, covered with : *alum*.

LARGE : Bry, Graph, Kali-c, Lac-d, Mag-m, nat-m, **Phos, Pyrog, Sel, Sulph,** thuj, **Verat**.
too large : **Graph, Sulph**.

LIENTERIC : abrot, **Bry, Chin, Ferr, Graph,** *mag-c*, **Podo, Olnd**.
milk, after, or milk passes undigested : *mag-c*, **Mag-m**.

LIGHT coloured : **Chel**, chin, **Dig**.

LIQUID : (See Thin).

LUMPY : Graph (lumps united by mucous threads), *plb*.

MEAT-like sediment with : **Podo**.

MEMBRANOUS : Canth, Colch.

MUCUS, slimy : aloe, **Arg-n,** *chel*,**Graph, Hell,** *ip*, *kali-bi*, **Merc, Merc-c,** tab, ter.
bloody : *canth, carb-ac*, **Colch**.
covered with : *alum*.
fluid : carb-ac.
frog spawn, like : hell.
green : **Arg-n,** *ip*, tab.
turning, on diaper : **Arg-n**.
involuntary passage of : *aloe*.
jelly-like : *aloe, hell, kali-bi*, podo.
lumpy : aloe (in masses or 'gobs') arg-n, asar.
red : **Canth**.
shreddy strips : arg-n, asar, colch, merc-c.
stringy : **Kali-bi**.
tenacious : **Canth, Hell, Kali-bi,** hydr.
transparent : aloe, **Hell**.
white : canth, colch, *hell*.

ODOUR, cadaveric : kreos.
carrion-like : (See Putrid).
cheese, rotten : **Bry, Hep,** *sanic*.
eggs, rotten : **Cham, Arn**.

offensive : **Ars**, **Bapt**, **Benz-ac**, *bism*, *carb-ac*, carb-v, *cham*, **Crot-h**, **Graph**, *lach*, **Merc-c**, mur-ac, **Nux-m**, **Op**, **Podo**, **Psor**, pyrog, rumx, *ter*, **Tub**, verat.

putrid : anthraci, **Ars**, **Bapt**, **Benz-ac**, *carb-ac*, carb-v, nux-m, **Podo**, **Psor**, **Pyrog**, sec, stram.

sour : **Calc**, **Hep**, *mag-c*, **Rheum**, **Sulph**, *sul-ac*.

washing cannot remove : sanic, **Sulph**, *sul-ac*.

PASTY, papescent : alum, bism, **Chel**, *plat*.

PIPE-STEAM, like : *dig*.

REDDISH (See Bloody) : *canth*.

RIBBON-like, from enlarged prostate or retroverted uterus : arn.

SAGO-LIKE particles : **Phos**.

SCANTY : *ars*, camph, *mag-m*, *merc-c*, **Nux-v**.

SCRAPING of intestine, like : **Canth**, *carb-v*, **Colch**.

SCRUMBLED eggs, like : sanic.

SHEEP-DUNG, like (See Balls) : **Alum**, **Chel**, **Mag-m**, nat-m, **Op**, **Plb**, verat.

SHINING : (See Fatty).

SHOOTING out : **Crot-h**, **Gamb**, **Grat**, **Podo**, thuj.

SHREDDY : *asar*, croc.

SMALL : **Alum**, **Ars**, **Mag-m**, **Nux-v**, *pyrog*.

SOFT : **Alum**.

STRINGY : *asar*.

TENACIOUS : **Hell**, med, phos, **Plat**.

THIN, liquid : bapt, **Benz-ac**, *carb-v*, **Crot-t**, **Graph**, mur-ac, sil.

brown : **Graph**.

formed, then thin : **Bov**, **Calc**, **Lyc**.

running right through diaper : *benz-ac*, **Podo**.

solid partly and fluid partly : ant-c, bry.

TOUGH : *caust*.

UNDIGESTED : (See Lienteric).

WATERY : aster, **Benz-ac**, *bism*, **Cham**, *chin*, crot-t, *hell*, *merc-sul*, petr, *ph-ac*, **Phos**, **Podo**, **Psor**, **Puls**, **Sec**, tab, ter, tub, **Verat**.

brown : aster.

clear : bry, podo.

dirty : podo.
  soaking napkin through : benz-ac, podo.
rice water : verat.
white : **Benz-c, Ph-ac**.
yellow : apis, calc, chin, *crot-t*, dulc, **Gamb**, *grat*.

WHITE : **Benz-ac**, *calc*, **Canth**, *chel*, chin, *colch*, *dig*, dol, *hell*, **Nux-m**, **Ph-ac**, podo.

YELLOW : aloe, **Chel**, chin, *crot-t*, *petr*, **Ph-ac**, *plb*, **Podo**, puls, tab.
  bright : **Chel**.
  greenish-yellow : **Grat**, puls, tab.
  gold, as : **Chel**.

Teeth

BITE, together, desire to : **Phyt,** *podo.*
    dentition, during ; **Phyt,** *podo.*

BLEEDING : (See Gum).

CRIES decayed, hollow : **Fl-ac,** *kreos,* **Merc, Mez, Staph.**
    appear, as soon as they : *kreos.*
    crown : **Merc.**
    edges, at : staph.
    gums, at edge of : syph, *thuj.*
    prevents : *coca.*
    rapid : *fl-ac.*
    roots : **Mez, Thuj.**
    sides : mez, staph, thuj.

CONVERGE at their tips : staph, syph.

CRUMBLING : *staph, thuj.*

CUPPED : syph.

DECAYED : (See Caries).

DENTITION, difficult, complicated : **Calc, Calc-p, Cham,** *kreos, podo, rheum.*
    delayed : **Calc, Calc-p.**
    slow : (See Delayed).

DISCOLOURED, black : **Staph.**
    dark streaks, in : staph.
    yellow : syph, *thuj.*

DWARFED : *syph.*

EDGE, feels as if on : **Am-c, Lach, Mez.**
    sets teeth on : **Rob, Sul-ac.**

ELONGATION, sensation of : cham, **Mez,** rat.

GRINDING : *cic, cina, podo, spig.*
    dentition, during : *cic.*
    sleep, during : **Cina,** *kali-br,* kali-p.

LOOSENESS of : **Carb-v.**

PAIN, toothache in general : am-c, bism, **Bry**, **Cham**, **Chin**, **Coff**, *kali-c*, *mag-c*, *mag-m*, *mag-p*, **Merc**, *mez*, *nat-s*, *puls*, rat, **Rhod**, spig, **Staph** (both in decayed and sound), *ther*, thuj.

evening : *merc*.

night : **Mag-c**, mag-p, **Merc**, *mez*.

air, cold : **Merc**, *spig*, *staph*.

amel : nat-s, **Puls**.

drawn in, amel : *mez*, *staph*.

autumn, in the : rhod.

biting teeth together : **Mez**.

blowing nose, on : thuj.

coffee, from : **Cham**.

cold, from : **Kali-c**, *mag-p*, *merc*.

cold water in mouth, from : *acon*, bell, *cham*, *kali-c*, nux-v, **Rhus-t**, spig.

amel : *bism*, **Bry**, *clem*, **Coff**, *ferr-p*, *nat-s*, **Puls**.

but returns when water becomes warm : *bism*, **Bry**, *caust*, **Coff**, *nat-s*, **Puls**, sep.

cold, anything : **Kali-c**.

drink, from : **Mag-p**, **Staph**, *ther*.

decayed teeth, in : *ant-c*, **Kreos**, mag-c.

damp weather : **Merc**.

eating, during : **Kali-c**, *mag-m*, mag-p.

after : **Staph**.

amel : plan, spig.

heat, amel : **Mag-p**.

of room, agg : *puls*.

intermittent : coff.

jerking : coff.

lying, agg : rat.

amel : spig.

masticating, from : *mag-m*.

menses, during : *am-c*, *cham*, **Sep**, **Staph**.

neuralgia : *spig*.

noise, agg : *ther*.

nursing the child, while : chin.

periodic : spig.

pregnancy, during : *cham*, *mag-c*, *rat*.

pressure, amel : *mag-p*.

rubbing cheek, amel : **Merc**.

spring, in the : **Lach**, **Rhod**.

tea-drinking : coff, *sel*, thuj.

thunderstorm : **Rhod**.

tobacco smoking : **Spig**.

thinking about it : *spig*.

touch, from : mag-m, **Sep**, *staph*.

 of food, from : mag-m (but not from biting or chewing).

 of tongue : **Ant-c**, *mez*.

walking, while amel : *rat*.

wandering : *mag-p*.

warm drink, from : bism, *bry*, **Cham**, **Coff**.

 things : **Kali-c**, *merc*, **Puls**.

warmth, external : **Coff**.

 amel : **Mag-p**.

 of bed : **Cham**, **Merc**.

warm room, agg : *cham*.

washerwomen's toothache : phos.

washing, after, cold water, with : kali-c.

weather, change : *rhod*.

  windy : **Rhod**.

winter, sharp : **Acon**, *rhod*.

extending to ear : **Merc**.

jerking : *coff*.

lacerating : merc.

neuralgia : **Bell**, **Coff**, *mez* (agg by eating or motion of jaw).

pressing : culx, thuj.

shooting : (See Stitching).

stitching : *merc*.

 extending to, ears : merc.

     face : merc.

tearing : **Merc**.

throbbing : *kali-c*, *merc*.

SERRATED : med, syph.

SORDES : Ars, Bapt, *carb-v*, Hyos, *mur-ac*, **Ph-ac**, **Rhus-t**.

❑❑❑

Throat

AFFECTIONS, of the, from suppressed, chancre : *syph*.

        foot sweat : bar-c, **Graph**, **Psor**, sanic, **Sil**.

ANAESTHESIA : *gels*, *kali-br*.

ANGINA : **Hydr** (syphilitic).

CHOKING, constricting (See Larynx) : anac, **Bell**, **Cham**, cina, **Ign**, **Naja**, med, ter.

        night : hydr, spig.

          from mucus from posterior nares : hydr, spig.

        drinking, when : anac, cann-s, nit-ac, pip-m.

        eating, when : *anac*, cann-s, nit-ac, pip-m.

        spasm of epiglottis, from : med.

        speaking, when : naja.

        swallowing in, when : anac, cann-s.

BURNING : (See Pain).

COLDNESS, sensation of : med.

COMPLAINTS : (See Affections).

DIPHTHERIA : (See Membrane).

DISCOLOURATION,

        dark : *bapt*.

        mottled : bapt.

        purple : **Lach**, naja.

        red : bapt, **Caps**, **Lyc**. *sulph*.

          brownish : **Lyc**.

          dark red : **Bapt**, *caps*, diph, *merc-cy*, merc-i-r, *phyt*.

        yellow or white patches : lac-c.

        tonsils : *bapt*.

          dark red : **Bapt**, *diph*.

          white or yellow patches : lac-c.

        uvula, translucent : kali-bi, phyt, rhus-t.

DROPSY : (See Swelling).

DRYNESS : **Aesc**, alum, *apis*, **Bell**, **Bry**, *dros*, **Nux-m**, *phyt*, **Rhus-t**. Sabad, *spong*, *stram*, **Sulph**, tarent.

menses, during : nux-m, tarent.
sleeping, when : *nux-m*, tarent.
thirst, without : nux-m, puls.

ELONGATED, uvula : *alum*, bar-c, *merc*, phyt.
cold, agg : *alum*, bar-c.

ENLARGEMENT of tonsils : *alum*, **Bar-c**, *hep*.
cold, agg : *alum*, **Bar-c**.

FISHBONE : (See Pain, as of Splinter).

FOOD, lodges in throat : *caust*, **Lach**, lyc, **Nit-ac**.
passes into nose : lyc, nit-ac.

GANGRENE : am-c, **Crot-h**, lach, merc-cy.
tonsils : *crot-h*.

GRASP the throat, child, when coughing : all-c, iod.

GLOBUS hystericus : (See Lump).

GRANULATIONS in the throat : **Arg-n**.

GURGLING, drinking, when, oesophagus : *Ars*, *cina*, *cupr*, *laur*, thuj.
coughing, when, as if water being poured from a bottle : *cupr*.

HAWK, disposition to : alum, *arg-met*, **Arg-n**, cor-r. **Hep**, **Kali-c**, Nat-c, *psor*.
reading aloud, when : *arg-met*.

HAWKS up cheesy lump : *agar*, kali-bi, **Kali-m**, *psor*.
carrion-like : **Ka-m**, **Psor**.
taste, disgusting : **Psor**.

INFLAMMATION : Acon, aesc, aloe, *bapt*, **Bar-c**, **Bell**, **Caps**, **Hep**, **Lach**, *lac-c*, *merc-i-r*, *merc-i-f*, psor, sabad, *rhus-t*.
night : **Bell**, **Lyc**, *merc-i-f*.
left : **Lach**, *merc-i-r*.
extending to right : *lac-c*, **Lach**, sabad.
chronic : *alum*, *arg-n*, bar-c, *hep*, *lyc*, plb, *psor*.
hypertrophy, with : **Bar-c**, *hep*, *lyc*, plb, *psor*.
cold, after : *bar-c*, *bell*.
erysipelatous : **Apis**.
follicular : *aesc*, **Bell**, **Hep**, *nat-m*.
hot-drink, agg : **Lach**.
mercury, after : *merc-d*.
painless : **Bapt**.
palate, soft : *bapt*.

pharynx : aesc, *merc-d*, *nat-m* (follicular, after silver nitrate).

tonsils : *acon*, *bapt*, **Bar-c**, **Bell**, *caps*, **Hep**, kali-m, **Lach**,
   Lac-c, *lyc*, **Merc**, merc-i-r, merc-i-f, **Nit-ac**, *psor*, *sabad*.

   left : **Lach**.

      extending to right : **Lach**, *lac-c*, *sabad*.

   right : **Lyc**.

      extendng to left : *lyc*.

   alternating sides : **Lac-c**.

   cold, least, after : *bar-c*, *bell*, dulc (damp cold).

   hot drink, agg : **Lach**.

   painless : **Bapt**.

   suppressed foot sweat, from : **Bar-c**.

   tendency to suppuration : *bar-c*, **Hep**, **Psor**.

uvula : **Apis**.

ITCHING : con, iod.

LIQUIDS, taken are forced into nose (See also Food) : **Arum-t**, **Lach**, **Lyc**.

LUMP, plug, etc, sensation of : aesc, *alum*, *arg-n*, *hep*, **Ign**, lach, lac-d, nit-
   ac, *phyt*, rumx.

   rising sensation : **Asaf**, *lac-d*, *kalm*.

   swallowing, returns after : *ign*, **Lach**, *rumx*.

MEMBRANE, exudation, diphtheria, etc : *acet-ac*, am-c, *bapt*, **Brom**, **Diph**,
   Kali-bi, **Lac-c**, **Lach**, **Lyc**, *merc*, *merc-cy*, merc-i-r, merc-i-f, *mur-
   ac*, **Phyt**, pyrog, sabad.

      right : *apis*, **Lyc**, merc-i-f.

         extending to left : **Lyc**.

      left : **Lach**, merc-i-r.

         extending to right : *lac-c*, **Lach**, *sabad*.

      alternating sides : **Lac-c**.

      ash-coloured : (See Gray).

      ascending or begining in bronchi, etc. and extending
         upwards: **Brom**.

      brownish-black : diph.

      borders, shred-like, adherent or free : merc.

      cold, drink agg : **Lyc**.

      descend from nose to right tonsil : **Lyc**.

      fibrinous : kali-bi.

      gray : phyt, merc.

         dark : diph.

malignant : *acet-ac, crot-h, diph,* **Lac-c**, *merc-cy*.

in the very begining when patient seems doomed : **Diph**.

painless : *diph*.

pearly : kali-bi, **Lac-c**.

prophylactic, when corresponds to genus epidemicus : **Merc-cy**.

pseudo-membranous : kali-bi, merc-cy.

putrid : merc-cy.

shining, glazed : **Lac-c**.

sleep agg : *lac*, lyc.

thick : diph, merc.

warm drink agg : *lach*.

white : **Lac-c**.

yellow : lac-c.

extending down to larynx and trachea : **Kali-bi**, lac-c, merc-cy.

to nose : brom.

fauces : merc-cy.

ash-coloured : phyt.

tonsils : *kali-bi, lac-c,* **Lach, Lyc, Phyt**.

right : *lyc*.

left : lach.

ash-coloured : phyt.

uvala : **Phyt**.

ash-coloured : phyt.

MUCUS : *chel,* **Kali-bi, Kali-c**, med, *merc-i-r, merc-i-f,* **Nat-c**, *psor*.

drawn from posterior nares : hydr, med, **Nat-c**.

dropping from posterior nares : **Nat-c**.

flies from throat when coughing : bad, *chel, kali-c*.

frothy : lyss.

gray : med.

greenish : merc-i-r.

jelly-like : aloe.

offensive : bapt, diph.

putrid : anthraci, carb-ac, **Psor**, *pyrog*.

tenacious, viscid : canth, **Kali-bi**, lyss, *merc-i-r, merc-i-f, psor*.

thick : **kali-bi**, med.

NUMBNESS (See Anaesthesia) : *kali-br*.

PAIN : am-c, arg-met, **Arg-n**, **Arum-t**, **Bapt**, **Caps**, *cupr*, *hep*, *ign*, kali-c,
lac-c, **Lach**, *lyc*, merc-i-r, merc-i-f, *nit-ac*, *phyt*, psor, *sabad*, *sulph*.

    right : **Lyc**, merc-i-f.

        then left : *lyc*.

    left : lac-c, **Lach**.

        then right : *lach*.

    cold drink, from : *lyc*.

    coughing, on : **Arg-met**, *arum-t*.

    putting out the tongue : *kali-bi*.

    swallowing, on : alum, **Arg-met**, **Arum-t**, *kali-c*, **Lac-c**, *lach*,
        Merc, *merc-i-r*, *merc-i-f*, *phyt*, psor, *sabad*.

        children refuses food and drink : *arum-t*, **Merc**.

        empty, on : *crot-h*, ign, **Kali-c**, *lac-c*, **Lach**, merc-i-r,
            merc-i-f.

        food : merc-i-r.

        liquid : **Bell**, bry, ign, **Lach**, merc-i-r.

        amel : bapt, *caps*, *ign*.

        when not or between acts of deglutation : **Caps**, **Ign**.

    warm drinks : **Lach**, merc-i-f.

    amel : **Ars**, **Hep**, **Lyc**.

    warmth in general : **Lach**.

PAIN, extending to ear : *hep*, kali-bi, *lac-c*, *phyt*.

                  swallowing, on : kali-bi, lach, *lac-c*, *phyt*.

    glands of neck : am-c.

    tonsils : am-c, caps, *hep*.

PAIN, burning : *aesc*, *ars*, bell, canth, **Caps**, **Caust**, *iris*, **Lyc**, *phyt*, psor,
Sang, **Sulph**.

    coal of fire, as from : **Ars**, phyt.

    cayenne pepper : **Caps**.

    red hot iron, as from : phyt.

    swallowing does not agg : caust.

    oesophagus : **Sang**.

    pharynx : **Sang**.

    cutting : merc-c.

        extending to ears, swallowing, on : psor.

    fish-bone sensation : (See Pain, Splinter, as From).

    rawness : *aesc*, alum, **Arg-met**, *arum-t*, **Caust**.

        coughing, on : **Arg-met**.

swallowing, on : **Arg-met**.

scalded as from : psor.

shooting, extending to ear : *lac-c*.

smarting : **Caps**.

sore : *am-c*, **Arg-met**, **Arum-t**, **Bapt**, *caps*, **Caust**, **Ign**, **Lach**, **Lyc**, *lyss*, mag-c, med, *phyt*, *psor*.

    right : **Lyc**.

    left : *lac-c*, **Lach**.

    alternating sides : **Lac-c**.

    clergyman's sore throat : *alum* (chronic), **Arum-t**, dros.

    coughing, on : **Arg-met**.

    menses, begins with : lac-c.

    menses, before : *lac-c*, *mag-c*.

            after : **Lac-c**.

    painless : bapt.

    splinters, as from : *alum*, **Arg-n**, **Dol**, **Hep**, **Kali-c**, **Nit-ac**, **Sil**.

    swallowing, on : (See Pain in General).

    sweats, after : **Spong**.

    warm food and drink amel : *alum*, **Hep**.

splinters as from : (See Pain Sore, Splinter as From),

stinging : *aesc*, **Apis**, *nit-ac*.

stitching : *aesc*, **Bell**, **Hep**, **Kali-c**, **Nit-ac**, *sabad*.

    swallowing, on : **Apis**, *bell*, **Bry**, **Calc**, **Hep**, kali-c, *sabad*.

    extending to ears : *lac-c*.

tearing, extending to ears, on swallowing : psor.

PARALYSIS pharynx, post-diphtheritic : *caust*, *diph*, *gels*.

PLUG : (See Lump).

QUINSY : (See Inflammation).

RAWNESS : *aesc*.

ROUGHNESS : dros.

SCRAPING : dros.

SKIN sensation of a, hanging in the throat, must swallow : sabad.

STIFFNESS : *nux-m*.

SUPPURATION, tonsils : *bar-c*, **Hep**, **Psor**.

SWALLOW, constant disposition : *aesc*, bell, **Caust**, cina, *lac-c*, *lyss*, **Merc**, phyt.

difficult : *bapt*, **Bar-c**, **Kali-c**, **Lach**, **Lyss**, merc-cy, *phyt*, *psor*, *sabad*, **Stram**.

food, warm, can swollour easily : *sabad*.

fluid only, can swallow, but solid food gags : *bapt*, bar-c, *sil*.

liquids : kali-n (due to short breathing), **Lach**, **Lyss**, **Stram**.

more difficult than solid : bell, bry, *ign*, *lach*.

regurgitate through nose : (See Liquid).

solid : **Bapt**, **Bar-c**.

impeded : *bapt*.

liquids only, can swallow, least food gags : *bapt*, bar-c.

impeded, liquids only can swallow, but has aversion to them: **Sil**.

impossible : *bapt*, bar-c, med, merc, **Stram**.

fluids vomited or returned by nose : *diph*.

liquids anything but : bapt, bar-c.

liquids, hot : **Lach**, *phyt*.

painless : diph.

SWELLING : aesc, **Bell**, crot-h, **Hep**, **Lach**, med, **Phyt**, psor.

tonsils : alum, *apis*, **Bapt**, **Bar-c**, caps, diph, *merc-i-r*, *merc-i-f*, **Phyt**, *psor*.

right : *merc-i-f*.

left : *merc-i-r*.

oedematous : crot-h.

uvula : *alum*, **Apis**, *kali-bi*, merc, *phyt*, rhus-t.

oedematous : **Apis**, **Kali-bi** (bladder-like appearance), phyt, rhus-t.

SYPHILITIC affections : *aur*, kali-bi, **Merc**.

THREAD hanging in, sensation of : *valer*.

TICKLING : (See Larynx).

ULCERS of throat : **Hep**, *kali-bi*, **Merc**, **Merc-c**, *merc-cy*, *merc-i-r*, *merc-i-f*.

phagedemic : merc-cy.

fauces : **Kali-bi**, merc-i-r.

syphilitic : **Kali-bi**.

tonsils : *am-c*, merc-i-f, merc-i-r.

gangrenous : *am-c*.

External-Throat

ABSCESS : Hep, Merc, Sil.

BAND, tight, intolerance of : **Lach**.

CLOTHING or collar agg, must loosen it : aml-ns, **Lach**, *sep*.

CONSTRICTION : alum, cact, **Lach, Stram**.

GOITRE : *brom* (light haired), **Iod** (dark haired, acts best when given after
full-moon or when moon is waning).

        hard, indurated : brom (after Iod failed), iod, *spong*.

INDURATION of glands : bar-c, **Bar-m, Calc, Carb-an, Con, Iod**.

        carotids : phyt.

            diphtheria after : phyt.

            scarlet fever, after : phyt.

        submaxillary : phyt.

PULSATION, carotids : *aml-ns, aur*, **Bell**, *cact*, chin, croc, **Glon**, *meli*.

SENSITIVE to slightest touch : **Lach**, *lac-c*.

SWELLING : *am-c, bell, iod*.

        cervical glands : **Bar-c**, *carb-an*, diph, *iod*, **Merc**, Merc-i-r,
        Merc-i-f, Rhus-t, Sil.

            suppurative : **Merc, Sil**.

        thyroid gland : brom, iod.

            stony hard : *brom*.

Urethra

AGGLUTINATION of meatus : *cann-s*, graph, *med*, *thuj*.
  morning : **Sep.**
CONSTRICTION : caps.
DISCHARG, acrid : **Arg-n**, **Merc-c**.
  bland : *puls*, sep.
  bloody : **Canth.**
  gleety : **Agn**, **Alum**, *calad*, cop, **Nat-m**, **Petros**, **Sel**, **Sep**,
    Sulph.
    morning : **Sep.**
    impotency, with : agn.
    long standing : *kali-i*, *sep*.
    painless : **Nat-m**, **Sep.**
    staining linen : *sep*.
  gluey : *graph*, sep,
    morning : sep.
  gonorrhoeal : **Cann-s**, **Canth**, *cop,cub*, **Merc**, **Merc-c** (second
    stage), **Nat-s**, **Petros**, *psor*.
    chronic : **Calc**, **Calc-s**, **Nat-m**, **Nat-s**, **Psor**, **Thuj.**
    suppressed : *nat-s*.
    torpid : *merc*.
  greenish : **Merc**, *merc-c*, nat-s, *kali-i*.
    night : **Merc**, *merc-c*.
    yellowish : **Merc**, **Nat-s.**
  jelly-like ; *kali-bi*.
  milky : **Cop.**
  painless : *nat-s*.
  purulent : *cann-s*, *cub*.
  stringy : *kali-bi*.
  thick : *cann-s*, *cub*, kali-i, *nat-s*, *puls*, thuj, sep.
  yellow : **Alum**, **Arg-n**, cann-s, *cub*, **Merc**, **Nit-ac**, **Puls**, **Sel**,
    Sep, **Thuj.**
    green : **Kali-s**, **Nat-s**, **Puls.**

HAEMORRHAGE : *canth*, **Merc-c**, *phos*.

        vicarious : *phos*.

INFLAMMATION : Cann-s (acute stage), *cub* (second stage), *petros*, *thuj*.

        chronic : *petros*.

        traumatic : petros.

ITCHING : canth, *petros*.

        voluptuous : **Petros**.

           fossa navicularis : caust, **Petros**.

           rub, must, with some rough article which amel : **Petros**.

NUMBNESS (See Sensation Absent) : **Caust**, kali-br.

PAIN : apis, cann-s, canth, *merc-c*, thuj.

        meatus : *cann-s*,

           extending backwards : **Cann-s**.

        urinating, when not : **Benz-ac**, *berb*, **Canth**, **Caust**.

        urination, during : **Canth**, **Caust**, *merc-c*.

           urging to stool, with : **Nux-v**.

           at close of : berb, *equis*, med, **Sars**, thuj.

        walk, cannot, with legs close together : cann-s.

PAIN biting : **Petros**.

        deep in urethra : **Petros**.

        fossa navicularis : **Petros**.

        meatus, urination, during : **Cann-s**.

      burning : **Berb**, **Cann-s**, **Canth**, **Caps** (as from red pepper), equis-h, **Merc**, *merc-c*, petros, *staph*, ter.

        urinating, when not : **Merc**, *staph*.

        urination, during : **Canth**, *equis*, kreos, **Merc-c**, **Sulph**.

           after : *cub*, kreos, nat-m, *staph*, sulph.

               in prostatic troubles of old men : staph.

           last few drops cause violent burning : *equis-h*, *merc*.

           forepart of urethra, during urination : *merc*.

      cutting : **Canth**, **Con**, *equis-h*, nat-m, thuj.

        urination, during : **Canth**, *equis-h*.

           after : **Canth**, **Nat-m**, *thuj*, sars.

           at close of : sars, **Thuj**.

      drawing : *berb*, *cann-s*, ter.

smarting : (See Burning).

soreness : caust, *cann-s*.

> pressure, to : cann-s.
>
> touch to : cann-s.
>
> walking erect, from : cann-s.

sticking, urinating, when : cann-s.

stitching : cann-s.

> urination, during : **Cann-s**.
>
> posteriorly : cann-s.

tearing : **Cann-s**.

> zig-zags : *cann-s*.

PRESSURE, sensitive to : *cann-s*.

REDNESS, meatus : *sulph*.

SENSATION absent, when urinating : **Caust**, kali-br. *sars*.

urination, after, as if urine trickling : thuj.

STRICTURE : Canth, Clem, *petros*.

TICKLING : (See Itching).

TINGLING : *petros*.

TOUCH, sensitive : *cann-s*.

□□□

Urine

ACRID : *apis*, canth, **Merc**, *sars*, **Sulph**.

ALBUMINOUS : Apis, Ars, *calc, canth*, colch, *dig,* **Glon, Hell,** *helon,* **Merc-c, Ter**.

   acute : helon, **Ter**.

   chronic : helon.

   cold and dampness, from exposure to : *calc*, ter.

   diphtheria : ter.

   pregnancy : **Apis,** *ars, helon*.

   scarlet fever, with : **Apis,** *hell, lach, ter*.

   typhoid : ter.

BLOODY : Apis, Cact, Calc, Canth, *colch,* cop, **Crot-h,** erig, **Ham, Ip,** *kreos*, lach, **Merc, Mill** (bloody cake forms at the bottom of vessel), ph-ac, **Phos,** *sars*, **Sec, Ter, Tril-p**.

CLOTS : colch.

   passive : *ham, kreos*.

BURNING : Apis, Ars, Canth, Hep, Merc-c, Sulph.

CASTS : ter.

   blood : *ter*.

CLEAR : equis-h, helon.

CLOUDY : Apis, Berb, Cina, Canth, Con, *lyc*, lyss, *nit-ac*, **Ter**.

   passed, when : *cina*.

   remains of a cider barrel-like : *nit-ac*.

   standing, on : *cina*.

    turns milky : *cina*.

     semi-solid : *cina*.

   white clouds : ph-ac.

COLD : *nit-ac*.

COLOUR, black : **Colch,** *hell*, **Ter**.

   ink-like : **Colch**.

   brown : **Benz-ac,** *colch*, **Merc-c**, ter.

    dark : **Benz-ac,** Chel, nit-ac.

   dark : **Benz-ac, Bry,** chin, **Colch,** nat-c, **Sel, Ter**.

greenish : berb, *ruta*,

pale : cham, cina, **Con**, kreos, *lac-d*, mag-m, mag-p, **Ph-ac**, sec.

lemon-coloured : chel.

red : **Benz-ac**, *berb*, hell, lob, *sel*, ter, verat-v.

> deep red : **Benz-ac**, lob.
>
> blood-red : *berb*.
>
> orange-red : lob.

smoky : (See Cloudy).

yellow, light : **Aur**, **Lach**, mag-m, plb, **Sep**.

yellow : chel.

COLORLESS : *ph-ac*, *sulph*.

COPIOUS (increased) : **Cina**, *equis-h*, *helon*, ign, kreos, lac-ac, *lac-d*, mag-p, **Merc**, **Ph-ac**, *sars*.

> night : *ph-ac*, **Sulph**, *ter*.
>
> in comparison with the amount of water drunk : *merc*.
>
> headache, during : lac-d.

DECOMPOSING, rapidly : ph-ac.

FLAKY, flocculent : (See Sediment).

HOT : **Merc-c**.

INVOLUNTARY : (See Urination).

JELLY-LIKE : coloc.

MILKY : *cina*, *dulc*, **Ph-ac**.

> standing, on : *cina*.

MUCUS : (See Sediment).

ODOUR, offensive : **Bapt**, **Benz-ac**, ind (after standing), coloc, **Nit-ac**, **Sep** (must be removed from the room), viol-o.

> ammoniacal : med.
>
> cat's urine, like : viol-o.
>
> horse's urine, like : **Nit-ac**.
>
> putrid : **Bapt**, *benz-ac*, sep.
>
> sourish : sep.
>
> strong : **Benz-ac**, **Nit-ac**.
>
> > intensely urinous : **Benz-ac**.
>
> violet, like : ter.

SCANTY : am-c, **Apis**, *apoc*, **Arum-t**, *bry*, **Canth**, **Colch**, coloc, **Hell**, lyss, **Merc-c**, **Nit-ac**, **Ruta**, **Sars**, **Sel**, verat-v.

SEDIMENT : *berb*, chin, **Lyc**, **Sars**, Sep, ter.

          adherent : **Sep**.

          blood : **Canth**, **Ph-ac**.

          brick-dust : (See Sand, Red).

          burnt, as if : sep.

          clay-coloured : berb, *sep*.

          coffee-ground, like : **Apis**, **Hell**, *ter*.

          copious : lob.

          flocculent : **Berb**, **Canth**, **Mez**, **Sars**.

          jelly-like : berb, *colch*, **Ph-ac**.

          lithic acid and lithates : caust.

          milky : *ph-ac*.

          mucous : **Berb**, cann-i, chin, cop, equis-h, *lith-c*, **Sars**.

              ropy : chim.

              thick slimy : *berb*, sars.

          phosphates : **Ph-ac**.

          red : *berb*, *lob*, *lyc*, **Sep**.

              renal calculi : **Benz-ac**, **Lith-c**, **Lyc**, **Sars**.

          sand : **Benz-ac**, borx, **Led**, **Lyc**, **Phos**, **Sars**, **Sel**.

              gravel (small calculi) : **Lyc**, **Sars**.

              coarse : *sel*.

              red (brick dust) : *benz-ac*, **Lob**, **Lyc**, **Merc-c**, oci, **Phos**, **Sel**.

              white : **Sars**.

          transparent : *berb*.

          turbid : berb.

          uric acid, excess : *benz-ac*, lith.

          white : **Berb**, calc, **Sars**.

SEMI-SOLID, standing on : **Cina**.

SUGAR : *colch*, **Helon**, **Lyc**, **Lyss**, *lac-ac*, (with rheumatic pain in joints).

THICK : *benz-ac*, coloc.

TURBID : (See Cloudy).

VISCID : coloc.

WATERY : equis-h, ign, *ph-ac*, *sec*.

❑❑❑

Vertigo

VERTIGO : Acon, Agar, *alum*, **Arg-n**, *bar-c*, **Bell**, borx, **Bry**, **Cocc**, *coloc*, **Con**, **Cycl**, eup-per, *ferr*, **Gels**, *kalm*, *mur-ac*, **Puls**, **Rhus-t**, Sil, *spig*, **Tab**, *ther*.

        morning : acon, *bry*, **Lach**, *nux-v*.

            rising, on : acon, **Bell**, **Bry**, **Phos**, **Puls**, **Rhus-t**.

        night : hyper.

AIR, open, in amel : **Tab**.

ALCOHOLIC liquors : **Coloc**.

ASCENDING, stairs : **Calc**.

BACK, comes up the : *sil*.

BALANCING, sensation : ferr.

        as if on water : ferr.

BED turned as if : con.

CLOSING eyes, on : *alum*, *arg-n*, **Lach**, **Ther**, *thuj*, stram.

        amel : **Tab**.

CROSSING a bridge : ferr, lyss.

        running water : ferr, *lyss*.

DIMNESS of sight, with : cycl, gels, nux-v.

DESCENDING, on : **Borx**, **Ferr**, sanic.

        stairs : **Borx**.

EATING, after : grat, nux-v, puls.

FAINTING, with : nux-v.

FALL, tendency to : coloc, *puls*, *sil*.

        looking down, on : kalm, **Spig**.

        backward : *bell*.

        forward : graph, rhus-t, sil.

        looking up, from : puls, *sil*.

        sideways : con, sulph.

        to left : eup-per.

            cannot turn the head to left for fear of falling : coloc.

FLOWERS, from odor of : nux-v, phos.

HIGH HOUSES, from sight of **: Arg-n**.

INTOXICATED, as if : *gels*, petr.

LEFT swaying toward : *eup-per*.

cannot turn the head to left for fear of falling : coloc.

LOOKING with eyes turned : **Spig**.

downward : *kalm*, phos, **Spig**, sulph.

upward : **Puls**, *sil, tab*.

LOSS of fluid : calc, chin, sep, sulph.

sleep : *cocc, nux-v*.

LYING down, on : rhus-t.

while : **Con**, *rhus-t*.

amel : apis.

LIE down, must : **Bry**, cocc, phos, puls.

MENSES, after suppressed : cycl, puls.

MOTION, from : **Bry**, *cocc*, gels, mill.

violent motion amel : mill.

MOVING the head : **Con** (must keep head perfectly still).

the eyes : **Con**.

NAUSEA, with : **Cocc**.

NOISE, from : **Ther**.

OBJECTS move : *cocc*.

OCCIPITAL : Gels, petr, **Sil**.

OLD people : **Bar-c**, *con*, dig, phos.

OPENING (See Closing Eyes) : **Tab**.

PAROXYSMAL : tab.

POSITION, change of : *bell*.

RIDING in a carraige, while : *bry, cocc*.

RISING, from seat : **Acon, Bry**, petr, phos, **Rhus-t, Tab**.

from bed, on : **Cocc** (as if intoxicated), bell, chel, *bry*, **Phyt**, *rhus-t*.

from stooping : **Bell**, *bry*.

ROCKING : borx, *coff*.

SEASICKNESS, like (See Rocking) : **Cocc**, petr.

SLEEP, after : **Lach**.

STAGGERING, with : arg-n, **Gels**, kali-br, nux-v, phos.

STANDING, while : rhus-t.

STOOPING, on : **Bell**, *bry*, *kalm*, rhus-t.
             on rising after stooping : **Bell**, *bry*.

STUDYING, while : nat-m.

TURNING, as if in a circle : **Con**.
          on : calc, *con*, kali-c.
          in bed, on : **Con**.
          on moving the head : *bry*, calc, **Con**.
               quickly turning the head : *coloc*, **Con**.
               to left : *coloc, con*.
          a street corner, afraid he will run against corner house : arg-n.

UTERINE and ovarian complaints, with : **Con**.

VISION, with blurred : gels.

VOMITING, amel : *tab*.

WALKING, while : agar, ferr, *rhus-t*, nat-m, nux-v, phos, puls.
            stumbles over everyting : *agar*.
            over a bridge : ferr.

WATER, crossing running ; *ferr*, *lyss*.
        seeing flowing : *ferr*.
        walking over : *ferr*.

WHIRLING, as if : bry, **Con**, cycl, puls.

WORMS, from : acon, cic, merc, sil.

❏❏❏

RELATIONSHIP
OF
REMEDIES

Relationship of Remedies

ABBREVIATIONS:

Compl, Complementary.
Ant, Antidote.
Inm, Inimical.
Incom, Incompatible.
Sim, Similar.
Com, Compare.

With Compl	Follows well	Followed by	Ant, Inm, Incom	Sim, Com.
ABROTANUM	(Acon, Bry), in pleurisy. Hep in boils.			
ACETICUM ACIDUM	Chin, in haemorrhage. Dig, in dropsy.			
ACONITUM NAP. Arn, in traumatism. Coff, in fever, pain, sleeplessness. Sulph in all cases. Acon is acute of sulh.	Arn, Coff, Sulph, Verat.	Arn, Ars, Bell, Bry, Hep, Sulph.	For abuse of Acon— Sulph. Ant— Alcohol, Nux-v, Sulph.	

With Compl	Follows well	Followed by	Ant, Inm, Incom	Sim, Com
ACTAEA RACEMOSA				Sim—Agar, Lil-t, Sep. Caul and Puls in uterine and rheumatic affections.
AESCULUS HIP. Coll.	Coll, Nux-v, Sulph in piles.			Sim—(Aloe, Coll, Ign, Mur-ac, Nux-v, Sulph). in haemorrhoids.
AETHUSA CYN. Calc.				Sim—Ant-c, Ars, Calc, Sanic.
AGARICUS MUS.				Sim— (Calc, Cann-i, Cimic. Hyos, Kali-p, Lach, Nux-v. Op. Stram), in delirium of alcoholism. (Myg, Tarent, Zinc), in chorea.
AGNUS CASTUS		(Calad, Sel) in sexual weakness, or impotency.		
ALLIUM CEPA Phos, Puls, Thuj.		(Calc, Sil) in polypus.		Sim—Euphr. but coryza and lachrymation are opposite.

With Compl	Follows well	Followed by	Ant, Inm, Incom	Sim, Com
ALOE SOCOTRINA			Sulph—when Aloe has been abused as purgatives.	Like Sulph in many chronic diseases, with abdominal plethora and congestion of portal circulation. Sim—Am-m, Gamb. Nux-v. Podo.
ALUMINA Bry. ferr. It is chronic of Bry. AMBRA GRISEA	Bry, Lach, Sulp.			Sim—(Bar-c, Con), in ailments of old people. Sim— Asaf, Cimic. Coca. Ign. Mosch, Phos. Valer.
AMMONIUM CARB.		Ant-c, Phos, Puls, Sanic.	Inm—to Lach. It antidotes poisoning with Rhus and stings of insects.	
AMMONIUM MUR.			Ant—Acet-ac for vapours.	
AMYLENUM NITROSUM				Sim—Bell, Cact, Coca, ferr, Glon, Lach.

With Compl	Follows well	Followed by	Ant, Inm, Incom	Sim, Com
ANACARDIUM ORIENT.	Lyc. Plat. Puls.	Plat.		Comp—Rhus-r, Rhus-t, Rhus-v.
ANTHRACINUM				Sim— (Ars. Carb-ac, Lach, Sec, Pyrog) in malignant and septic conditions. Comp—Euphr in terrible pains of cancer, carbuncle or erysipelas, when Ars. fails.
ANTIMONIUM CRUDUM Squila.	Merc, Puls. Sulph.			Sim—(Bry, Ip, Lyc, Puls). in gastric complaints.
ANTIMONIUM TART.	Ip—when lungs seem to fail.			Sim—Lyc but motion of alae is replaced by dilated nostrils. Verat in diarrhoea, cloic, vomiting, coldness.

With Compl	Follows well	Followed by	Ant, Inm, Incom	Sim, Com
				Ip but has more drowsiness ;nausea but amel. vomiting.
				Hep in cough when children not easily impressed.
				(Thuj, Sil), after vaccination.
				Sil, in dyspnoea from foreign body.
				Puls, in suppressed gonorrhoea.
				Ter, from damp basement.
APIS MELLIFICA Nat-m.	(Canth, Dig, Hell) in albuminuria.	Ars, Puls.	Massive doses, poisoning, and stings are antidoted by Nat-m (crude salt solution and potencies), onion. Disagrees, when used before or after Rhus.	

With Compl	Follows well	Followed by	Ant, Inm, Incom	Sim, Com
APOCYNUM CAN.				Sim—(Acet-ac, Apis (no thirst), Ars, Chin, Dig, (in dropsical affections).
ARGENTUM MET.	Alum.			Sim—Stann in cough excited by laughing.
ARGENTUM NIT.	Bry, Caust (urethral affections).	Kali-c, Lyc, Sep.	Ant—Nat-m (hemical and dynamic).	Sim— Aur, Cupr, Lach Nat-m, Nit-ac.
ARNICA MONT. Acon, Ip.	Acon, Apis, Ham, Ip, Verat.	Sul-ac.		Sim—(Bapt, Chin, Phyt, Pyrog, Rhus-t, Ruta, Staph), in soreness as if bruised. Com—Hyper in spinal concussion.
ARSENICUM ALB. All-c, Carb-v, Phos. Pyrog.	Acon, Bell.	Apis, Calc, Hep. Lyc, Nux-v. Rhus-t follows well in skin affections.	Ant—Bapt, (when Ars has been improperly used in typhoid).	

With Compl	Follows well	Followed by	Ant, Inm, Incom	Sim, Com
ARUM TRIPHYLLUM	(Hep, Nit-ac), in dry, hoarse, croupy cough. (Caust, Hep), in morning hoarseness and deafness, and in scarlatina.		—Chemical, animal charcoal, hydrated perioxide of iron, lime water, magnesia. —Dynamic, opium. Brandy and stimulants if there is depression and collapse. If poisonous doses —milk, albumen; emetics-zinc sulp. castor oil, as purgative.	

With Compl	Follows well	Followed by	Ant, Inm, Incom	Sim, Com
ASARUM EUROPAEUM				Sim—Caust in modalities. (Aloe, Arg-n, Merc, Podo, Puls, Sulph), in stringy shreddy stools.
ASTERIAS RUBENS				Sim—Murx, Sep. Com—(Carb-an, Con, Sil) in mammary cancer. —(Bell, Calc, Sulph), in epilepsy.
AURUM METALLICUM	Syph.	Syph.		Sim—(Asaf, Calc, Plat, Sep, Tarent, Ther), in one and uterine disease.
BAPTISIA TINCT.		(Crot, Ham, Nit-ac, Ter) in haemorrhage of typhoid and typhus.	It antidotes improper use of Ars in typhoid.	Sim—(Arn, Ars, Bry, Gels), in early stages of fever with drowsiness and muscular weakness.
BARYTA CARB. Dulc.	Psor, Sulph, Tub.	Psor, Sulph, Tub.	Incom—after Calc.	Sim—Alum, Calc, Dulc, Fl-ac, Iod, Sil.

With Compl	Follows well	Followed by	Ant, Inm, Incom	Sim, Com
BELLADONNA Calc.				Sim—Acon, Bry, Cic, Gels, : Glon, Hyos. Meli, Op, Stram.
BENZOICUM ACIDUM	Colch–in gout. Cop–in suppressed gonorrhoea.		Incom—Wine which aggravates urinary, gouty and rheumatic affections. It antidotes abuse of Cop.	Sim—(Cop, ferr, Nier, Thuj) in enuresis. —(Berb, Lith-c), in arthritic complaints.
BERBERIS VULG.	(Arn, Bry, Kali-bi, Rhus-t, Sulph), in rheumatic affections.			Sim—(Canth, Lyc, Sars, Tab) in renal colic.
BLATTA ORIENTALIS	(Apis, Apoc, Dig), in general dropsy.			
BORAX	Calc, Psor, Sanic, Sulph.	Ars, Bry, Lyc. Phos. Sil.	Incom—Acet-ac, vinegar, wine.	
BOVISTA	Rhus (seemed indicated but failed), in chronic urticaria.		It antidotes local application of tar, and suffocation from gas.	Com—Am-c, Bell, Calc, Mag-s, Sep), in menstrual irregularities.

With Compl	Follows well	Followed by	Ant, Inm, Incom	Sim, Com
BROMIUM	Iod (after failed) in goitre. (Hep, Iod, Phos, Spong) in after failure, in croup.			Com—(Chlor, Hep, Iod, Spong) in croup and croupy affections.
BRYONIA ALBA Alumina, Rhus-t. Alumina is chronic of Bry.	Acon, Nux-v, Rhus-t, Sulph.	Alum., Kali-c, Nux-v, Phos, Rhus-t, Sulph.	Ant—Chel, when Bry is abused in hepatic complaints.	Sim—(Bell, Hep), for hasty speech and hasty drinking. —Ran-b, in pleurisy and rheumatism of chest. —Ptelea, in aching heaviness in hepatic region.
CACTUS GRAND.				Com—Acon, Dig, Gels, Kali-c, Lach, Tab. Com—Con, Glon, Lith-c, Puls, Nux-v.
CALCAREA ARS.	Con—in lymphatic, psoric or tubercular persons.			
CALCAREA OSTR. Rhus-t.	(Nit-ac, Puls, Sulph), especially, if pupils are dilated.	Lyc, Nux, Phos, Sil, Kali-bi, in nasal catarrh.	Should not be used before Nit-ac., Sulph.	

With Compl	Follows well	Followed by	Ant, Inm, Incom	Sim, Com
CALCAREA PHOS. Ruta, Tril-p.	Ars, Iod, Tub.	Iod, Psor, Sanic, Sulph.		Sim—Calc, Calc-fl, Carb-an, Fl-ac, Ka-p. Psor, in debility after acute disease. Sil, but sweat of head is wanting.
CALENDULA Hep, Sal-ac.	Ars.	Ars, Arn, Bry, Hep, Rhus-t.	Ant—Arn.	Sim—Hyper, when nerves injured. Arn, in traumatism without laceration of soft tissues. (Calc-p, Symph) for non-union of bones. (Rhus-t, Ruta) in strains or injuries, of single muscle. Sal-ac, in preventing suppuration and gangrene. Sul-ac, in gangrenous wounds.

With Compl	Follows well	Followed by	Ant, Inm, Incom	Sim, Com
CAMPHORA			It antidotes alomost all vegetable medicines, also tobacco, fruits containing prussic acid; poisonous mushrooms.	Com—Carb-an, Op, Sec, Verat.
CANNABIS INDICA				Comp—Bell, Hyos, Stram.
CANNABIS SATIVA				Sim—(Canth, Caps, Gels, Petros) in early stages of specific urethrities.
CANTHRIS				Sim—Apis, Ars, Equis-h, Merc.
CAPSICUM		Cina, in intermittent fever.		Com—Apis, Bell, Bry, Calad, Puls.
CARBO ANIMALIS Calc-p.		Ars, Nit-ac, Phos, Puls, Sulph.		Sim—Bad, Brom, Carb-v, Phos, Sep, Sulph.
CARBO VEGETABILIS Chin, Dros, Kali-c.		Ars, Chin, Dros, Kali-c, Lyc, Nux-v, Puls, Sep, Sulph.		Com—Ant-t, in threatened paralysis of lungs. (Chin, Plb), in neglected pneumonia.

With Compl	Follows well	Followed by	Ant, Inm, Incom	Sim, Com
				(Op, Valer), in lack of reaction. Phos, in bleeding ulcers. Puls, in fat food and pastry. Sulph, in acrid-smelling menstrual flow and erysipelas of mammae.
CARBOLICUM ACIDUM			Ant—Dilute cider vinegar internally or externally when acid has been swallowed.	Com—(Ars, Kreos) in burns. (Gels, Merc, Sulph), in ulcers with unhealthy, offensive discharge.
CAULOPHYLLUM				Sim—Bell, Cimic, Lil-t, Puls, Sec, Thlas, Vib. Puls, in labor pains, but mental condition opposite. Sep, in 'moth patches' and reflex symptoms from uterine irregularities.

With Compl	Follows well	Followed by	Ant, Inm, Incom	Sim, Com
CAUSTICUM Coloc, Carb-v, Petros. Merc-c (assists the action of Caust, and vice versa).			Incom—Phos, acids, coff. It antidotes-paralysis from lead poisoning, also abuse of Merc and Sulph in scabies.	Comp—Arn, must swallow mucus. (Gels, Graph, Sep) in ptosis, (Carb-v, Rumx), in hoarseness. Sulph, in chronic aphonia.
CHAMOMILLA Mag-c, Puls, Bell. In children's disease: Bell-cranial nerves, Cham-abdominal nerves.			It anidotes-cases spoiled by Op. or morphia in complaints of children.	Comp—Bell, Borx, Bry, Coff, Puls, Sulph.
CHELIDONIUM MAJUS	Bry (if abused in hepatic complaints).	Ars. Lyc. Sulph.	It antidotes abuse of Bry in hepatic complaints.	Comp—Acon, Bry, Lyc. Merc, Nux-v, Sang. Sep. Sulph.
CICUTA VIROSA				Comp—Hydr-ac, Hyper, Nux-v. Stry.
CHINA Fe.	Calc-p in hydrocephaloid.	Calc-p. Ferr. Ph-ac.	Incom—after Dig. Sel. It antidotes excessive tea drinking or when haemorrhage results.	Comp—Chinin-s, in intermittent fever

With Compl	Follows well	Followed by	Ant, Inm, Incom	Sim, Com
CINA	Ant-t. Dros, in pertussis. (Acon, Phos, Spong) in aphonia, after they had failed.			Com—(Ant-c, Ant-t, Bry, Cham, Kreos, Sil, Staph), in irritability of children.
COCA				Com—Stram, desires light and company. Coca, desires darkness and solitude.
COCCULUS	Nux-v in umbilical hernia with obstinate constipation.			Com—(Ign, Nux-v), in chorea and paralytic symtoms. —Ant-t. in sweat of affected part.
COFFEA CRUDA			Incom—Canth, Caust, Cocc, Ign.	Com—Acon, Cham, Ign, Sulph.
COLCHICUM	(Apis, Ars) in dropsy.			Com—Bry, in rheumatic gout with serous effusions.
COLLINSONIA CAN.	(Coloc, Nux-v) fail in colic, when.			Com—Aesc, Aloe, Cham, Nux-v, Sulph. Consult—Coll, when Cact, Dig, fail in

With Compl	Follows well	Followed by	Ant, Inm, Incom	Sim, Com
				heart disease complicated with haemorrhoids.
COLOCYNTHIS Merc. in dysentery.		Bell, Bry, Caust, Cham, Merc, Nux-v.		Com—Gnaph, in sciatica. —Staph, diseases from bad effects, in of anger, indignation, silent grief.
CONIUM MAC.		Psor, in tumors of mammae.		Com—(Arn, Rhus-t) in contusion. —(Ars. Aster) in cancer. —(Calc, Psor), in glandular swelling.
CROCUS SATIVUS		(Nux-v, Puls) in nearly all complaints.		Com—Ust., in menstrual disorder.
CROTALUS HOR.				Com—Elaps. Lach. Naja, Pyrog. —Elaps. affections of right lung. expectoration of black blood.

With Compl	Follows well	Followed by	Ant, Inm, Incom	Sim, Com
				—Lach. skin cold and dry.
CROTON TIGLIUM				Com—(Kali-br. Phos) in chronic infantile diarrhoea. —Sil. in pain from nipple through to back when nursing.
				Com—(Ars, Verat) in cholera and cholera morbus.
CUPRUM MET. Calc, Gels, in an over-worked brain. Zinc, in hydrocephalus from suppressed eruption.		(Apis, Zinc), in convulsions from suppressed eruptions. Verat. in whooping cough and cholera.	Ant.—Bell.	
CYCLAMEN EUR.				Com—(Chin, Ferr, Puls) in anaemia and chlorosis. —(Croc, Thuj) in, as if something alive in abdomen.

With Compl	Follows well	Followed by	Ant, Inm, Incom	Sim, Com
DIGITALIS			Ant—Chin. Nit-ac.	
DIOSCOREA VILL.				Com—Coloc, Phos, Podo, Rhus-t, Sil.
DROSERA ROT.	Samb, Sulph, Verat.	Calc, Puls, Sulph.		Comp—(Chin, Cor-r, Cupr. Ip. Samb) in spasmodic cough.
DULCAMARA Bar-c.	Bry, Calc, Lyc, Rhus-t, Sep.		Incom—Acet-ac, Bell. It antidotes abuse of mercury.	Sim—Kali-s, the chemical analogue. —Merc, in ptyalism, glandular swellings, bronchitis, diarrhoea.
EQUISETUM		Nat-m, Sep.		Com—Apis, Canth, Ferr-p, Puls, Squil.
EUPATORIUM PERF.				Com—(Chel, Podo, Lyc), in jaundiced conditions. —Bry, has free sweat, and quiet patient. —Eup-per, has scanty sweat and a restless patient.

With Compl	Follows well	Followed by	Ant, Inm, Incom	Sim, Com
EUPHRASIA		Chin, in nearly all diseases.		Sim—Puls, affections of eyes. Reserve of All-c, in coryza and lachrymation.
FERRUM MET.		Chin, in nearly all diseases, acute or chronic.		
FLUORICUM ACIDUM. Coca. Sil.	Ars—in ascites of drunkards. Kali-c—in hip disease. (Coff, Staph) in sensitive teeth. Ph-ac. in diabetes. (Sil, Symph) in bone diseases. Spong, in goitre.			
GELSEMIUM				Com—Bapt, in typhoid. —Ip, in ague after suppression of quinine.

With Compl	Follows well	Followed by	Ant, Inm, Incom	Sim, Com
GLONOINUM				Comp—Aml-ns, Bell, Ferr, Gels, Meli, Stram.
GRAPHITES	Lyc. Puls. Calc, in fat women. Sulph, in skin disease. Sep, in gushing leucorrhoea.			Sim—(Lyc, Puls) in menstrual troubles.
HAMAMELIS Ferr, in haemorrhage.				Com—(Arn, Calen) in traumatism.
HELLEBORUS NIGER				Com—(Apis, Apoc, Ars, Bell, Bry, Dig, Lach, Sulph, Tub, Zinc) in brain or meningeal affections.
HELONIAS DIOICA				Comp—Alet, Ferr, Lil-t, Ph-ac. Sim—Alet, in debility.
HEPAR SULPHURIS Calen, in injury.	Acon, Arn, Bell, Lach, Merc, Nit-ac.	Acon, Arn, Bell, Bry, Iod, Lach, Merc, Nit-ac. Sulph.	It antidotes Merc and other metals. iodine, iodide of potash, cod liver oil.	Com—in skin afections, Sulph, dry, itching, and not sensitive.

With Compl	Follows well	Followed by	Ant, Inm, Incom	Sim, Com
				Hep, moist, unhealthy, suppurating and sensitive.
HYOSCYAMUS NIGER	Bell, in deafness after apoplexy.	Phos in lasciviousness.		Com—Bell, Stram, Verat. (Nux-v, Op), in haemoptysis of drunkards.
HYPERICUM. Arn.				
IGNATIA			Ant—Puls, for bad effects of Ign.	Com—Arn, Calen, Ruta, Staph.
IODIUM	Hep, Merc.	Kali-bi in croup.	Incom—Coff, Nux-v, Tab.	
IPECACUANHA Cupr.		Ars, in influenza, chill, croup, debility, cholera.		Com—(Acet-c, Brom, Con, Kali-bi, Spong) in membranous croup and croupy affections.
				Sim—(Ant-c, Puls), in gastric troubles.

With Compl	Follows well	Followed by	Ant, Inm, Incom	Sim, Com
KALIUM BICHROMICUM	(Canth, Carb-ac) in dysentery. Iod in croup. Calc in nasal catarrh.	Ant-t, in foreign body in larynx. Ant-t in catarrhal affections and skin disease.		Com—(Brom, Hep, Iod), in croupy affections.
KALIUM BROMATUM	Eugenia jambos in acne.		It antidotes lead poisoning	
KALIUM CARB. Carb-v.	(Kali-s, Phos, Stann) in loose rattling cough. Nat-m, when it fails to bring menses.			Com—Bry, Lyc, Nat.m, Nit-ac, Stann.
KALMIA LAT.	Spig in heart disease.			Sim—(Led, Rhod, Spig), in rheumatic and gouty affections.
KREOSOTUM		(Ars, Phos, Sulph), in malignant disease.	Inm—Carb-v.	
LACHESIS Hep, Lyc, Nit-ac.		Nat-m in intermittent fever when type changes.	Incom—Acet-ac, Carb-ac.	

With Compl	Follows well	Followed by	Ant, Inm, Incom	Sim, Com
LAC CANINUM				Sim—Apis, Con, Kali-bi, Lach, Murx, Puls, Sep, Sulph.
LEDUM PAL.				Com—(Arn, Belli, Crot-t, Ham, Ruta) in traumatism. Con in lasting affects of injury.
LILIUM TIG.				Com—Agar, Cact, Helon, Cimic, Murx, Nat-p, Plat, Sep, Spig, Tarent.
LOBELIA INFLATA				Com—Ant-t, Ars, Ip, Tab, Verat.
LYCOPODIUM CLAV. Chel, Iod, Lach. Ip, in capillary bronchitis.	Calc, Carb-v, Lach, Sulph.	Bell, Lach.		
LYSSINUM.				Comp—(Bell, Canth, Hyos, Stram), in hydrophobia.
MAGNESIUM MUR.				Comp—Cham in diseases of children.

With Compl	Follows well	Followed by	Ant, Inm, Incom	Sim, Com
MAGNESIUM PHOS.				Com—Bell, Caul, Coloc, Lac-c, Lyc, Puls. Cham, is its vegetable analogue.
MEDORRHINUM				Comp—Ip, in dry cough. (Camph, Sec, Tab, Verat), in collapse. (Pic-ac, Gels), in inability to walk. (Aloe, Sulph), in morning diarrhoea.
MELILOTUS ALBA				Com—(Aml-ns, Ant-c), in epistaxis after headache. (Bell, Glon, Sang) in congestive headache, red face, hot head.
MENYANTHES	Caps, Lach, Lyc, Puls, Rhus-t, Verat.			Comp—Cact, Calc, Gels, Mag-m, Pari, Sep.

With Compl	Follows well	Followed by	Ant, Inm, Incom	Sim, Com
MERCURIUS Bad.	Bell. Hep. Lach. Sulph.	Ars, Bell, Calc, Nit-ac, Sulph.	Ant—Aur, Hep, Lach, Mez, Nit-ac, Sulph, and high potency of Merc.	Com—Mez, its vegetable analogue
MERCURIUS SULPH.				Com—Ars, Cimb, Dig, Sulph.
MEZEREUM				Com—Caust, Guaj, Phyt, Rhus-t.
MILLEFOLIUM	(Acon, Arn) in haemorrhage.			Com—Erech, in epistaxis and haemoptysis, blood bright red.
MUREX PURPUREA				Com—(Lil-t, Plat) in nymphomamia. Sep, in bearing-down sensation but has no sexual erethism.
MURIATICUM ACIDUM	Bry, Merc, Rhus-t.		It antidotes excessive use of opium and tobacco, in muscular weaknes	
NAJA TRIPUDIANS				Com—Ars, Cact, Crot-h, Lach, Mygal, Spig.

With Compl	Follows well	Followed by	Ant, Inm, Incom	Sim, Com
NATRIUM CARB.	Sep. in bearing-down.			Com—Nat-s for yeast-like vomiting. Calc, Sep.
NATRIUM MUR. Apis, Sep.	Apis, Ign.	Apis. Sep, Thuj.	Ant—Ars for bad effects of sea bathing.	
NATRIUM SULPH.				Com—Nat-m, Sulph. (Merc, Thuja), in syphilis and sycosis, in hydrogenoid constitutions.
NITRICUM ACIDUM Ars. Calad.	Aur in abuse of mercury. Calc. Carb-an in bubo. Hep in throat affections. Kali-c, in phthisis. Mez in secondary syphilis. Nat-c, Puls, Sulph, Thuj.	Arn in collapse of dysentery.	Inm—Lach. It antidotes abuse of mercury, and bad effects of Dig.	Sim—Ars in morbid fear of cholera. Merc suits light-haired. Nit-ac suits black-haired.

With Compl	Follows well	Followed by	Ant, Inm, Incom	Sim, Com
NUX MOSCHATA			It antidotes mercurial inhalation, lead colic, oil of turpentine, spirituous (especially bad beer).	
NUX VOMICA Dros, Sulph.	Ars, Ip, Phos, Sep, Sulph.	Bry, Phos, Puls, Sulph.	Inm—Zinc.	
OPIUM			Ant—(Strong coffee, Nux-v, Kali-perm and constant motion) for poisonous doses. —Potencies, for opium drugging.	Com—Apis, Bell, Hyos, Stram, Zinc.
PETROLEUM			It antidotes lead poisoneing.	
PETROSELINUM				Com—(Cann-s, Canth, Merc), in sudden urging to urinate.

With Compl	Follows well	Followed by	Ant, Inm, Incom	Sim, Com
PHOSPHORICUM ACIDUM	Chin, in colliquative sweat, diarrhoea, debility. Nux-v in fainting after meal.	Chin, in colliquative sweat, diarrhoea, debility. Calc-p, Ferr, Kali-p, Phos, Lyc, Sulph.		Com—Phos, Pic-ac, Puls, Sil. Mur-ac, in typhoid.
PHOSPHORUS All-c, Ars.	Calc, Chin.		Incom—Caust. Removes bad effects of Iodium and excessive use of table salt.	
PHYSOSTIGMA				Com—Bell, Con, Cur, Gels, Hyper, Stry.
PHYTOLACCA				It occupies a position between Bry and Rhus, cures when these fail, though apparently indicated.
PODOPHYLLUM	(Ip, Nux), in gastric affections. (Calc, Sulph), in liver disease.		It antidotes bad effects of Merc.	Com—Aloe, Chel, Coll, Lil-t, Merc, Nux-v, Sulph.

With Compl	Follows well	Followed by	Ant, Inm, Incom	Sim, Com
PICRICUM ACIDUM				Com—Arg-n, Gels. Kali-p. Ph-ac, Phos. Petr, Sil.
PLATINAUM MET.				Com—Aur, Croc, Ign, Kali-p, Puls, Sep, Stann. Valer, is its vegetable analogue.
PLUMBUM MET.			Ant—Alum, Petr, Plat, Sul-ac, Zinc.	Com—(Alum, Plat, Op) in colic. Podo, in retraction of navel. Nux-v, in strangulated hernia. Podo is its vegetable analogue.
PODOPHYLIUM (See above)				
PSORINUM Sulph, Tab.	Lac-ac in vomiting of pregnancy. Arm in traumatic affections of ovaries.	Alum, Borx. Hep. Sulph, Tub. Sulph, in mammary cancer.		

With Compl	Follows well	Followed by	Ant, Inm, Incom	Sim, Com
PULSATILLA Kali-s, Kali-m, Lyc, Sil, Sul-ac. Kali-s and Sil are its chronic.	Kali-bi, Kali-m, Lyc, Sep, Sil, Sulph.	Kali-m.	It antidotes iron, quinine, tonics, resulting in anaemia and chlorosis. It antidotes abuse of Chamomilla, mercury, tea drinking, Sulphur.	
PYROGENUM				Com—Ars, Carb-ac, Carb-v, Op, Psor, Rhus-t, Sec, Verat.
RATANHIA				Com—Canth, Carb-ac, Iris, Sulph, Thuj.
RANUNCULUS BULB.			Incom—Staph, Sulph.	Com—Acon, Arn, Bry, Clem, Euph, Mez.
RHEUM Mag-c.	Mag-c.			Com—Cham, Coloc, Hep, Ip, Mag-c, Podo, Staph, Sulph.
RHODODENDRON				Com—Bry, Calc, Con, Led, Lyc, Rhus-t, Sep.

With Compl	Follows well	Followed by	Ant, Inm, Incom	Sim, Com
RHUS TOX. Arn, Bry, Calc.		Arn, Ars, Bell. Con.	Inm—Apis. Ant—Anac.	Com—Arn, Bry, Nat-s, Rhod. Sulph.
RUMEX CRISPUS				Com—Bell, Caust, Dros, Hyos, Phos, Sang, Sulph.
RUTA GRAVEOLENS	Arn in joint affections. Symph in injuries of bones.			Com—Arn, Arg-n, Con, Euphr, Phyt, Rhus-t, Symph.
SABINA	Thuj in condylomata and sycotic affections.			Com—Calc, Croc, Mill, Sec, Tril-p.
SABADILLA	(Bry, Ran-b) in pleurisy.			Com—(Coloc, Colch, Lyc) in 4 to 8 p.m. agg. (Puls, Sabin), in open air amel.
SAMBUCUS NIGRA			It antidotes abuse of Ars.	Com—Chin, Chlor, Ip, Meph, Sulph.

With Compl	Follows well	Followed by	Ant, Inm, Incom	Sim, Com
SANGUINARIA	Bell in scarlatina		It antidotes narcosis of opium.	Com—(Bell, Iris, Meli) in sick headache. (Lach, Sulp), in climacteric affections. (Chel, Phos, Sulph, Verat-v), in chronic bronchitis.
SANICULA				Related to—Abrot, Alum, Borx, Calc, Graph, Nat-m, Sil.
SARSAPARILA Merc, Sep.			It antidotes abuse of Merc.	Com—Berb, Lyc, Nat-m, Phos.
SECALE CORNUTUM				Com—Cinnamon, in post-partum haemorrhage. Sim—Ars, but cold and heat opposite. Resembles Colch, in cholera morbus.

With Compl	Follows well	Followed by	Ant, Inm, Incom	Sim, Com
SELENIUM	(Calad, Nat-m, Staph, Ph-ac) in sexual weakness.		It antidotes suppressed itch by mercurials and Sulphur.	Com—Phos, in genito-urinary and respiratory symptoms. —(Arg-met, Stann), in laryngitis of singers and speakers. — Alum, hard stool. Sim—(Lach, Sang, Ust), in climacteric irregularities.
SEPIA Nat-m.	Sil, Sulph.		Inm—Lach. Puls.	Com—Gettysbery, Hep, Hyper, Kali-p, Pic-ac, Ruta, Sanic.
SILICEA Fl-ac, Puls, Sanic, Thuj.	Calc, Graph. Hep, Nit-ac, Phos.	Fl-ac, Hep, Lyc, Sep.		
SPIGELIA				Cam—(Acon, Ars, Cact, Dig, Kali-c, Kalm, Naja, Spong) in heart affections.
SPONGIA TOSTA	(Acon, Hep) in cough and croup when dryness prevails.	Hep when mucus commences to rattle.		Com—(Arn, Caust, Iod, Lach, Nux-m) sputa loosened but must be swallowed again.
STANNUM MET. Puls.				

With Compl	Follows well	Followed by	Ant, Inm, Incom	Sim, Com
STAPHYISAGRIA	Coloc. (Caust, Coloc staph), follow well in the order named.	Coloc.		Com—Caust, Coloc, Ign, Lyc, Puls.
STRAMONIUM	Bell, Cupr, Hyos, Lyss.	Sec, in metrorrhagia from ratained placenta, after failure of Stram.	It antidotes overaction of Bell in whooping cough:	
SULPHUR Aloe, Psor. Acon, Puls, Nux-v. It is chronic of last three. Sulph complements Rhus-t in paralysis.	(Sulph, Calc, Lyc) follow in order. (Ant-t, Ip) in lung affections esply left side.	Acon, Alum, Ars, Bell, Bry, Calc, Graph, Lyc, Merc, Nit-ac, Nux-v, Phos, Puls, Sars, Sep.	Ant—Camph, Merc, Puls. It antidotes abuse of metals generally.	
SULPHURICUM ACIDUM Puls.	(Arn, Con, Led, Ruta) in injury. Arn in injury.	Arn, Calc, Con, Lyc, Sulph.	Ant—Ip, Puls.	Com—Ars, Borx, Calen, Led, Rheum, Ruta, Symph.
SYMPHYTUM				Com—Arn, Calen, Calc-p, Fl-ac, Hep, Sil.

With Compl	Follows well	Followed by	Ant, Inm, Incom	Sim, Com
SYPHILINUM				Comp—(Aur, Asaf, Kali-i, Merc, Phyt) in bone disease and syphililic affections.
TABACUM			Ant—Ars for bad affect of tobacco chewing. (Clem, Plan) for tobacco toothache. Gels for occipital headache and vertigo. Ign for hiccough. Ip for nausea and vomiting. Lyc for impotence. Nux for gastric sympoms. Phos for palpitation, tobacco-heart, sexual weakness. Puls for hiccough. Sep for neuralgia of right side of face.	

With Compl	Follows well	Followed by	Ant, Inm, Incom	Sim, Com
TARANTULA			Spig for heart affections. Tab (200 or 1000) for craving when discontinuing its use.	Sim—Apis, Crot-h, Lach, Mygal, Naja, Plat, Ther.
TEREBINTHINE				Com—Alumn, Ars. Canth, Lach. Nit-ac.
THERIDION	Calc, Lyc.			Com—Sin-n, Tril-p, Vib, Ust.
THLASPI BURSA PAST.				Com—Cann-s, Canth, Caps, Staph.
THUJA OCC. Med, Sabin, Sil.	Med, Merc, Nit-ac.			Com—Bell, Chin, Kali-c, Lach, Mill Sep, Sulph, Thlas, Ust.
TRILLIUM PENDULUM				

With Compl	Follows well	Followed by	Ant, Inm, Incom	Sim, Com
TUBERCULINUM Psor, Sulph.	Psor as a constitutional remedy. Bell in acute atacks occuring in tuberculous diseases.	Hydr to fatten patient cured with Tub.		
VALERIANA			It antidotes abuse of Chamomile tea.	Com—Asaf, Asar, Croc, Ign, Lac-c, Spig. Sulph. —Agar, Caust, Cyel, Lob, Meny, Phyt.
VERATRUM ALBUM	Arn, Ars, Chin, Camph in cholera and cholera morbus. (Am-c, Carb-v, Bov) in dysmenorrhoea with vomiting and purging.			
ZINCUM MET.		Ign.	Inm—Cham, Nux-v.	Com—(Hell, Tub) in incipient brain diseases from suppressed eruptions.

Remedies and their Abbreviations

Abies-n., Abies nigra.

Abrot., Abrotanum.

Absin., Absinthium.

Acet-ac., Aceticum acidum.

Acon., Aconitum nepellus.

Aesc., Aesculus hippocastanum.

Aeth., Aethusa cynapium.

Agar., Agaricus muscarius

Agn., Agnus castus.

Ail., Ailanthus.

Alet., Aletris farinosa.

All-c., Allium cepa.

Aloe, Aloe.

Alum., Alumina.

Alumn., Alumen.

Ambr., Ambra grisea.

Ammc., Ammoniacum.

Am-c., Ammonium carbonicum.

Am-m., Ammonium muriaticum.

Aml-ns., Amylenum nitrosum.

Anac., Anacardium orientale.

Anag., Anagallis.

Ang., Angustura.

Anis., Anisum stellatum.

Anthraci., Anthracinum.

Ant-c., Antimonium crudum.

Ant-t., Antimonium tart.

Apis, Apis mellifica.

Apoc., Apocynum cannabinum.

Apom., Apomorphinum.

Aral., Aralia racemosa.

Aran., Aranea diadema.

Arg-met., Argentum metallicum.

Arg-n., Argentum nitricum.

Arn., Arnica montana.

Ars., Arsenicum album.

Ars-i., Arsenicum iodatum.

Art-v., Artemesia vulgaris.

Arum-t., Arum triphyllum.

Asaf., Asa foetida.

Asar., Asarum europaeum.

Aster., Asterias rubens.

Aur., Aurum metallicum.

Aur-m., Aurum muriaticum.

Aur-m-n., Aurum muriaticum natronatum.

Bad., Badiaga.

Bals-p., Balsam peru.

Bapt., Baptisia tinctoria.

Bar-c., Baryta carbonica.

Bar-m., Baryta muriatica.

Bell., Belladonna.

Bell-p., Bellis perennis.

Benz-ac., Benzoicum acidum.

Berb., Berberis vulgaris.

Bism., Bismuthum.

Blatta, Blatta orientala.

Borx., Boraxveneta.

Bov., Bovista.

Brom., Bromium.

Bry., Bryonia.

Bufo., Bufo rana.

Cact., Cactus.

Cadm., Cadmium sulphuratum.

Calad., Caladium.

Calc-ar., Calcarea arsenicosa.

Calc., Calearea carbonica.

Calc-fl., Calcarea fluorica.

Calc-i., Calcarea iodata.

Calc-p., Calcarea phosphorica.

Calc-hp., Calcarea hypophos.

Calc-s., Calcarea sulphurica.

Camph., Camphora.

Cann-i., Cannabis indica.

Cann-s., Cannabis sativa.

Canth., Cantharis.

Caps., Capsicum.

Carb-ac., Carbolicum acidum.

Carb-an., Carbo animalis.

Carb-v., Carbo vegetabilis.

Card-m., Carduus marianus.

Casc., Cascarilla.

Castm., Castoreum.

Caul., Caulophyllum.

Caust., Causticum.

Cean., Ceanothus americanus.

Cedr., Cedron.

Cham., Chamomilla.

Chel., Chelidonium majus.

Chenop., Chenopodium.

Chim., Chimaphila.

Chin., China.

Chinin-s., Chininum sulphuricum

Cholor., Chlorum.

Cic., Cicuta virosa.

Cimic., Cimicifuga racemosa.

Cimx., Cimex.

Cina, Cina.

Cinnb., Cinnabaris.

Cist., Cistus canadensis.

Clem., Clematis erecta.

Cob., Cobaltum.

Coca, Coca.

Cocc., Cocculus.

Coc-c, Coccus cacti.

Coch., Cochlearia armoracia.

Cod., Codeinum.

Coff., Coffea cruda.

Colch., Colchicum.

Coll., Collinsonia.

Coloc., Colocynthis.

Com., Comocladia.

Con., Conium.

Conv., Convallaria majalis.

Cop., Copaiva.

Cor-r., Corrallium rubrum.

Croc., Crocus sativus.

Crot-h., Crotalus horridus.

Crot-t., Croton tiglium.

Cub., Cubeba.

Cund., Cundurango.

Cupr., Cuprum metallicum.

Cur., Curare.
Cycl., Cyclamen.
Daph., Daphne indica.
Dig., Diagitalis.
Dios., Discorea.
Dol., Dolichos pruriens.
Dor., Doryphora.
Dros., Drosera.
Dulc., Dulcamara.
Echi., Echinacea angustifalia.
Elaps, Elaps.
Elat., Elaterium.
Epig., Epigea repens.
Epiph., Epiphegus.
Equis-h., Equisetum.
Erig., Erigeron.
Erio., Eriodictylon.
Eup-per., Eupatorium perfotiatum.
Eup-pur, Eupatorium purpureum.
Euphr., Euphrasia.
Ferr., Ferrum metallicum.
Ferr-p., Ferrum phosphoricum.
Fl-ac., Fluoricum acidum.
Gamb., Gambogia.
Gels., Gelsemium.
Glon., Glonoinum.
Gnaph., Gnaphalium.
Graph., Graphites.
Grind., Grindelia.
Grat., Gratiola.
Guaj. Guajacum.
Ham., Hamamelis.
Hecla, Hecla lava.

Hell., Helleborus niger.
Helon., Helonias dioica.
Hep., Hepar sulphuris calcareum.
Hydr., Hydrastis.
Hydro., Hydrocotyle.
Hyos., Hyoscyamus.
Hyper., Hypericum neger.
Ign., Ignatia.
Ind., Indium metallicum.
Indg., Indigo.
Iod., Iodium.
Ip., Ipecacuanha.
Iris, Iris versicolor.
Jab., Jaborandi.
Jal., Jalapa.
Jatr., Jatropha.
Kali-ar., Kalium arsenicosum.
Kali-bi., Kalium bichromicum.
Kali-br., Kalium bromatum.
Kali-c., Kalium carbonicum.
Kali-ch., Kali chloricum.
Kali-i., Kalium iodatum.
Kali-m., Kalium muriaticum.
Kali-n., Kalium nitricum.
Kali-p., Kalium phosphoricum.
Kali-s., Kalium sulphuricum.
Kalm., Kalima.
Kreos., Kreosotum.
Lac-c., Lac caninum.
Lac-d., Lac vaccinum defloratum.
Lach., Lachesis mutus.
Lachn., Lachnanthes.
Lac-ac., Lacticum acidum.

Lap-a, Lapis albus.

Laur., Laurocerasus.

Led., Ledum palustre.

Lil-t., Lilium tigrinum.

Lith-c., Lithium carbonicum.

Lob., Lobelia inflata.

Lyc., Lycopodium.

Lys., Lyssinum.

Mag-c., Magnesium carbonicum.

Mag-m., Magnesium muriaticum.

Mag-p., Magnesium phosphoricum.

Mag-s., Magnesium sulphuricum.

Maland., Malandrinum.

Mang-act., Manganum aceticum.

Mang-m., Manganum muriaticum.

Med., Medorrhinum.

Mell., Melilotus alba.

Meny., Menyanthes.

Merc., Mercurius solutions.

Merc-c., Mercurius corrosivus.

Merc-cy., Mercurius cyanatus.

Merc-d., Mercurius dulcis.

Merc-i-f., Mercurius iodatus flavus.

Merc-i-r., Mercurius iodatus ruber.

Merc-sul., Mercurius sulphuricus.

Mez., Mezereum.

Mill., Millefolium.

Mosch., Moschus.

Murx., Murex.

Mur-ac., Muriaticum acidum.

Mygal., Mygale lasiodora.

Myrt., Myrtus communis.

Myos., Myosotis.

Naja, Naja.

Nat-c., Natrium carbonicum.

Nat-m., Natrium muriaticum.

Nat-p., Natrium phosphoricum.

Nat-s., Natrium sulphuricum.

Nit-ac., Nitricum acidum.

Nux-m., Nux moschata.

Nux-v., Nux vomica.

Oci., Ocimum canum.

Olnd., Oleander.

Ol-an., Oleum animale.

Ol-j., Oleum jecoris aselli.

Onos., Onosmodium.

Op., Opium.

Orig., Origanum majorana.

Osm., Osmium.

Ox-ac., Oxalicum acidum.

Pareir., Pareira brava.

Par., Paris quadrifolia.

Petr., Petroleum.

Petros., Petroselinum.

Phel., Phellandrinum.

Ph-ac., Phosphoricum acidum.

Phos., Phosphorus.

Phys., Physostigma.

Phyt., Phytolacca decandra.

Pic-ac., Picricum acidum.

Pix-l., Pix liquida.

Plan., Plantago.

Plat., Platinum.

Plb., Plumbum.

Pod., Podophyllum.

Psor., Psorinum.

Ptel., Ptelea trifoliata.
Puls., Pulsatilla.
Pyrog., Pyrogenium.
Ran-b., Ranunculus bulbosus.
Ran-s., Ranunculus sceleratus.
Raph., Raphanus.
Rat., Ratanhia.
Rheum, Rheum.
Rhod., Rhododendron.
Rhus-t., Rhus toxicodendron.
Rhus-r., Rhus radians.
Rhus-v., Rhus venenata.
Rob., Robinia.
Rumx., Rumex crispus.
Ruta, Ruta.
Sabad., Sabadilla.
Sabin., Sabina.
Sal-ac., Salicylicum acidum.
Samb., Sambucus nigra.
Sang., Sanguinaria.
Sanic., Sanicula aqua.
Sars., Sarsaparilla.
Sec., Secale cornutum.
Sel., Selenium.
Senec., Senecio.
Seneg., Senega.
Sep., Sepia.
Sil., Silicea terra.
Sin-n., Sinapis nigra.
Spig., Spigelia
Spong., Spongia.
Squil., Squilla.
Stann., Stannum metallicum.

Staph., staphfsagria.
Stict., Sticta pulmonaria.
Still., Stillingia.
Stront-c., Strontium carbonicum.
Stram., Stramonium.
Stry., Strychninum.
Sulph., Sulphur.
Sul-ac., Sulphuricum acidum.
Sumb., Sumbucus.
Syph., Syphilinum.
Symph., Symphytum.
Tab., Tabacum.
Tarax., Taraxacum.
Tarent., Tarentula.
Tell., Tellurium.
Ter., Terebinthinea.
Teucr., Teucrium narum verum.
Ther., Theridion.
Thuj., Thuja.
Trill., Trillium pendulum.
Tub., Tuberculinum.
Uran., Uranium nitricum.
Urt-u., Urtica urens.
Ust., Ustilago maydis.
Vac., Vaccininum.
Valer., Valeriana.
Verat., Veratrum album.
Verat-v., Veratrum viride.
Verb., Verbascum thapsus.
Vib., Viburnum opulus.
Viol-o., Viola odorata.
Zing., Zingiber officinale.
Zinc., Zincum metallicum.